Controversies in General Surgery

Editor

SEAN J. LANGENFELD

SURGICAL CLINICS
OF NORTH AMERICA

www.surgical.theclinics.com

Consulting Editor
RONALD F. MARTIN

December 2021 • Volume 101 • Number 6

ELSEVIER

1600 John F. Kennedy Boulevard • Suite 1800 • Philadelphia, Pennsylvania, 19103-2899

http://www.surgical.theclinics.com

SURGICAL CLINICS OF NORTH AMERICA Volume 101, Number 6
December 2021 ISSN 0039–6109, ISBN-13: 978-0-323-83544-2

Editor: John Vassallo, j.vassallo@elsevier.com

Developmental Editor: Arlene Campos

Surgical Clinics of North America (ISSN 0039–6109) is published bimonthly by Elsevier Inc., 360 Park Avenue South, New York, NY 10010-1710. Months of publication are February, April, June, August, October, and December. Business and Editorial Offices: 1600 John F. Kennedy Blvd., Suite 1800, Philadelphia, PA 19103-2899. Periodicals postage paid at New York, NY and additional mailing offices. Subscription prices are $443.00 per year for US individuals, $1198.00 per year for US institutions, $100.00 per year for US & Canadian students and residents, $547.00 per year for Canadian individuals, $1270.00 per year for Canadian institutions, $536.00 for international individuals, $1270.00 per year for international institutions and $250.00 per year for foreign students/residents. To receive student/resident rate, orders must be accompanied by name of affiliated institution, date of term, and the *signature* of program/residency coordinator on institution letterhead. Orders will be billed at individual rate until proof of status is received. Foreign air speed delivery is included in all *Clinics* subscription prices. All prices are subject to change without notice. POSTMASTER: Send address changes to *Surgical Clinics*, Elsevier Health Sciences Division, Subscription Customer Service, 3251 Riverport Lane, Maryland Heights, MO 63043. **Customer Service (orders, claims, online, change of address): Telephone: 1-800-654-2452 (U.S. and Canada); 314-447-8871 (outside U.S. and Canada). Fax: 314-447-8029. E-mail: journalscustomerservice-usa@elsevier.com (for print support); journalsonlinesupport-usa@elsevier.com (for online support).**

Reprints. For copies of 100 or more, of articles in this publication, please contact the Commercial Reprints Department, Elsevier Inc., 360 Park Avenue South, New York, New York 10010-1710. Tel. 212-633-3874, Fax: 212-633-3820, E-mail: reprints@elsevier.com.

The Surgical Clinics of North America is also published in Spanish by McGraw-Hill Interamericana Editores S.A., P.O. Box 5-237 06500 Mexico D.F. Mexico; and in Portuguese by Interlivros Edicoes Ltda., Rua Comandante Coelho 1085, CEP 21250, Rio de Janeiro, Brazil; and in Greek by Paschalidis Medical Publications, Athens Greece.

The Surgical Clinics of North America is covered in *MEDLINE/PubMed (Index Medicus), EMBASE/Excerpta Medica, Current Contents/Clinical Medicine, Current Contents/Life Sciences, Science Citation Index,* and *ISI/BIOMED.*

Contributors

CONSULTING EDITOR

RONALD F. MARTIN, MD, FACS
Colonel (Retired), United States Army Reserve, Department of General Surgery and
Surgical Oncology, Madigan Army Medical Center, Tacoma, Washington

EDITOR

SEAN J. LANGENFELD, MD, FACS, FASCRS
Chief, Colon and Rectal Surgery, Associate Professor, Department of Surgery, University
of Nebraska Medical Center, Omaha, Nebraska

AUTHORS

SHAHRIAR ALIZADEGAN, MD, FACS
Assistant Professor of Surgery, Division of Vascular and Endovascular Surgery, Medical
College of Wisconsin, Milwaukee, Wisconsin

SULLIVAN A. AYUSO, MD
Gastrointestinal and Minimally Invasive Surgery, Department of Surgery, Carolinas
Medical Center, Charlotte, North Carolina

KEVIN F. BAIER, MD
Complex Abdominal Wall Reconstruction Fellow, Cleveland Clinic Foundation, Cleveland,
Ohio

SARAH BAKER, MD
Georgia Colon and Rectal Surgical Associates, Northside Hospital, Atlanta, Georgia

STEPHANIE BONNE, MD
Associate Professor, Department of Surgery, Division of Trauma and Surgical Critical
Care, Rutgers, New Jersey Medical School, Newark, New Jersey

KELLIE R. BROWN, MD, FACS, DFSVS
Professor of Surgery, Division of Vascular and Endovascular Surgery, Medical College of
Wisconsin, Milwaukee, Wisconsin

MILOŠ BUHAVAC, MD
Assistant Professor, Department of Surgery, Texas Tech University Health Sciences
Center, Lubbock, Texas

DAVID C. CHEN, MD
Professor of Clinical Surgery, Department of Surgery, David Geffen School of Medicine at
UCLA, Lichtenstein Amid Hernia Clinic at UCLA, Santa Monica, California

PAUL D. COLAVITA, MD
Gastrointestinal and Minimally Invasive Surgery, Department of Surgery, Carolinas
Medical Center, Charlotte, North Carolina

KYLE G. COLOGNE, MD
Division of Colon and Rectal Surgery, Department of Surgery, Keck School of Medicine of USC, Los Angeles, California

SHARMILA DISSANAIKE, MD
Professor, Department of Surgery, Texas Tech University Health Sciences Center, Lubbock, Texas

ALI ELSAADI, MD
Department of Surgery, Texas Tech University Health Sciences Center, Lubbock, Texas

OLUWADAMILOLA M. FAYANJU, MD, MA, MPHS, FACS
The Helen O. Dickens Presidential Associate Professor and Chief of Breast Surgery, Penn Medicine, Philadelphia, Pennsylvania

ABBEY FINGERET, MD, MHPTT
Assistant Professor, Department of Surgery, Division of Surgical Oncology, University of Nebraska Medical Center, Omaha, Nebraska

MATTHEW A. FUGLESTAD, MD
Department of Surgery, University of Nebraska Medical Center, Omaha, Nebraska

CPT SAMUEL GRASSO, DO
Department of General Surgery, William Beaumont Army Medical Center, El Paso, Texas

LILY GUTNIK, MD, MPH
Breast Surgical Oncology Fellow, Duke University School of Medicine, Durham, North Carolina

ALEXANDER T. HAWKINS, MD, MPH
Section of Colon and Rectal Surgery, Department of Surgery, Assistant Professor of Surgery, Colon and Rectal Surgery, Section of Surgical Sciences, Vanderbilt University Medical Center, Nashville, Tennessee

B. TODD HENIFORD, MD
Gastrointestinal and Minimally Invasive Surgery, Department of Surgery, Carolinas Medical Center, Charlotte, North Carolina

CHRISTINE HSIEH, MD
Division of Colon and Rectal Surgery, Department of Surgery, Keck School of Medicine of USC, Los Angeles, California

AIMAL KHAN, MD
Section of Colon and Rectal Surgery, Department of Surgery, Assistant Professor of Surgery, Colon and Rectal Surgery, Section of Surgical Sciences, Vanderbilt University Medical Center, Nashville, Tennessee

ERIN KING-MULLINS, MD
Faculty/Research Director, Colon and Rectal Surgery Fellowship, Georgia Colon and Rectal Surgical Associates, Northside Hospital, Atlanta, Georgia

JENNIFER A. LEINICKE, MD, MPHS, FACS, FASCRS
Assistant Professor of Surgery, University of Nebraska Medical Center, Omaha, Nebraska

YANG LU, MD
Resident Physician, Department of Surgery, David Geffen School of Medicine at UCLA, Los Angeles, California

IAN T. MACQUEEN, MD
Assistant Clinical Professor, Department of Surgery, David Geffen School of Medicine at UCLA, Lichtenstein Amid Hernia Clinic at UCLA, Santa Monica, California

KIMBERLY MILLER-HAMMOND, MD
Atlanta Surgery Associates, Atlanta, Georgia

VEESHAL H. PATEL, MD, MBA
Department of Surgery, University of Washington, Department of Surgery, University of Washington Medical School, Seattle, Washington

KEELY REIDELBERGER, BS, MS
University of Nebraska Medical Center College of Medicine, Omaha, Nebraska

JORDAN N. ROBINSON, MD
Gastrointestinal and Minimally Invasive Surgery, Department of Surgery, Carolinas Medical Center, Charlotte, North Carolina

MICHAEL J. ROSEN, MD, FACS
Professor of Surgery, Center for Abdominal CoreHealth, Medical Director, Cleveland Clinic Foundation, Cleveland, Ohio

FARIHA SHEIKH, MD
Assistant Professor, Department of Surgery, Division of Trauma and Surgical Critical Care, Rutgers, New Jersey Medical School, Newark, New Jersey

ELISABETH L. TRACEY, MD
Department of Surgery, University of Nebraska Medical Center, Omaha, Nebraska

LTC AVERY WALKER, MD
Department of General Surgery, William Beaumont Army Medical Center, El Paso, Texas

ANDREW S. WRIGHT, MD
Department of Surgery, University of Washington Medical School, Center for VideoEndoscopic Surgery Endowed Professor, University of Washington, Seattle, Washington

Contents

Incisional hernia remains a common complication following abdominal surgery, and its incidence can be reduced with standardized wound closure techniques. Robust evidence exists to support certain fascial closure methods, such as using a small bites, 4-to-1, continuous slow absorbable suture technique for elective midline laparotomies. On the other hand, there are other common surgical practices that lack quality data to support their routine use, such as abdominal binders, negative-pressure wound therapy, and reapproximation of subcutaneous tissue.

Surgical site infection (SSI) remains an important complication of surgery. SSI is estimated to affect 2% to 5% of all surgical patients. Local and national efforts have resulted in significant improvements in the incidence of SSI. Familiarity with evidence surrounding high-quality SSI-reduction strategies is desirable. There exists strong evidence for mechanical and oral antibiotic bowel preparation in colorectal surgery, smoking cessation before elective surgery, prophylactic antibiotics, chlorhexidine-based skin antisepsis, and maintenance of normothermia throughout the perioperative period to reduce SSI. Use of other practices should be determined by the operating surgeon and/or local hospital policy.

Diverticulosis of the sigmoid colon is common in the developed world, affecting approximately 33% of persons older than 60 years. Up to 15% of these patients will develop diverticulitis at some point in their lifetime. The incidence of diverticulitis has increased in the last decade, accounting for nearly 300,000 US hospital admissions and $1.8 billion in annual direct medical costs. With such a wide prevalence and diverse spectrum of clinical presentation, there are bound to be multiple controversies regarding disease management. This article will serve to educate the reader on several important areas to consider when treating this ubiquitous disease.

(CPM) in the United States despite uncertain benefit, (2) indications for and use of neoadjuvant chemotherapy (NACT) and endocrine therapy (NET), and (3) staging and treatment of the axilla, particularly after neoadjuvant systemic therapy. We discuss the patient populations for whom CPM may or may not be beneficial, indications for NACT and NET, and the trend toward de-escalation of locoregional axillary treatment.

This article highlights the quagmire of the surgeon who encounters a small bowel obstruction in the absence of previous abdominopelvic surgery. Historic literature implies urgent surgical intervention is required; however, there is no current standard of care to guide management. Key principles of general surgery apply, and definitive management is based on the provider's clinical judgment after synthesizing key clinical history and additional diagnostic imaging studies.

Laparoscopic cholecystectomy is a common operation; approximately 20 million Americans have gallstones, the most common indication. Surgeons who operate on the biliary tree must be familiar with the presentations and treatment options for acute and chronic biliary pathology. We focus on the difficult "bad" gallbladder. We explore the available evidence as to what to do when a gallbladder is too inflamed, too technically challenging, or a patient is too sick to undergo standard laparoscopic cholecystectomy. We discuss whether or not open cholecystectomy is a relevant tool and what can be done to manage common bile duct stones found unexpectedly intraoperatively.

Inguinal hernias represent one of the most common pathologic conditions presenting to the general surgeon. In surgical practice, several controversies persist: when to operate, the utility of a laparoscopic versus open approach, the applicability of robotic surgery, the approach to bilateral hernias, management of athletic-related groin pain ("sports hernia"), and the role of tissue-based repairs in modern hernia surgery. Ideally, surgeons should approach each patient individually and tailor their approach based on patient factors and preferences. The informed consent process is critical, especially given increasing recognition of the risk of long-term chronic pain following hernia repair.

Incidental findings are common in the evaluation of surgical patients. Understanding the appropriate assessment and management of these frequent occurrences is important for the provision of comprehensive

SURGICAL CLINICS
OF NORTH AMERICA

SERIES OF RELATED INTEREST

Advances in Surgery
https://www.advancessurgery.com/
Surgical Oncology Clinics
https://www.surgonc.theclinics.com/
Thoracic Surgery Clinics
http://www.thoracic.theclinics.com/

THE CLINICS ARE AVAILABLE ONLINE!
Access your subscription at:
www.theclinics.com

SURGICAL CLINICS
OF NORTH AMERICA

Foreword

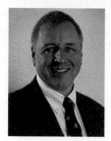

Ronald F. Martin, MD, FACS
Consulting Editor

Should it be necessary that controversies be controversial? I realize the actual question is a bit tautologic. I realize the very semantics of the matter would lead many to an obvious answer. Yet, I don't believe for one second that controversies should be controversial, at least not in the sense that controversial matters divide us. To me, a proper controversy is simply our collective recognition that some matters we have not fully sorted out; more specifically, we have not sorted it out to our collective agreement. What makes the topic *controversial* includes how we respond to it emotionally. There certainly will be times when we have a concept well enough sorted out for divisions of thought (who frequently feel they have sorted it definitively) to have developed into entrenched camps. I might submit that when we have almost reached an understanding of something we are at our most precarious and dangerous portion of our journey to wisdom.

Controversy or difference of opinion should lead us to a greater desire to resolve questions. Ideally, controversy should fuel our desire to further question ourselves. Sadly, controversy more frequently causes us to retreat to our respective corners, declare intellectual victory rather than continue the hard work of inquiry, and question those who oppose us.

Those in positions of power too often declare that "enough is enough," and all must listen. These are the owners of dogma. Those out of power often pronounce how they "believe" it should be and point out that any attempt to resist the "enlightenment" offered is a sign of either rigidity or senility. These are the owners of pretense. Those who have neither the position to benefit from dogma nor the appetite for rebelliousness generally keep their heads down until the dust clears. In the final analysis, our desire for affirmation frequently leads to confirmation bias and hinders our ability to elevate our knowledge.

This "where one stands depends upon where one sits" mentality is nothing new. People have always done their best to champion what they believe to beneficial—whether to others or to themselves. What perhaps may be somewhat new is that we have witnessed a generational shift in how we scrutinize ourselves in surgery. There

Surg Clin N Am 101 (2021) xiii–xv
https://doi.org/10.1016/j.suc.2021.09.008
0039-6109/21/© 2021 Published by Elsevier Inc.

was a time when a paper written or presented was intentionally attacked at its core, sometimes mercilessly, usually by some wise elder or editor, in the belief that if the thinking proposed withstood that level of scrutiny that it must be of value. Some of that was probably good, but perhaps as much of it was to prolong a preexisting viewpoint rather than refine or change it. The editors, the chairs, the professors, and others of the inner circles not only controlled the flow of information but also controlled the conclusions that were allowed to see the light of day. In more recent times, the idea of openly criticizing a paper, or worse, the presenter, is a bit more frowned upon. Most likely that represents progress as a society, but it comes at a price. We all too often fawn over some topic that is poorly presented or poorly supported rather than risk offense by questioning its validity.

In an excellent book published in 2018, *The Coddling of the American Mind*, Lukianoff and Haidt[1] describe a generational shift in thinking. Their original interest in the topic was in part due to a desire to understand a recent increase in the demand of college students to "disinvite" speakers who may present views that were antithetical to their beliefs. Also in the book, they describe a general sense among some students, that ideas being presented that were at odds with their firmly held beliefs represented a threat to their safety, for which they felt they had a right to counter this threat with physical violence. The book is a truly fascinating read, and I highly recommend that anyone who is involved with younger physicians (particularly in a training capacity) reviews this material. Obviously, it does not describe everybody, nor does it claim to, but it does give one insight into a changing set of perspectives and expectations. Many of the points described involve the concepts of "safe" zones and "triggering" events, as well as how people handle topics that make them uncomfortable.

Which brings us back to controversy. We surgeons need controversy. We need to understand that our answers are rarely, if ever, perfect. We need the awkward sensation in our limbic systems that we could and should improve our imperfect conceptions. Those of us who have been around for a while need our authority questioned. The corollary is also true: those of us who are questioning authority need to listen to the answers when they are given. That is not to suggest that the answer *must* be believed, but it *must* be heard. Whatever dissonance arises from that is fertile ground for inquiry and investigation. At the end of the day, developing better questions is almost always more useful than slightly altering answers.

This issue of the *Surgical Clinics* was conceived with the specific aim to select a series of topics that carry with them much in the way of strong beliefs, though not always with strong support (ie, controversies). I am deeply indebted to Dr Sean Langenfeld for his tireless work on behalf of the series and to his colleagues for their excellent contributions. They have given us a collection of articles that is designed to be provocative. One may or may not agree with all the viewpoints, that is just fine. There are some propositions in this issue that I would debate, not necessarily because I disagree with the material or the analysis per se, but rather that I think the conclusions described may not incorporate a long enough timescale to be as definitive as they may be portrayed. As I stated earlier, further opportunity for refinement.

We surgeons must focus on what is safest for our patients. To do that, we must learn the profession, science, and art required to be a surgeon. Much of that education involves having to learn how to deal with situations that make us uncomfortable and challenge us at our core. Much of our learning is done in less-than-private settings where our knowledge deficits are laid bare before our peers. Pretty much all our operative learning is done in front of an audience, in which most everybody in the room is judging the performance the way that some would watch a sporting event or a play. No doubt, it can be quite stressful. Still, there are limits to how many alternatives there are to learn the craft. We must embrace controversy, and we must embrace that our reasoning and debate will be judged by others.

I might submit there are two things that any surgeon can do to reduce stress at work. First, be as prepared as is humanly possible by understanding what your patient needs and how you can provide that. The second is to understand that we all fall short of perfect in that quest, but we should never allow that as an excuse to stop trying to improve. These articles will provide you a basis to consider what you know and what you believe. I leave it to you to decide what to do with what you are provided.

It is hoped that respectful and civil disagreement and discourse will lead to mutual growth and understanding. Only discussing matters that allow us to feel safe and don't risk challenging our beliefs, no matter how firmly held, will impede our growth. Seek common ground and seek uncommon ground. Our collective futures rely on our ability to do this and do it well.

Ronald F. Martin, MD, FACS
Colonel (retired), United States Army Reserve
Department of General Surgery and Surgical Oncology
Madigan Army Medical Center
9040 Jackson Avenue
Tacoma, WA 98431, USA

E-mail address:
rfmcescna@gmail.com

REFERENCE

1. Lukianoff G, Haidt J. The coddling of the American mind: how good intentions and bad ideas are setting up a generation for failure. New York: Penguin Press; 2018.

Preface

Controversies in General Surgery

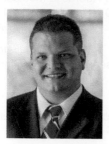

Sean J. Langenfeld, MD, FACS, FASCRS
Editor

A well-trained chief resident has experience that spans across multiple organs and diseases. However, about 80% of graduating residents pursue fellowship and ultimately have a narrowed focus of practice.[1] Even those who remain in general surgery are most likely going to gravitate toward certain procedures over time. For this reason, it's easy to fall behind on the latest advances in subspecialty surgery. The purpose of this issue was to bring the readers up-to-date on areas of controversy and clinical equipoise that exist outside of their typical scope of practice.

This is my third opportunity to be a guest editor for *Surgical Clinics*. In my first two endeavors, I was given topics in which I have clinical expertise: colorectal cancer and inflammatory bowel disease. This time, however, I operated far outside of my wheelhouse, which is why it's great that I'm not actually the author on any of these articles. My understanding of controversies in areas such as vascular surgery and trauma is superficial and outdated, and I have *just enough* self-awareness to know when to step aside and let the experts speak.

Thankfully, I was able to recruit a diverse group of subspecialty surgeons to assist with this issue. I was blown away by their depth of understanding of these complex topics, as well as their ability to explain things in a way that I could understand well. I feel uniquely confident that you'll find this issue interesting and educational.

I would like to thank the wonderful authors for their time and expertise. I would also like to thank the Elsevier publishing team for their ongoing support and organization. Last, I would like to thank Dr Ronald Martin for his leadership, vision, and dedication

Surg Clin N Am 101 (2021) xvii–xviii
https://doi.org/10.1016/j.suc.2021.06.001
0039-6109/21/© 2021 Published by Elsevier Inc.

surgical.theclinics.com

to surgical education. I'm very lucky to be surrounded by such wonderful collaborators.

Sean J. Langenfeld, MD, FACS, FASCRS
Department of Surgery
University of Nebraska Medical Center
983280 Nebraska Medical Center
Omaha, NE 68198-3280

E-mail address:
sean.langenfeld@unmc.edu

REFERENCE

1. Coleman JJ, Esposito TJ, Rozycki GS, et al. Early subspecialization and perceived competence in surgical training: are residents ready? J Am Coll Surg 2013;216(4): 764–71 [discussion: 771–3].

The Voodoo that We Do: Controversies in General Surgery

Yang Lu, MD[a], Ian T. Macqueen, MD[b], David C. Chen, MD[b],*

KEYWORDS

- Wound closure • Laparotomy • Incisional hernia • Wound complications • Small bite
- Prophylatic mesh • Prophylaxis • Abdominal binder

KEY POINTS

- Use a non-midline laparotomy incision wherever possible.
- For elective laparotomy, close the midline fascia, using a slowly absorbable suture in a continuous fashion.
- Use a small bites technique by taking 5-mm to 8-mm bites of fascia and spacing the stitches every 5 mm.
- Use a suture–to–wound length ratio of at least 4 to 1.
- Prophylactic mesh augmentation should be considered in high-risk patients undergoing elective midline laparotomy.
- Laparoscopic fascial defects greater than or equal to 10 mm should be closed.

INTRODUCTION

Laparotomies are among the most common surgical approaches used to access the abdominal cavity (**Table 1**). With more than 2 million laparotomies performed in the United States annually, incisional hernias are a frequent complication (approximately 26%) and pose a major health care problem because they are associated with significant morbidity to the patient, frequent reoperation, and increased costs to the medical system and society.[1,2] More than 300,000 incisional hernia operations are performed each year in the United States, costing the national health care system more than $3 billion in expenditures.[1] Furthermore, recurrence rates exponentially increase with each subsequent hernia repair, placing the emphasis on prevention to effectively lower the overall burden of incisional hernias. Another frequent complication following laparotomies is surgical site occurrences, which include surgical site

[a] Department of Surgery, David Geffen School of Medicine at UCLA, 10833 Le Conte Avenue, 72-227 CHS, Los Angeles, CA 90095, USA; [b] Department of Surgery, David Geffen School of Medicine, Lichtenstein Amid Hernia Clinic at UCLA, 1304 15th Street, Suite 102, Santa Monica, CA 90404, USA
* Corresponding author.
E-mail address: DCChen@mednet.ucla.edu

Surg Clin N Am 101 (2021) 939–949
https://doi.org/10.1016/j.suc.2021.08.001
0039-6109/21/© 2021 Elsevier Inc. All rights reserved.

surgical.theclinics.com

Table 1
Summary of practical points for surgeons on evidence-based wound closure techniques

Statement	Quality of Evidence	Strength of Recommendation
Use a non-midline laparotomy incision wherever possible.	Moderate	Strong
For midline fascial closure, use a slowly absorbable suture material and employ continuous suturing technique.	Low/moderate	Strong
Use a small bites technique by taking 5-mm to 8-mm bites of fascia and placing stitches every 5 mm.	Moderate	Weak
Use a suture–to–wound length ratio of at least 4:1.	Low	Weak
Prophylactic mesh augmentation for elective midline laparotomy in a high-risk patient should be considered	Moderate	Weak
For single-incision laparoscopic surgery, closure of the fascial incision is recommended.	Moderate	Weak
For laparoscopic surgery, closure of fascial defects greater than or equal to 10 mm is recommended.	Low	Weak

Adapted from 2015 European Hernia Society guidelines on the closure of abdominal wall incision.[7]

infections and wound dehiscence.[3] These are potentially preventable outcomes associated with significant morbidity, mortality, longer hospitalization, greater readmission rates, and increased health care costs.[4,5] Although various patient-related risk factors and individual pathology play a significant role in incisional hernia rates and wound complications, modifying surgical technique may lower complication rates[6] and the quality and methodology of suture technique in fascial closure is associated with better outcomes.[7,8]

HOW TO LOWER THE RISK OF INCISIONAL HERNIAS AND WOUND COMPLICATIONS

There are well-established patient risk factors associated with development of incisional hernias and surgical site occurrences that are intrinsic (age, contamination, and urgency of the repair) or modifiable (smoking, body mass index, nutritional status, glycemic control, immunosuppression, and other modifiable comorbidities).[9,10] The urgency of the laparotomy and circumstance of the patient dictate whether it is feasible to modify these patient risk factors prior to embarking on the intended operation. If an operation can be delayed without major undue risk, then it is a surgeon's duty to help optimize patients perioperatively and offer anticipatory counsel regarding elevated risk for development of incisional hernias and wound complications following abdominal surgery. In addition to managing medical comorbidities, there is growing evidence in the surgical literature that supports standardized wound closure techniques, choice of incision location and orientation, minimally invasive surgical approaches. and perioperative care bundles to reduce incisional hernias and wound complications.[7,8,11] The focus of this section is to explore the evidence, as well as the lack thereof, behind the technical aspects of wound closure techniques and how they modulate the risk of hernia development and surgical site occurrences.

FASCIAL CLOSURE

Traditionally, surgeons have closed fascia based on personal preference, what they have learned in training, or habit influenced by available resources within their current practice environment. The tradition of suturing the midline fascia with 1-cm bites and

1-cm advances using a robust diameter number 0 or number 1 suture on a large-gauge needle remains surgical dogma for many. The perception of this standard closure as being robust along with the generally insidious nature of development for most incisional hernias have made changing existing surgical technique—"the voodoo that we do"—a true challenge. There are robust data, however, to support a standardized method of closing fascia for elective laparotomies.[8] Thus, optimizing surgical technique to close laparotomy incisions using evidence-based methods has the potential to reduce patient suffering from incisional hernias and lower health care and societal costs in the long term.

Choice of Laparotomy Incision

Laparotomy incisions are chosen based on the type of abdominal operation performed and vary depending on the exposure that is needed. When feasible and available, minimally invasive approaches to the abdomen generally minimize the risk and extent of incisional hernia development. For open operations, a variety of midline, transverse, oblique, or paramedian incisions can be used to access the abdomen.[12] Two large meta-analyses of randomized studies comparing incisional hernia rates among different laparotomy incisions recommend using non-midline incisions, such as paramedian and transverse incisions, whenever feasible because they are associated with a lower incidence of incisional hernias (midline vs paramedian; relative risk [RR] 3.41; midline vs transverse, RR 1.77).[13,14] A study by Bickenbach and colleagues[13] demonstrated an additional quality-of-life benefit, with transverse incisions reducing perioperative narcotics use, finding a difference of approximately 23 mg of morphine equivalents between the 2 groups. Furthermore, a single-center randomized controlled trial of 150 female patients undergoing open cholecystectomy compared midline versus transverse laparotomy incisions and showed a lower incidence of incisional hernias (2% vs 14%, respectively) with shorter skin incisions associated with a more pleasing appearance in the transverse laparotomy group.[15] When there is a choice to utilize a non-midline laparotomy incision that does not hinder the intended abdominal operation, current evidence supports avoiding a midline incision to reduce rates of incisional hernias. Needless to say, for many abdominal operations, a midline incision still provides the best exposure compromise should not be made in these situations.

Specimen Extraction Site

Minimally invasive approaches to abdominal surgery continue to rise in prevalence, and the decision of where to extract a specimen from the abdomen becomes increasingly important as it pertains to incisional hernia risk. There still are few prospective data available on this question. A single-center randomized controlled trial of 165 patients in Canada undergoing laparoscopic colectomy assigned patients to transverse or midline specimen extraction and found a higher incidence of incisional hernias in the midline extraction group (15% vs 2%, respectively) in the per protocol analysis of the trial and supports using a transverse extraction technique for laparoscopic colectomy.[16] More recently, a prospective cohort study performed in Korea of 4276 colorectal cancer patients undergoing laparoscopic or robotic-assisted colectomy compared clinical data between those who had transverse versus midline extractions found a higher incidence of incisional hernia in the midline extraction group (3.5% versus 1.7%, respectively).[17] This difference did not bear out in the multivariate analysis, however, where location of specimen extraction was no longer significant between groups and transfusion requirement became the strongest predictor of incisional hernias.[17] At this point, larger studies and longer patient follow-up are needed to be able to better establish patient outcomes and incisional hernia rates related to specimen extraction sites.

Standardized Fascial Closure Technique for Midline Laparotomies

There is a large body of literature published on the impact of fascial closure techniques. Interpretation of this evidence can be challenging given its immense heterogeneity, because many of the prospective studies compare several different variables across multiple study arms, which add confounders to data interpretation. Closure techniques can be split into discrete components that include use of continuous versus interrupted sutures, closure versus nonclosure of peritoneum, suture–to–wound length ratio, suture material, absorbability, and needle type, addressed later. The literature behind the current recommendations is well summarized in the European Hernia Society guidelines, published in 2015.[8] The strength of evidence varies greatly between each component and each is addressed individually.

A meta-analysis performed by Diener and colleagues[18] in 2010 concluded that continuous sutures are associated with lower incisional hernia rates in elective laparotomies (odds ratio [OR] 0.59; $P = .001$). This meta-analysis, however, included many studies that employed rapidly absorbable multifilament sutures in the interrupted suture arm and nonabsorbable or slowly absorbable monofilament sutures in the continuous suture arm.[18] An earlier meta-analysis from 2002 included both elective and emergency cases and found no difference in incisional hernia formation between interrupted and continuous suturing groups.[19] Faster closure times were reported, however, in the continuous group, which confers obvious benefit in emergency cases because it reduces operative time. An updated meta-analysis in 2016 reached the same conclusion that a slowly absorbable monofilament suture using a continuous/running technique offers the highest efficacy with regards to reducing the incidence of incisional hernia rates after elective midline laparotomy.[20] Gurusamy and colleagues,[21] in a Cochrane review published in 2013 that included 5 randomized controlled trials and 836 patients undergoing laparotomy, examined the relationship between peritoneum closure and risk of developing incisional hernias and burst abdomen. The study concluded no benefit of performing closure of the peritoneum with a separate layer of sutures.[21]

In 2009, a single-center RCT of 737 patients undergoing laparotomy via a midline incision were randomized to fascial closure using a continuous, single-layer of monofilament suture and self-locking anchor knots to either short stitch length or long stitch length groups.[22] In the long stitch group, stitches were placed at least 1 cm from wound edge using a 1-0 polydioxanone (PDS) on a TP-1 needle and, in the short stitch group, stitches were placed 5 mm to 8 mm from the wound edge using a 2-0 PDS suture on an MH-1 needle. The study found increased surgical site infection (10.2% vs 5.2%, respectively, at 4 weeks) and incisional hernia rates (18% vs 5.6%, respectively, at 12 months) in the long stitch group at the expense of a slightly longer closing time in the operating room (14 minutes vs 18 minutes, respectively).[22] The explanation for these findings is substantiated in separate studies that examine tissue integrity, demonstrating that the longer stitches compress and devitalize more tissue in the wound, which in turn increases the opportunity for infection. Over time, tissue devitalization contributes to redundancy and loss of tension in the suture, leading to a higher rate of incisional hernias.

In 2015, another landmark multicenter randomized controlled trial (STITCH) from the Netherlands examined 560 patients undergoing midline laparotomy and split patients into small bite (5-mm tissue bites with 5-mm travel between sutures) and large bite groups (1-cm tissue bites with 1-cm travel between sutures) and found a decrease in incisional hernias (21% vs 13%, respectively) in the small bite group at 1-year follow-up.[23] Special attention should be paid to emphasizing the important concept of suture–to–wound length ratio, which refers to the quotient between the amount of suture used to the fascial defect. A suture–to–wound length ratio of at least 4 was associated with lower rate of incisional hernia development (11.3% vs 25.9%, respectively).[22] Suture material also is an important consideration. In a 2011 systematic review comparing slowly absorbing versus nonabsorbable sutures, no differences in incisional hernia rates were found between both groups; however, there was an increased risk of postoperative pain and sinus formation in the nonabsorbable suture group.[24] There was no direct comparison between using monofilament versus multifilament sutures, but this may be a moot point because all slowly absorbable sutures are monofilament. Multifilament suture, however, is associated with a higher rate of surgical site infection because bacteria can embed in the suture material and escape phagocytosis.

There is not enough direct evidence on either needle type or the need for retention sutures during elective midline laparotomy closures. The use of smaller, noncutting needles is thought to contribute to the benefits seen with short stitch technique using smaller diameter suture. Finally, antibiotic-impregnated sutures have been shown, in a 2014 meta-analysis by Diener and colleagues,[25] to be associated with reduced surgical site infections.

To briefly summarize the European Hernia Society guidelines from 2015, it currently is recommended that midline laparotomy incision be closed with a slowly absorbable monofilament suture in a single layer aponeurotic closure method.[8] The suture–to–wound length should be at least 4:1 and application of small bites technique of 5 mm by 5 mm should be the standard closure method.[8] These same recommendations are echoed in the most recent recommendations published by the Progress on Prevention Surgical Group, which also recommends that, across all specialties performing abdominal operations, surgeons should aim for an incision hernia rate of less than 10% as a target benchmark.[26]

Prophylactic Mesh

Another important consideration in incisional hernia prophylaxis during elective laparotomies is the placement of prophylactic mesh to augment fascia closure. The European Hernia Society Guidelines Development Group reviewed the data on the outcomes of incisional hernias, seromas, and surgical site infections after placement of prophylactic mesh and found its use to be effective in the prevention of incisional hernias (RR 0.17; CI, 0.08–0.37).[8] At the time of publication, the strength of the recommendation is classified as weak given the relative scarcity of robust prospective trials and the heterogeneity of mesh type, position, and methods of fixation. Since that publication, an updated meta-analysis by Borab and colleagues[27] in 2017 reviewed prophylactic mesh augmentation in elective midline laparotomies and reported 85% RR reduction in formation of incisional hernias, at the expense of an increased risk of seroma formation (1.95%), more prevalent after an onlay technique, and increased chronic wound pain (1.70%). The HULC trial is an ongoing multicenter randomized controlled trial designed to provide more robust evidence to address the looming question of whether onlay mesh augmentation in addition to small stitched fascial closure provides benefit of preventing incisional hernia formation compared with small stitched fascial closure alone in elective laparotomies.[28]

There currently are few data to make conclusions regarding the efficacy and safety of prophylactic mesh augmentation in the emergency laparotomy setting.[29] At present, prophylactic mesh augmentation should be considered in high-risk patient populations undergoing elective midline laparotomies.[27]

In practice, surgeons still are slow to adopt new closure techniques and mesh augmentation into practice and there remains significant variation in clinical practice. Various surgical societies worldwide have attempted creative methods to disseminate these standardized guidelines to currently practicing surgeons. For example, the Turkish Hernia Society sent educational letters to specialty societies to present on closure techniques.[30] The Americas Hernia Society launched the Stop the Bulge campaign to raise awareness of the current guidelines and made educational slides readily available online.[30] In addition, despite the growing body of evidence, there still are few long-term prospective data on the utility of these closure techniques in domestic studies with representative American patient cohorts as well as in unique situations, such as emergency laparotomies and select patient population, such as the obese.

Trocar Size and Port Closure

Closure of trocar sites deserves special attention as the incidence of laparoscopic and robotic-assisted approaches to abdominal operations continue to rise in popularity. Helgstrand and colleagues[31] in 2011 conducted a systematic review of trocar-site hernias after laparoscopic surgery and found a risk reduction of hernia rates with suture closure for trocar diameters larger than 10 mm. Although the overall incidence was low (0.5%–2%), trocar-site hernia occurred most often at port sites greater than 10 mm and in the periumbilical region (82%).[31] There are few data regarding routine prophylactic mesh use in augmenting port site closures. A 2014 randomized clinic trial of 106 patients with elevated comorbid risk factors for incisional hernia (age >65, diabetes, chronic obstructive pulmonary disease, and body mass index >30 kg/m^2) undergoing laparoscopic cholecystectomy randomized patients to primary closure with a nonabsorbable suture versus coverage with intraperitoneal polypropylene mesh.[32] The study found that periumbilical trocar site incisional hernias were higher in the primary closure only group (31.9% vs 4.4%, respectively; $P < .001$) without a significant difference in wound infection rates (8.5% vs 0%, respectively; $P = .045$) and advocated for the routine use of prosthetic closure of the umbilical trocar site.[33] A meta-analysis showed a rare incidence but higher risk of incisional hernias in single-port surgery (OR 4.94; 95% CI, 1.26–19.4) and recommend fascial closure in these cases.[34]

Abdominal Binders

Postoperative abdominal binders frequently are given to patients following a laparotomy. The actual utility in preventing wound dehiscence and symptomatic benefit of these binders, however, have been called into question in a systematic review by Bouvier and colleagues[33] published in 2014, which summarized 4 clinical trials and also conducted a national survey in France examining this common practice. The study found that most surgeons routinely use abdominal binders because it was the practice during their surgical training and there is a perceived benefit of binders preventing abdominal wall dehiscence and an improvement in patient comfort and postoperative pain following laparotomy.[33] To date, however, there is no robust prospective clinical trial that definitively supports improved pain, incisional hernia, or wound dehiscence outcomes after routine application of an abdominal binder.

How Are Surgeons Currently Closing Laparotomies?

A 2021 study by Paulsen and colleagues[35] reviewed abdominal wall closure techniques in lower transverse laparotomy incisions by colorectal surgeons and obstetricians/gynecologists and found that practice varies significant across surgical specialties. For example, approximately 98% of the colorectal surgeons and 66% of the obstetricians/gynecologists used a monofilament suture when closing the fascia. Although a majority of colorectal surgeons report using continuous suture and small bites technique, only half of the obstetricians/gynecologists practiced this technique. Approximately two-thirds of the colorectal surgeons and one-third of the obstetricians/gynecologists used a suture length–to–wound length ratio greater than 4:1.[35] This study highlights both the need for more conclusive evidence for standardized fascial closure techniques for different types of laparotomy incisions—midline, transverse, paramedian, and oblique—as well as the need for better education and dissemination of information to practicing providers and surgeons-in-training. The Progress on Prevention Surgical Group published a report in 2021 that strongly advocates for collaboration among an interdisciplinary group of abdominal surgeons, including general, vascular, gynecologic, urologic, colorectal, and hepatopancreatobiliary surgeons to adhere to the principles of standardized closure techniques during elective laparotomies in effort to jointly minimize the incidence of incisional hernias to a goal rate of less than 10% across all disciplines.[26]

SUBCUTANEOUS WOUND CLOSURE

Aside from fascial closure, there are controversy and variation among surgeons in the manner by which subcutaneous wounds are addressed during laparotomy. In the obstetric population, reapproximation of subcutaneous tissue has been shown to reduce frequency of wound disruption. A 2017 meta-analysis, including 10 studies and 3696 female patients undergoing caesarean section, found that reapproximation of the subcutaneous tissue significantly reduced the odds of developing any type of wound complication (OR 0.66; 95% CI, 0.47–0.93) and reduced the incidence of seroma (OR 0.53; 95% CI, 0.33–0.84).[36] Obliteration of dead space via a subcutaneous stitch seems to be associated with decreased rate of postoperative seroma formation,[37] although the quality of the existing data remains poor.

NEGATIVE-PRESSURE WOUND THERAPY

Frequently following laparotomies where wound contamination is a major concern, the wound is left open to heal by secondary intention. Here the surgeon has a choice between various wound care modalities. Currently, the evidence for the use of negative-pressure wound therapy (NPWT) on postoperative wound outcomes remains equivocal. The most recent Cochrane review on this topic conducted in 2019 reported no significant differences in wound dehiscence, mortality, reoperation rates, seroma or hematoma formation, and quality-adjusted life years between NPWT and conventional dressing.[38] The investigators acknowledged a small reduction in the rate of surgical site infections (RR 0.67; 95% CI, 0.53–0.85) and more cost-effectiveness compared with standard dressings.[38] The quality of the existing evidence overall, however, is poor and may be at risk for bias.[38]

Since the 2019 Cochrane review, newer trials have been published that compared NPWT to conventional dressings. A randomized controlled trial published in 2021 examined patients undergoing elective laparotomy for presumed gynecologic malignancies who randomized to standard gauze NPWT and found similar rate of wound complications (17.3% vs 16.3%, respectively) and an increased rate of blister formation (13% vs 1.2%, respectively) in the NPWT group.[39] A multicenter randomized clinical trial evaluating obese women (average body mass index 39.5) undergoing elective or urgent cesarean deliveries randomized patients to NPWT and standard gauze dressing and also reported no difference in surgical site infections (3.6% vs 3.4%, respectively) and other wound complications (6.5% vs 6.7%, respectively).[40] Finally, a multinational, multicenter observer-blinded randomized clinical trial (SAWHI) compared 539 patients undergoing laparotomies to NPWT versus conventional wound treatment and found that the mean time to wound closure was shorter (36 days vs 39 days, respectively) and wound closure rate at 42 days (35.9 vs 21.5%, respectively) in the NPWT group; however, this is offset by the higher wound-related adverse events (RR 1.51; 95% CI, 0.99–2.35) in the intervention group.[41] The study concluded that NPWT may be better than conventional dressing in achieving complete closure of subcutaneous abdominal wounds but is associated with more wound related adverse events.[41] Due to the heterogeneity and short follow-up intervals present in existing studies, no definitive conclusions can be made on the benefit of routine use of NPWT for contaminated laparotomy wounds.

SUMMARY

Incisional hernias are common complications following laparotomies and contribute to significant patient morbidity, high reoperation rates, and increased health care costs. There currently are robust data to support standardized wound closure techniques to reduce incisional hernia rates. These include small bites suture technique (5-mm by 5-mm suture distance) with a greater than or equal to 4:1 suture–to–wound length, prophylactic mesh augmentation in high-risk patients and closure of trocar site defects greater than 10 mm in minimally invasive surgery. Although high-quality evidence exists for these techniques, other common practices in abdominal surgery, such as abdominal binder usage, NPWT, and reapproximation of subcutaneous tissue, still lack quality evidence to support their routine use in abdominal surgery. At this point, larger studies and longer patient follow-up are needed to better establish patient outcomes related to these commonplace yet evidence-deficient wound closure techniques in abdominal surgery.

DISCLOSURE

The authors have nothing to disclose.

REFERENCES

1. Poulose BK, Shelton J, Phillips S, et al. Epidemiology and cost of ventral hernia repair: making the case for hernia research. Hernia 2012;16:179–83.
2. Bucknall TE, Cox PJ, Ellis H. Burst abdomen and incisional hernia: a prospective study of 1129 major laparotomies. Br Med J (Clin Res Ed) 1982;284(6320): 931–3.
3. Leaper DJ, van Goor H, Reilly J, et al. Surgical site infection—a European perspective of incidence and economic burden. Int Wound J 2004;1(4): 247–73.
4. Keenan JE, Speicher PJ, Thacker JK, et al. The preventive surgical site infection bundle in colorectal surgery: an effective approach to surgical site infection reduction and health care cost savings. JAMA Surg 2014;149(10): 1045–52.

5. Petrosillo N, Drapeau CM, Nicastri E, et al. Surgical site infections in Italian Hospitals: a prospective multicenter study. BMC Infect Dis 2008;8:34.

6. Aga E, Keinan-Boker L, Eithan A, et al. Surgical site infections after abdominal surgery: incidence and risk factors. A prospective cohort study. Infect Dis (Lond) 2015;47(11):761–7.

7. Muysoms FE, Antoniou SA, Bury K, et al. European Hernia Society guidelines on the closure of abdominal wall incisions. Hernia 2015;19(1):1–24.

8. Israelsson LA, Jonsson T. Closure of midline laparotomy incisions with polydioxanone and nylon: the importance of suture technique. Br J Surg 1994;81(11): 1606–8.

9. Hoer J, Lawong G, Klinge U, et al. Factors influencing the development of incisional hernia. A retrospective study of 2,983 laparotomy patients over a period of 10 years. Chirurg 2002;73:474–80.

10. Antoniou GA, Georgiadis GS, Antoniou SA, et al. Abdominal aortic aneurysm and abdominal wall hernia as manifestations of a connective tissue disorder. J Vasc Surg 2011;54:1175–81.

11. Pop-Vicas AE, Abad C, Baubie K, et al. Colorectal bundles for surgical site infection prevention: a systematic review and meta-analysis. Infect Control Hosp Epidemiol 2020;41(7):805–12.

12. Burger JW, van't Riet M, Jeekel J. Abdominal incisions: techniques and postoperative complications. Scand J Surg 2002;91:315–21.

13. Bickenbach KA, Karanicolas PJ, Ammori JB, et al. Up and down or side to side? A systematic review and meta-analysis examining the impact of incision on outcomes after abdominal surgery. Am J Surg 2013;206(3):400–9.

14. Brown SR, Goodfellow PB. Transverse verses midline incisions for abdominal surgery. Cochrane Database Syst Rev 2005;(4):CD005199.

15. Halm JA, Lip H, Schmitz PI, et al. Incisional hernia after upper abdominal surgery: a randomised controlled trial of midline versus transverse incision. Hernia 2009; 13(3):275–80.

16. Lee L, Mata J, Droeser RA, et al. Incisional hernia after midline versus transverse specimen extraction incision: a randomized trial in patients undergoing laparoscopic colectomy. Ann Surg 2018;268(1):41–7.

17. Choi HB, Chung D, Kim JS, et al. Midline incision vs. transverse incision for specimen extraction is not a significant risk factor for developing incisional hernia after minimally invasive colorectal surgery: multivariable analysis of a large cohort from a single tertiary center in Korea. Surg Endosc 2021. https://doi.org/10.1007/s00464-021-08388-z.

18. Diener MK, Voss S, Jensen K, et al. Elective midline laparotomy closure: the inline systematic review and meta-analysis. Ann Surg 2010;251:843–56.

19. van't Riet M, Steyerberg EW, Nellensteyn J, et al. Meta-analysis of techniques for closure of midline abdominal incisions. Br J Surg 2002;89:1350–6.

20. Heger P, Pianka F, Diener MK, et al. Current standards of abdominal wall closure techniques: conventional suture techniques. Chirurg 2016;87(9): 737–43.

21. Gurusamy KS, Cassar Delia E, Davidson BR. Peritoneal closure versus no peritoneal closure for patients undergoing non-obstetric abdominal operations. Cochrane Database Syst Rev 2013;2013(7):CD010424.

22. Millbourn D, Cengiz Y, Israelsson LA. Effect of stitch length on wound complications after closure of midline incisions: a randomized controlled trial. Arch Surg 2009;144(11):1056–9.

23. Deerenberg EB, Harlaar JJ, Steyerberg EW, et al. Small bites versus large bites for closure of abdominal midline incisions (STITCH): a double-blind, multicentre, randomised controlled trial. Lancet 2015;386(10000):1254–60.
24. Sajid MS, Parampalli U, Baig MK. A systematic review on the effectiveness of slowly-absorbable versus non-absorbable sutures for abdominal fascial closure following laparotomy. Int J Surg 2011;9(8):615–25.
25. Diener MK, Knebel P, Kieser M, et al. Effectiveness of triclosan-coated PDS Plus versus uncoated PDS II sutures for prevention of surgical site infection after abdominal wall closure: the randomised controlled PROUD trial. Lancet 2014; 384:142–52.
26. Garcia-Urena MA, POP (Progress On Prevention) Surgical Group. Preventing incisional ventral hernias: important for patients but ignored by surgical specialties? A critical review. Hernia 2021;25(1):13–22.
27. Borab ZM, Shakir S, Lanni MA, et al. Does prophylactic mesh placement in elective, midline laparotomy reduce the incidence of incisional hernia? A systematic review and meta-analysis. Surgery 2017;161(4):1149–63.
28. Heger P, Feibt M, Krisam J, et al. Hernia reduction following laparotomy using small stitch abdominal wall closure with and without mesh augmentation (the HULC trial): study protocol for a randomized controlled trial. Trial 2019; 20(1):738.
29. Burns FA, Heywood EG, Challand CP, et al. Is there a role for prophylactic mesh in abdominal wall closure after emergency laparotomy? A systematic review and meta-analysis. Hernia 2020 Jun;24(3):441–7.
30. Yheulon C, Davis SS. Adopting the STITCH Trial: crossing the chasm from publication to practice. JAMA Surg 2019;154(12):1087–108.
31. Helgstrand F, Rosenberg J, Bisgaard T. Trocar site hernia after laparoscopic surgery: a qualitative systematic review. Hernia 2011;15(2):113–21.
32. Armañanzas L, Ruiz-Tovar J, Arroyo A, et al. Prophylactic mesh vs suture in the closure of the umbilical trocar site after laparoscopic cholecystectomy in high-risk patients for incisional hernia. A randomized clinical trial. J Am Coll Surg 2014;218(5):960–8.
33. Bouvier A, Rat P, Drissi-Chbihi F, et al. Abdominal binders after laparotomy: review of the literature and French survey of policies. Hernia 2014;18(4):501–6.
34. Milas M, Devedija S, Trkulja V. Single incision versus standard multiport laparoscopic cholecystectomy: up-dated systematic review and meta-analysis of randomized trials. Surgeon 2014;12:271–89.
35. Paulsen CB, Zetner D, Rosenberg J. Variation in abdominal wall closure techniques in lower transverse incisions: a nationwide survey across specialties. Hernia 2021;25(2):345–52.
36. Pergialiotis V, Prodromidou A, Perrea DN, et al. The impact of subcutaneous tissue suturing at caesarean section on wound complications: a meta-analysis. BJOG 2017;124(7):1018–25.
37. Aho JM, Nickerson TP, Thiels CA, et al. Prevention of postoperative seromas with dead space obliteration: A case-control study. Int J Surg 2016;29:70–3.
38. Webster J, Liu Z, Norman G, et al. Negative pressure wound therapy for surgical wounds healing by primary closure. Cochrane Database Syst Rev 2019;3(3): CD009261.
39. Leitao MM Jr, Zhou QC, Schiavone MB, et al. Prophylactic negative pressure wound therapy after laparotomy for gynecologic surgery: a randomized controlled trial. Obstet Gynecol 2021;137(2):334–41.

40. Tuuli MG, Liu J, Tita ATN, et al. Effect of prophylactic negative pressure wound therapy vs standard wound dressing on surgical-site infection in obese women after cesarean delivery: a randomized clinical trial. JAMA 2020;324(12):1180–9.

41. Seidel D, Diedrich S, Herrle F, et al. Negative pressure wound therapy vs conventional wound treatment in subcutaneous abdominal wound healing impairment: the SAWHI randomized clinical trial. JAMA Surg 2020;155(6):469–78.

Evidence-based Prevention of Surgical Site Infection

Matthew A. Fuglestad, MD, Elisabeth L. Tracey, MD, Jennifer A. Leinicke, MD*

KEYWORDS

- Surgical site infection • SSI • Enhanced recovery after surgery • SSI bundles

KEY POINTS

- Despite significant progress in reducing the incidence of surgical site infection, infectious complications remain a challenging and costly complication of surgery.
- There is strong evidence to support the use of mechanical and oral antibiotic bowel preparation in colorectal surgery, smoking cessation before elective surgery, prophylactic antibiotics, chlorhexidine-based skin antisepsis, and maintenance of normothermia throughout the perioperative period. These measures should be strongly considered during development of local surgical site infection reduction bundles.
- Interventions such as surgical caps, use of surgical jackets, preoperative bathing with antibiotic-containing soaps, adhesive surgical barriers, iodine-impregnated adhesive drapes, hyperoxia, and hair removal before surgery have inconsistent levels of evidence to provide strong recommendations for or against their use. Decisions regarding these practices should be deferred to institution and/or surgeon preference using a common-sense approach.

INTRODUCTION

Surgical site infection (SSI) remains a frequent and challenging complication of surgery. SSI accounts for greater than 20% of all health care–associated infections, rivaling pneumonia as the most common nosocomial infection.[1] SSI affects an estimated 160,000 to 300,000 individuals annually with an associated financial cost that may exceed $3.5 billion.[2–6] The high morbidity and costs associated with SSI have resulted in a concerted effort to precisely define and study SSI in order to limit infectious complications after surgery.[2]

There has been significant progress in reducing the incidence of SSI through a variety of local and national programs, including the American College of Surgeons (ACS) National Surgical Quality Improvement Program (NSQIP).[7–10] Despite this, SSI continues to affect 2% to 5% of all surgical patients.[4] The medical and surgical community

Department of Surgery, University of Nebraska Medical Center, 983280 Nebraska Medical Center, Omaha, NE 68198-3280, USA
* Corresponding author.
E-mail address: jennifer.leinicke@unmc.edu

Surg Clin N Am 101 (2021) 951–966
https://doi.org/10.1016/j.suc.2021.05.027

has responded with high-quality SSI-reduction research, clinical practice guidelines, and development of multifaceted SSI-prevention bundles with encouraging results.[6,9–16] In addition, surgeons have looked to the past and reincorporated older practices as new data have provided insight into the benefits of their use.[7,15–17] With the wide range of available strategies to reduce the risk of SSI, familiarity with the evidence behind their use is desirable.

This article reviews common SSI-reduction strategies and provides an evaluation of the data for their use. It highlights high-quality interventions that are easily incorporated into practice and have been shown to reduce SSI. It also discusses practices that have limited evidence to strongly support or refute their use and encourages these practices to be left to the discretion of the operating surgeon or hospital system.

DEFINING SURGICAL SITE INFECTION AND WOUND CLASSIFICATIONS

The United States Centers for Disease Control and Prevention (CDC) National Healthcare Safety Network (NHSN) has provided precise criteria and definitions for SSI.[2,18] For the purposes of this article, SSI is defined according to CDC NHSN definitions as infection occurring within or around the surgical site within 30 days of the index procedure or within 90 days of a procedure with implantation of prosthetic material.[2] Further, SSI is subcategorized by the location of infection, including superficial SSI, deep SSI, and organ/space SSI (**Table 1**).

Wound classification continues to be used to categorize surgical wounds in the literature, although there is some debate regarding its ability to predict development of SSI. Surgical wounds are classified into clean, clean contaminated, contaminated, or dirty/infected, with a presumed higher risk of SSI as the degree of contamination increases. This article focuses primarily on data relating to elective clean and clean-contaminated cases.

EVIDENCE-BASED REDUCTION OF SURGICAL SITE INFECTION
Smoking Cessation

Up to 50.6 million US adults are actively using tobacco products.[19] Current and former smokers are at increased risk for poor wound healing and development of postoperative complications.[20–24] A meta-analysis of 140 studies comparing smokers with non-smokers in elective surgery showed that the risk of SSI was nearly doubled in active smokers.[20] These findings were similarly shown in patients undergoing elective colorectal surgeries using the ACS-NSQIP database.[21] After adjusting for a variety of SSI risk factors, both current and former smoking was independently associated with an increased risk of SSI (odds ratio [OR], 1.32 and 1.27 respectively). For this reason, smoking cessation before elective surgery is recommended by multiple societies.[6,11,12]

The optimal duration of smoking cessation before elective surgery is unclear. Sorensen and colleagues[22] reported a randomized trial investigating the effect of smoking cessation on the development of SSI after creation of a series of identical wounds. Smokers were compared with a cohort of never-smokers. Active smokers developed wound infections at a rate of 12%. Both never-smokers and smokers who had abstained for 4 weeks had significantly lower rates of SSI compared with active smokers (2% and 1% respectively). The investigators concluded that 1 month of smoking cessation may be sufficient to reduce the development of SSIs.[22]

Another widely cited study has suggested that a 6-week to 8-week time frame preoperatively is desirable.[23] However, smoking cessation on the day of surgery alone may reduce the rate of SSI.[24] When possible, smoking cessation should occur at least

Table 1
United States Centers for Disease Control and Prevention National Healthcare Safety Network classification of surgical site infection[2]

Superficial Incisional SSI	The date of event occurs within 30 d after any NHSN operative procedure
	And
	Involves only skin and subcutaneous tissue of the incision
	And
	The patient has at least 1 of the following:
	  1. Purulent drainage from the superficial incision
	  2. An organism is identified from an aseptically obtained specimen from the superficial incision or subcutaneous tissue by a culture-based or non–culture-based microbiological testing method that is performed for purposes of clinical diagnosis or treatment
	  3. Superficial incision that is deliberately opened by a surgeon, physician, or physician designee and culture-based or non–culture-based testing of the superficial incision or subcutaneous tissue is not performed, and the patient has at least 1 of the following signs or symptoms: localized pain or tenderness, localized swelling, erythema, or heat.
	  4. Diagnosis of a superficial incisional SSI by a physician or physician designee

Deep Incisional SSI	The date of event occurs within 30 or 90 d after the NHSN operative procedure
	And
	Involves deep soft tissues of the incision (eg, fascial and muscle layers)
	And
	The patient has at least 1 of the following:
	  1. Purulent drainage from the deep incision
	  2. Deep incision that spontaneously dehisces, or is deliberately opened or aspirated by a surgeon, physician, or physician designee
	And
	An organism is identified from the deep soft tissues of the incision by a culture-based or non–culture-based microbiologic testing method that is performed for purposes of clinical diagnosis or treatment
	And
	The patient has at least 1 of the following signs or symptoms:
	  1. Fever(>38°C); localized pain or tenderness
	  2. An abscess or other evidence of infection involving the deep incision that is detected on gross anatomic or histopathologic examination, or imaging test

Organ Space SSI	Date of event occurs within 30 or 90 d after the NHSN operative procedure
	And
	Involves any part of the body deeper than the fascial/muscle layers that is opened or manipulated during the operative procedure
	And
	The patient has at least 1 of the following:
	  1. Purulent drainage from a drain that is placed into the organ/space (eg, closed suction drainage system, open drain, T-tube drain, computed tomography–guided drainage)
	  2. An organism identified from fluid or tissue in the organ/space by a culture-based or non–culture-based microbiologic detecting method that is performed for purposes of clinical diagnosis or treatment
	  3. An abscess or other evidence of infection involving the organ/space that is detected on gross anatomic or histopathologic examination, or imaging test evidence suggestive of infection
	And
	Meets at least 1 criterion for a specific organ/space infection site as defined by CDC/NHSN

4 weeks before an elective operation. Given the evidence for SSI reduction and the associated health benefits, smoking cessation should be pursued in all patients before elective surgery.

Perioperative Showering/Bathing

In an effort to further reduce the incidence of SSI, investigators have evaluated the utility of perioperative bathing/showering with chlorhexidine-based products in an effort to maximally decolonize skin before surgery. In theory, reduction of bacterial colonization would be anticipated to decrease SSI development. However, the effect on SSIs has been variable, with some studies suggesting potential harm.[25–27]

A 2015 meta-analysis of randomized controlled trials (RCTs) showed no significant benefit to preoperative washing with chlorhexidine compared with placebo (relative risk [RR], 0.91; confidence interval [CI], 0.80–1.04).[25] Similarly, compared with bar soap, washing with chlorhexidine did not significantly reduce the incidence of SSI (RR, 1.02; CI, 0.57–1.84). However, data were limited for the comparison with bar soap, and these findings should be interpreted with caution because the largest individual study included in the meta-analysis did find a reduction in SSI.[26] In the trials reporting adverse skin and allergic reactions, the incidence was low (0.0%–0.5%) and was comparable with placebo (0.6%). The meta-analysis advised that there was no clear benefit to the use of preoperative chlorhexidine washing compared with other wash products.

Prabhu and colleagues[27] reviewed 3924 patients undergoing ventral hernia repair in the Americas Hernia Society Quality Collaborative data registry from 2013 to 2016. Patients who received a prehospital chlorhexidine gluconate (CHG) scrub were compared with those who did not receive prehospital CHG scrub. Results of the multivariate regression modeling showed prehospital CHG was associated with an increased risk of SSI (OR, 1.49; CI, 1.05–2.11). These findings persisted after propensity score modeling. The investigators acknowledged that the administration of CHG scrub was not standardized, but suggested that their findings may approximate real-world use of CHG scrub before surgery. The investigators cautioned against indiscriminate use of CHG scrub before surgery without proven benefit, especially in the setting of concern for development of antibiotic-resistant organisms.

These data do not suggest that perioperative hygiene is not an important component of preparation for surgery. Patients should shower/bathe before surgery, as is generally recommended. However, with the current limitations in available data, and no clear benefit to preoperative showering/bathing with chlorhexidine-based products, the authors do not routinely use these products as part of our preoperative preparation of patients.

Bowel Preparation in Elective Colorectal Surgery

Data regarding the benefits of combined oral antibiotic and mechanical bowel preparation (CBP) in colorectal surgery were in part brought to light by Nichols and colleagues[17] in 1972, who reported a reduction in wound infections with the addition of neomycin-erythromycin base to mechanical bowel preparation (MBP). In the years following, various studies have reported conflicting results regarding the benefits of bowel preparation before colorectal surgery.[7,15,16,28–31] This culminated in a Cochrane Review that reported no significant benefit to MBP in 2011, and resulted in an overall movement away from preoperative bowel preparation.[31] However, through strong evidence provided by large statewide and national datasets, full mechanical and oral antibiotic bowel preparation before elective colorectal surgery has again entered the mainstream and is currently recommended in clinical practice guidelines by multiple surgical societies.[6,7,13,15,16]

Englesbe and colleagues[7] reported the results of the multi-institution Michigan Surgical Quality Collaborative investigation of bowel preparation in elective open and laparoscopic colectomy. After propensity score matching, CBP was associated with fewer SSIs overall, superficial SSI, and organ space SSI (4.6% vs 12.4%, 2.4% vs 8.6%, and 1.6% vs 4.3% respectively). The rate of *Clostridioides difficile* colitis was similar (1.9% vs 3.0%) in CBP versus MBP. The investigators concluded that there was a strong association with CBP and reduction in SSI, although a causal relationship was unable to be determined given the observational study design.

In 2017, Ohman and colleagues[15] reported the results of implementation of an infection prevention bundle. Use of this bundle decreased the rate of SSI from 19.7% to 8.2%. Patients who received an MBP, plus oral neomycin and Flagyl, had a lower rate of SSI compared with all other forms of bowel preparation (2.7% vs 15.8%). MBP and oral antibiotic–only bowel preparation resulted in similar rates of SSI compared with no bowel preparation. Only CBP was independently associated with a reduction in SSI, which persisted after multivariate analysis (adjusted OR, 0.2; CI, 0.1–0.6).

Similarly, Klinger and colleagues[16] evaluated the effect of bowel preparation on development of SSI in elective colorectal surgery using the 2012 to 2015 ACS-NSQIP data. Use of CBP resulted in a lower proportion of patients developing both superficial and organ space SSI compared with no bowel preparation within 30 days of surgery (OR, 0.39 and OR, 0.56 respectively). Further, MBP was compared with CBP. MBP was associated with an increased proportion of patients developing superficial and organ space SSI compared with CBP (ORs, 2.25 and 1.64 respectively). Anastomotic complications were less frequent in the CBP cohort, with similar rates of *C difficile* colitis between the two groups. Although SSI-prevention bundles and bowel preparation formulations before surgery were not standardized, the investigators concluded with a recommendation in favor of CBP.[16]

The optimal combination of oral antibiotic and mechanical preparation remains unknown. Additional studies are needed to delineate the optimal CBP before elective colorectal surgery. Further, to date there has been no RCT directly comparing CBP with oral antibiotic–only preparation. This omission will be evaluated in the upcoming ORALEV2 study, which is anticipated to be completed in 2022.

With the preponderance of data supporting the use of CBP, the authors are in favor of a combined mechanical and oral antibiotic preparation for all elective colorectal surgery in patients in whom it is safe and feasible.

Perioperative Surgical Attire

Perioperative surgical attire is an important component of patient and surgical staff safety. However, there are limited data to suggest optimal surgical dress, leaving much of operating room policy regarding surgical attire to be decided by expert consensus.[32] Definitions of appropriate surgical attire have become particularly relevant during periods of personal protective equipment shortage. Surgical attire standards have been tested by the scarcity of resources during the coronavirus disease 2019 (COVID-19) pandemic, causing some investigators to reevaluate the data behind former practices.

The use of disposable bouffant caps versus scrub caps as a way to reduce SSI has been an area of controversy, with strong proponents on either side of the issue. Despite limited data to show benefit to more stringent surgical attire, major medical centers have enacted large-scale changes to surgical attire policy in an effort to reduce SSI.[33,34]

Wills and colleagues[33] completed a retrospective cohort study of all inpatient cases at a single institution comparing no requirement for either bouffant or surgical jacket, the use of surgical jackets only, and mandatory use of both surgical jackets and bouffant with the primary end point of incidence of SSI. There was no significant difference in SSI risk between these 3 groups (1.01% vs 0.99% vs 0.83% respectively) and no significant difference in the secondary outcomes of mortality, postoperative sepsis, or wound dehiscence. These findings suggest that use of bouffant caps and surgical jackets is unlikely to have a meaningful impact on SSI development compared with other high-quality SSI-reduction interventions.

Similarly, Farach and colleagues[34] published the results of a series of strict surgical attire regulations in 2 teaching hospitals across the United States. In total, 6517 patients were analyzed across the 9 months before and after implementation. They reported no difference in the overall rate of SSI in clean and clean-contaminated cases between the two time periods (0.7% vs 0.8%). Multivariate analysis did not find these policies to be independently associated with the risk of SSI. The investigators then calculated that a sample size of 485,154 patients would be needed to appropriately power a future study to detect a 10% decrease in SSI in clean-contaminated cases at their institution, showing the impracticality of attempting to perform a large RCT. This hypothetical study would be associated with a number needed to treat of 1429 patients.

The choice of surgical headwear and its effect on incidence of SSI and contamination of the surgical field have been evaluated in multiple studies.[35–37] A retrospective review of the Americas Hernia Society Quality Collaborative Database performed by Haskins and colleagues[35] evaluated the relationship between the type of surgical hat worn and the development of SSI after hernia repair. Surgeons who had submitted at least 10 patients into the database were surveyed regarding their choice of surgical hat (disposable skull cap, cloth skull cap, cloth bouffant, disposable bouffant with ears exposed, disposable bouffant with ears covered, or other surgical headgear). Sixty-eight surgeons (79.1% of those surveyed) responded, resulting in 6210 cases being available for analysis. Surgeons most commonly wore a disposable skull cap (55.3%) or disposable bouffant (34.8%). The overall incidence of SSI was 4.0% (251 patients). There was no significant difference in the distribution of surgical headwear between cases with and without SSI on univariate analysis. In addition, multivariate logistic regression found that, compared with disposable bouffant with ears covered, surgeon choice of headwear was not independently associated with development of SSI. The investigators concluded that there was no association between the type of surgical hat and the incidence of postoperative wound events following ventral hernia repair and that surgical hats may be chosen at surgeon discretion.

Using data from a previously published prospective RCT, Kothari and colleagues[36] investigated the effect of bouffant and skull caps on SSI rates. A total of 1543 patients were included, encompassing a variety of surgery types, including colorectal, hernia, biliary, and foregut surgery. Sixty-one percent of surgeons wore skull caps and 39% wore bouffant. SSIs occurred more frequently in cases where a bouffant was worn (8.1% with bouffant vs 5.0% with skull cap). When adjusting for type of operation and surgical approach, multivariate modeling did not show skull caps to be an independent risk factor for SSI. Again, surgeon preference was recommended when deciding the optimal headwear for surgery.

Material and microbial analysis of bouffant-style caps has brought into question the presumed benefits of over-the-ear bouffant caps.[37] Markel and colleagues[37] performed a 1-hour mock surgical procedure using both bouffant hats and skull caps, hypothesizing that bouffant-style hats would have similar permeability, particle transmission, and pore size. Bouffant hats had a significantly higher microbial shed rate, as measured by passive settle plate analysis. Interestingly, no human hair was detected on any of the settle plates following the procedures. Further, bouffant hats had significantly higher median permeability compared with both disposable and cloth skull caps. These findings may in part be explained by the porosity of bouffant caps. Both average pore diameter and maximum pore diameter were significantly larger in bouffant caps compared with skull caps as measured by electron microscopy. The results of this study run contrary to the assumption that disposable bouffant hats provide optimal protection against microbial contamination and provide a mechanistic explanation as to why disposable or cloth skull caps are an acceptable alternative to bouffant caps.

Given the impracticality of performing a definitive RCT regarding these matters and some data to suggest skull caps may provide enhanced protection, the authors recommend using a common-sense approach when creating surgical attire guidelines because flexibility in surgical caps or other surgical attire does not seem to have significant impact on perioperative outcomes. The data suggest that the focus on enforcing specific types of surgical headwear does not play a significant role in SSI. Resources are better used to focus on interventions that have been shown to reduce SSI.

Perioperative Hyperoxia and Supplemental Oxygen

Increased fraction of inspired oxygenation (Fio_2) has been studied as a method to reduce SSI and is included in many perioperative bundles and organizational guidelines.[6,11,38–41] Hypoxemia is thought to lead to impaired wound healing and may increase the risk of infection. Wound hypoxia can be caused by decreased systemic oxygen delivery or local wound trauma, resulting in interruption of blood flow to the wound. By increasing Fio_2, systemic oxygen delivery is increased and may prevent wound hypoxia, thereby reducing the incidence of SSI.

Belda and colleagues[38] randomized 300 patients undergoing elective, open colorectal resection to either 30% or 80% Fio_2 intraoperatively and for 6 hours postoperatively. Patients underwent similar bowel preparation and antibiotic prophylaxis before surgery. The rate of SSI was 24.4% in the 30% Fio_2 arm and 14.9% in the 80% Fio_2 arm. After adjustment for covariates, the use of 80% Fio_2 remained independently associated with a reduction in SSI (RR, 0.46; CI, 0.22–0.95). The investigators recommended, given the low cost and few risks to the patients, that higher Fio_2 supplemental oxygen be considered as part of ongoing quality improvement activities.

A meta-analysis of 5 RCTs performed by Qadan and colleagues[39] affirmed the benefits of higher Fio_2 in the perioperative period. Hyperoxia was associated with an overall reduction in the rate of infection from 12.0% to 9.0%, with a number needed to treat of 33. Considering colorectal procedures specifically, hyperoxia resulted in a larger reduction in SSI (RR, 0.556; CI, 0.383–0.808). Hyperoxia was not associated with a significant increase in pulmonary complications in the included trials. These findings provided further evidence that supplemental oxygenation plays an important role in reducing SSIs and, again, suggested that these effects are particularly noticeable in colorectal procedures.

However, not all studies have shown benefit of hyperoxia. The PROXI trial assessed the effects of hyperoxia on development of SSI as well as pulmonary complications.[40] Meyhoff and colleagues[40] randomized patients undergoing laparotomy to either 80% or 30% Fio_2 during surgery and for 2 hours postoperatively. Their findings showed no significant difference in SSI rates between the two groups (19.1% in the 80% Fio_2 arm and 20.1% in 30% Fio_2 arm; OR, 0.94; CI, 0.72–1.22). Although hyperoxia did not seem to reduce SSI, it notably did not lead to an increased rate of pulmonary complications. Specifically, atelectasis was identified in 7.9% of high Fio_2 versus 7.1% of low Fio_2, pneumonia in 6% versus 6.3, respiratory failure in 5.5% versus 4.4% (4.4%), and 30-day mortality in 4.4% versus 2.9%.

Although the data regarding the effect of perioperative hyperoxia on SSI have been controversial, it does not seem to cause significant harm to patients.[40,41] As with other measures taken to reduce SSI, it does seem to have more effect on subsets of populations, particularly patients undergoing colorectal surgeries. With the low cost and limited risks to patients, the authors agree with major societies in recommending use of supplemental oxygen in the perioperative period.[6,11,12]

Skin Preparation Before Elective Surgery

Antiseptic preparation of the skin is foundational to SSI prevention and is routinely performed before elective surgery. There are many commercially available preparations; however, most exist as a combination of povidone-iodine or chlorhexidine and a solubilizing agent. Both the antiseptic and solubilizing agent play an important role in SSI reduction.

Darouiche and colleagues[42] reported a multicenter RCT on the effect of chlorhexidine-alcohol–based versus povidone-iodine based skin preparation in clean-contaminated cases. All patients received appropriate preoperative intravenous antibiotics and similar proportions received preoperative showering. The overall rate of SSI was significantly lower in the chlorhexidine-alcohol group versus the povidone-iodine cohort (9.5% vs 16.1%, respectively). Specifically, superficial SSI (RR, 0.48) and deep SSI (RR, 0.33) saw a significant reduction; however, there was no difference in organ space infection or sepsis relating to SSI. These differences in overall rate of SSI persisted in a subgroup analysis specifically evaluating intra-abdominal surgery (12.5% vs 20.5% respectively).

A recent meta-analysis comparing chlorhexidine-based versus povidone-iodine–based skin preparation for surgical skin antisepsis has shown similar findings.[43] Specifically, chlorhexidine-based skin preparation was found to be associated with a significant reduction in SSI in clean-contaminated patients (RR, 0.58). Chlorhexidine-based preparation was also superior to povidone-iodine in clean patients (RR, 0.81). Adverse skin reactions occurred at a similar rate between the two skin preparations. The investigators cautiously concluded by suggesting chlorhexidine-based skin antisepsis is superior to povidone-iodine but acknowledged current limitations in the surgical literature and recommended further high-quality studies.

Tuuli and colleagues[44] evaluated the effect of chlorhexidine-alcohol and iodine-alcohol preoperative skin preparation before cesarean delivery on the incidence of wound-related complications. This RCT was performed at a single center with the primary outcome of superficial and deep SSI within 30 days of delivery. A total of 1147 patients were included in the intention-to-treat analysis. Among those with complete follow-up (94.3% of patients), SSI was diagnosed in 23 patients (4.3%) within the chlorhexidine-alcohol group and in 42 patients (7.7%) within the iodine-alcohol group (RR, 0.55). There was no significant difference in hospital readmissions for infection-related complications or hospital length of stay, but patients treated with chlorhexidine-alcohol preparations had significantly fewer office visits for wound complications. These data suggest that chlorhexidine provided a modest improvement in SSI-related outcomes compared with iodine antisepsis even when both skin preparations were alcohol based.

The finding of improved SSI rates in chlorhexidine-based skin preparations has not been replicated in all studies.[45] A nonrandomized, prospective study was performed by Swenson and colleagues[45] that compared the use of povidone-iodine scrub paint, 2% chlorhexidine/70% isopropyl alcohol, and iodine povacrylex/isopropyl alcohol skin preparations before surgery. The primary outcome was development of SSI at 6 months following the index operation. Each of these preparations was used as the preferred skin preparation modality for all general surgery procedures for a set period of time during the study. A total of 3209 operations were included. SSI rates were the lowest when DuraPrep was the preferred agent (3.9%) compared with Betadine (6.4%) and ChloraPrep (7.1%). Furthermore, their results showed significantly decreased SSI rates when either Betadine or DuraPrep was used (4.8%) compared with ChloraPrep (8.2%). The investigators suggested that iodophor-based compounds may be superior to chlorhexidine in the general surgery population.

Given the preponderance of data suggesting improvement in rates of SSI when chlorhexidine is used, the authors recommend preoperative skin antisepsis with a chlorhexidine-based product as directed by manufacturer instructions in all patients without sensitivity or allergy to chlorhexidine. In addition, we recommend use of an alcohol-based solubilizing agent when available because use of alcohol-based skin preparations may independently improve the overall rate of SSI.[44,45]

In the past, it has been recommended that skin preparations be applied in concentric circles radiating outward from the site of incision.[46] However, some guidelines more recently have suggested that a back-and-forth application may be preferable. At present, there are no compelling data to suggest a superior method of delivering skin antisepsis, whether that is a circular or back-and-forth application. Either preference is acceptable if a complete preparation of the operative site is ensured.

Hair Clipping Before Elective Surgery

Hair removal before surgery is widely practiced despite recommendations against routine removal. Results of a 2015 meta-analyses and a 2011 Cochrane Review have shown no benefit to hair removal (by clipping or chemical depilation), with preoperative shaving noted to increase the rate of SSI.[47,48] However, because practice patterns regarding hair removal before surgery are unlikely to change, recent studies have attempted to establish noninferiority of clipping.[49]

Kowalski and colleagues[49] reported the results of a noninferiority study comparing clipping with no hair clipping in 1678 elective general surgery operations. In line with previous studies, in the per-protocol analysis, the overall rate of SSI was 6.1% versus 6.3% in the clipped and nonclipped cohorts respectively. Although hair clipping did not reach the prespecified noninferiority limit, the investigators concluded that there is unlikely to be any clinically significant difference in SSI rate with clipping and that the decision to remove hair should be up to surgeon discretion.

An important consideration in the discussion of hair removal is the use of alcohol-based skin preparations. Manufacturers recommend a 3-minute dry time for hairless areas, but up to an hour's dry time for areas with hair. With evidence suggesting that chlorhexidine-alcohol skin antisepsis is superior to povidone-iodine preparations for reducing SSI, hair clipping is likely to remain widely practiced.

If hair removal is desired before surgery, hair should be removed by hair clippers rather than shaving. Care should be taken to avoid unnecessary injury to the surrounding skin, and clipping limited to the potential areas of interest.

Maintenance of Normothermia

Maintenance of intraoperative normothermia is routinely included in measures to reduce SSI.[6,11,12] It is thought that hypothermia leads to a higher incidence of SSI by way of vasoconstriction, reduced oxygen delivery, as well as impaired tissue immunity.[50] Early studies in patients undergoing colorectal surgery provided strong evidence for the benefits of maintaining normothermia.[50]

Kurz and colleagues[50] showed the benefits of normothermia in their double-blinded study of colorectal patients who underwent a standardized anesthesia and antibiotic administration and were placed into either the hypothermia (mean temperature, 34.7°C) or normothermia (mean temperature, 36.6°C) groups.[50] Within the hypothermic group, 19% developed SSI, whereas only 6% of normothermia group developed infection. Likewise, the hypothermic group's hospitalization was increased by 2.6 days.

Building on the evidence in favor of normothermia for colorectal patients, other specialties have also sought to identify whether temperature regulation can improve SSI rates universally. Seamon and colleagues[51] performed a retrospective study of all patients with trauma having laparotomy at a level 1 trauma center who survived at least 4 days postoperatively. The primary outcome was diagnosis of SSI within 30 days of surgery. Overall, 36.1% of these patients developed an SSI during the study. Patients who developed infection were found to have a lower mean intraoperative temperature nadir. The investigators determined that a temperature of 35°C was most predictive of SSI development. They also found that a single temperature measurement less than 35°C was an independent risk factor for SSI. These data suggest that the trauma population also benefits from tight temperature control as a means to reduce SSI.

However, temperature regulation and avoidance of intraoperative hypothermia do not seem to affect all populations equally. SSI data and temperature data for ventral hernia repairs were collected between 2005 and 2012 at a single institution.[52] The investigators found the mean temperature nadir to be 35.7°C and this was not associated with SSI (OR, 0.93; CI, 0.778–1.131). Likewise, they found the length of time spent at the temperature nadir did not increase the risk of SSI (OR, 1.471; CI, 0.983–2.203).

Maintenance of normothermia has variable benefit in differing surgical populations; however, it is an easy measure to implement. The authors advocate maintenance of normothermia in all surgical procedures, in agreement with other societies.[6,11,12]

Use of Adhesive Dressings After Skin Preparation

After appropriate skin cleansing, use of adhesive drapes or iodine-impregnated drapes after skin antisepsis has been theorized to reduce the risk of SSI by preventing wound contamination and bacterial migration. A recent study in patients undergoing open joint-preservation procedures showed a significant reduction in the incidence of bacterial colonization of the surgical incision at the conclusion of the operation when an iodine-impregnated dressing was applied before surgery compared with standard draping (12% vs 27.5% respectively).[53] The investigators did not go on to evaluate subsequent development of SSI, but suggested that reduction of bacterial colonization is desirable in patients undergoing operations with implantable prosthetic joints.

Adhesive drapes have also been investigated in clean and clean-contaminated abdominal surgery. Moores and colleagues[54] reported a nonrandomized comparison of a single surgeon's experience comparing the use of Ioban (3M, Maplewood, MN) before complex ventral hernia repair with mesh. All patients underwent a standardized perioperative regimen to optimize patient risk factors and received similar preoperative antibiotics. All patients underwent an open retrorectus and/or preperitoneal placement of large-pore polypropylene mesh. The incidence of SSI was 4% and 1% in the draped and nondraped cohorts respectively. The investigators concluded that there was no additional benefit of an iodine-impregnated drape and advised against routine use of iodine-impregnated drapes in open ventral hernia repairs in the setting of a clean wound.

Similarly, use of the microbial sealant InteguSeal (Kimberly-Clark, Irving, TX) did not reduce the incidence of SSI in elective colorectal surgery.[55] Patients undergoing open or laparoscopic colorectal procedures were randomized to use of a microbial sealant versus standard draping. Preoperative bowel preparation and perioperative care were the same between groups. The overall incidence of SSI was similar with or without microbial sealant (11% vs 16% respectively). No significant differences were noted in the open or laparoscopic subgroups. The investigators concluded that InteguSeal did not show additional SSI-reduction benefit in clean-contaminated colorectal procedures.

A 2015 meta-analysis of 7 RCTs including 4195 patients comparing the use of adhesive drapes concluded that there was added benefit to their use.[56] Specifically, in the 5 RCTs evaluating adhesive drapes without iodine impregnation, the SSIs were increased 13.7% versus 11.2% (RR, 1.23; CI, 1.02–1.48). Two RCTs involving 1113 patients investigating iodine-impregnated adhesive drapes showed no significant difference in SSI rate on pooled analysis (RR, 1.03; CI, 0.66–1.60). The investigator concluded that the available evidence suggests adhesive drapes are unlikely to reduce the rate of SSI and may in some instances increase their risk.

Given the limited evidence for their use in abdominal surgery, the authors do not use adhesive drapes, whether plain or iodine impregnated, as part of our SSI-reduction strategy and therefore recommend that the use of adhesive drapes be left to surgeon preference.

Preoperative Intravenous Antibiotics

Surgical antibiotic prophylaxis (SAP) is an effective and strongly evidence-supported practice.[57] Parenteral antibiotics should be tailored to the operation performed, and, in all cases, coverage for skin and viscus-specific flora should be considered. Comprehensive guidelines for antibiotic selection before surgery have been provided by multiple societies, including the Infectious Diseases Society of America.[58] Administration of a first-generation or second-generation cephalosporin is generally recommended for patients without allergy or adverse reaction that prohibits use. However, in select cases, specific SAP regimens may be more effective.[58]

Whenever possible, antibiotics should be administered before incision, should take into consideration the patient's weight, and should be redosed to achieve adequate tissue concentrations for prophylaxis.[6,11,58,59] Antibiotic administration within 1 hour of incision is most commonly recommended. This window should be extended in antibiotics such as vancomycin because of prolonged administration times. However, there are conflicting data on the exact time within the 60-minute window during which antibiotics should be given, or whether extending the window to 120 minutes before surgery influences SSI-related outcomes.[57,60–62]

In a prospective observational study of visceral, vascular, and trauma surgeries Weber and colleagues[60] investigated the effect of timing of antibiotic administration on subsequent development of SSI. The investigators reviewed 3836 cases that were predominantly class I wounds. Incisions were followed for a minimum of 30 days. After adjusting for SSI-related risk factors, antibiotic administration within the final 30 minutes before surgery was associated with significant increase in SSI compared with administration between 2 hours and 30 minutes before surgery (OR, 1.66; CI, 1.2–2.3). When subdivided into 15-minute intervals, administration 59 to 45 minutes before surgery was associated with the lowest incidence of SSI. From the results of this study, the investigators suggested prophylaxis be administered between 30 to 60 minutes before surgery.

In a later study, Weber and colleagues[61] randomized 5580 patients undergoing surgery to early versus late administration of antibiotic prophylaxis (in anesthesia room vs in operating room respectively). Median administration time was 42 minutes (interquartile range [IQR], 30–55 minutes) and 16 minutes (IQR, 10–25 minutes) in the early and late administration arms. Overall rate of SSI at 30 days with 88.8% of patients completing follow-up was similar in the 2 groups at 4.9% versus 5.3%. The investigators concluded that their study did not support narrowing the antibiotic administration window.

Multiple additional studies have provided conflicting results on the best timing of antibiotic administration, with each study possessing limitations that prohibit generalized recommendations.[57,60–62] At present, there is no compelling evidence to suggest that any specific time within the 1-hour window is superior to another. The authors continue to recommend antibiotic administration with a 1-hour window as recommended by a variety of medical and surgical societies.

Many surgeons continue antibiotics for 24 hours after clean-contaminated surgeries. However, there is level 1a evidence that prophylactic intravenous antibiotics do not need to be continued after wound closure, because it does not affect subsequent SSI.[63]

SUMMARY

SSIs continue to be a major source of postoperative morbidity and remain a costly complication of surgery. Accordingly, significant effort has been placed into identifying methods to reduce their incidence. There is strong evidence that oral antibiotics and MBP before colorectal surgery, smoking cessation before any elective surgery, prophylactic intravenous antibiotics, maintenance of normothermia, and chlorhexidine-based skin preparation are effective measures to help reduce SSI and should be strongly considered during development of SSI-reduction strategies. Other interventions, including choice of surgical attire (cap, jackets), hyperoxia, preoperative bathing, hair removal, surgical barriers, and iodine-impregnated drapes, have variable levels of evidence to promote their use or have differing efficacy in specific surgical populations, limiting their generalized use. With regard to these measures, discretion should be left up to individual surgeons or hospital systems when creating local guidelines.

CLINICS CARE POINT

- There is strong evidence that a mechanical bowel prep with oral antibiotics before colorectal surgery, smoking cessation before any elective surgery, prophylactic intravenous antibiotics, maintenance of normothermia, and alcohol/chlorhexidine based skin preparation are effective measures to prevent SSI.

DISCLOSURE

The authors have nothing to disclose.

REFERENCES

1. Magill SS, Edwards JR, Bamberg W, et al. Multistate point-prevalence survey of health care-associated infections. N Engl J Med 2014;370(13): 1198–208.

2. Centers for Disease Control and Prevention. National healthcare safety network patient safety component manual chapter 9: surgical site infection (SSI) event. Available at: https://www.cdc.gov/nhsn/pdfs/pscmanual/pcsmanual_current.pdf. Accessed February 26, 2021.

3. Magill SS, O'Leary E, Janelle SJ, et al. Changes in prevalence of health care-associated infections in U.S. hospitals. N Engl J Med 2018;379(18):1732–44.

4. Anderson DJ, Podgorny K, Berríos-Torres SI, et al. Strategies to prevent surgical site infections in acute care hospitals: 2014 update. Infect Control Hosp Epidemiol 2014;35(6):605–27.

5. Scott RD. The direct medical costs of healthcare-associated infections in U.S. hospitals and the benefits of prevention. Atlanta: Centers for Disease Control and Prevention; 2009. Available at: http://www.cdc.gov/hai/pdfs/hai/scott_costpaper.pdf. Accessed February 26, 2021.

6. Ban KA, Minei JP, Laronga C, et al. American college of surgeons and surgical infection society: surgical site infection guidelines, 2016 update. J Am Coll Surg 2017;224(1):59–74.

7. Englesbe MJ, Brooks L, Kubus J, et al. A statewide assessment of surgical site infection following colectomy: the role of oral antibiotics. Ann Surg 2010;252(3):514–9 [discussion: 519–20].

8. Cohen ME, Liu Y, Ko CY, et al. Improved surgical outcomes for ACS NSQIP hospitals over time: evaluation of hospital cohorts with up to 8 years of participation. Ann Surg 2016;263(2):267–73.

9. Cima R, Dankbar E, Lovely J, et al. Colorectal surgery surgical site infection reduction program: a national surgical quality improvement program–driven multidisciplinary single-institution experience. J Am Coll Surg 2013;216(1):23–33.

10. Weiser MR, Gonen M, Usiak S, et al. Effectiveness of a multidisciplinary patient care bundle for reducing surgical-site infections. Br J Surg 2018;105(12):1680–7.

11. Leaper DJ, Edmiston CE. World Health Organization: global guidelines for the prevention of surgical site infection. J Hosp Infect 2016;95(2):135–6.

12. Carmichael JC, Keller DS, Baldini G, et al. Clinical practice guidelines for enhanced recovery after colon and rectal surgery from the American society of colon and rectal surgeons and society of American gastrointestinal and endoscopic surgeons. Dis Colon Rectum 2017;60(8):761–84.

13. Migaly J, Bafford AC, Francone TD, et al. The American society of colon and rectal surgeons clinical practice guidelines for the use of bowel preparation in elective colon and rectal surgery. Dis Colon Rectum 2019;62(1):3–8.

14. Hoang SC, Klipfel AA, Roth LA, et al. Colon and rectal surgery surgical site infection reduction bundle: to improve is to change. Am J Surg 2019;217(1):40–5.

15. Ohman KA, Wan L, Guthrie T, et al. Combination of oral antibiotics and mechanical bowel preparation reduces surgical site infection in colorectal surgery. J Am Coll Surg 2017;225(4):465–71.

16. Klinger AL, Green H, Monlezun DJ, et al. The role of bowel preparation in colorectal surgery: results of the 2012-2015 ACS-NSQIP data. Ann Surg 2019;269(4):671–7.

17. Nichols RL, Broido P, Condon RE, et al. Effect of preoperative neomycin-erythromycin intestinal preparation on the incidence of infectious complications following colon surgery. Ann Surg 1973;178(4):453–62.

18. Berríos-Torres SI, Umscheid CA, Bratzler DW, et al. Centers for disease control and prevention guideline for the prevention of surgical site infection, 2017. JAMA Surg 2017;152(8):784–91.

19. Cornelius ME, Wang TW, Jamal A, et al. Tobacco product use among adults — United States, 2019. MMWR Morb Mortal Wkly Rep 2020;69:1736–42.
20. Sorensen LT. Wound healing and infection in surgery, the clinical impact of smoking and smoking cessation: a systematic review and meta-analysis. Arch Surg 2012;147(4):373–83.
21. Sharma A, Deeb AP, Iannuzzi JC, et al. Tobacco smoking and postoperative outcomes after colorectal surgery. Ann Surg 2013;258(2):296–300.
22. Sorensen LT, Karlsmark T, Gottrup F. Abstinence from smoking reduces incisional wound infection: a randomized controlled trial. Ann Surg 2003;238(1):1–5.
23. Møller AM, Villebro N, Pedersen T, et al. Effect of preoperative smoking intervention on postoperative complications: a randomised clinical trial. Lancet 2002; 359(9301):114–7.
24. Nolan MB, Martin DP, Thompson R, et al. Association between smoking status, preoperative exhaled carbon monoxide levels, and postoperative surgical site infection in patients undergoing elective surgery. JAMA Surg 2017;152(5): 476–83.
25. Webster J, Osborne S. Preoperative bathing or showering with skin antiseptics to prevent surgical site infection. Cochrane Database Syst Rev 2015;(2):CD004985.
26. Hayek LJ, Emerson JM. Preoperative whole body disinfection–a controlled clinical study. J Hosp Infect 1988;11(Suppl B):15–9.
27. Prabhu AS, Krpata DM, Phillips S, et al. Preoperative chlorhexidine gluconate use can increase risk for surgical site infections after ventral hernia repair. J Am Coll Surg 2017;224(3):334–40.
28. Cao F, Li J, Li F. Mechanical bowel preparation for elective colorectal surgery: Updated systematic review and meta-analysis. Int J Colorectal Dis 2012;27(6): 803–10.
29. Nicholson GA, Finlay IG, Diament RH, et al. Mechanical bowel preparation does not influence outcomes following colonic cancer resection. Br J Surg 2011;98(6): 866–71.
30. Hata H, Yamaguchi T, Hasegawa S, et al. Oral and parenteral versus parenteral antibiotic prophylaxis in elective laparoscopic colorectal surgery (JMTO PREV 07-01): a phase 3, multicenter, open-label, randomized trial. Ann Surg 2016; 263(6):1085–91.
31. Güenaga KF, Matos D, Wille-Jørgensen P. Mechanical bowel preparation for elective colorectal surgery. Cochrane Database Syst Rev 2011;2011(9):CD001544.
32. Link T. Guidelines in practice: surgical attire. AORN J 2020;111(4):425–39.
33. Wills BW, Smith WR, Arguello AM, et al. Association of surgical jacket and bouffant use with surgical site infection risk. JAMA Surg 2020;155(4):323–8.
34. Farach SM, Kelly KN, Farkas RL, et al. Have recent modifications of operating room attire policies decreased surgical site infections? an american college of surgeons NSQIP review of 6,517 patients. J Am Coll Surg 2018;226(5):804–13.
35. Haskins IN, Prabhu AS, Krpata DM, et al. Is there an association between surgeon hat type and 30-day wound events following ventral hernia repair? Hernia 2017;21(4):495–503.
36. Kothari SN, Anderson MJ, Borgert AJ, et al. Bouffant vs skull cap and impact on surgical site infection: does operating room headwear really matter? J Am Coll Surg 2018;227(2):198–202.
37. Markel TA, Gormley T, Greeley D, et al. Hats off: a study of different operating room headgear assessed by environmental quality indicators. J Am Coll Surg 2017;225(5):573–81.

38. Belda FJ, Aguilera L, García de la Asunción J, et al. Supplemental perioperative oxygen and the risk of surgical wound infection: a randomized controlled trial. JAMA 2005;294(16):2035–42.

39. Qadan M, Akça O, Mahid SS, et al. Perioperative supplemental oxygen therapy and surgical site infection: A meta-analysis of randomized controlled trials. Arch Surg 2009;144(4):359–66 [discussion: 366–7].

40. Meyhoff CS, Wetterslev J, Jorgensen LN, et al. Effect of high perioperative oxygen fraction on surgical site infection and pulmonary complications after abdominal surgery: the PROXI randomized clinical trial. JAMA 2009;302(14):1543–50.

41. Mattishent K, Thavarajah M, Sinha A, et al. Safety of 80% vs 30-35% fraction of inspired oxygen in patients undergoing surgery: a systematic review and meta-analysis. Br J Anaesth 2019;122(3):311–24.

42. Darouiche RO, Wall MJ Jr, Itani KM, et al. Chlorhexidine-alcohol versus povidone-iodine for surgical-site antisepsis. N Engl J Med 2010;362(1):18–26.

43. Chen S, Chen JW, Guo B, et al. Preoperative antisepsis with chlorhexidine versus povidone-iodine for the prevention of surgical site infection: a systematic review and meta-analysis. World J Surg 2020;44(5):1412–24.

44. Tuuli MG, Liu J, Stout MJ, et al. A randomized trial comparing skin antiseptic agents at cesarean delivery. N Engl J Med 2016;374(7):647–55.

45. Swenson BR, Hedrick TL, Metzger R, et al. Effects of preoperative skin preparation on postoperative wound infection rates: a prospective study of 3 skin preparation protocols. Infect Control Hosp Epidemiol 2009;30(10):964–71.

46. Stonecypher K. Going around in circles: is this the best practice for preparing the skin? Crit Care Nurs Q 2009;32(2):94–8.

47. Lefebvre A, Saliou P, Lucet JC, et al. Preoperative hair removal and surgical site infections: Network meta-analysis of randomized controlled trials. J Hosp Infect 2015;91(2):100–8.

48. Tanner J, Norrie P, Melen K. Preoperative hair removal to reduce surgical site infection. Cochrane Database Syst Rev 2011;11:CD004122.

49. Kowalski TJ, Kothari SN, Mathiason MA, et al. Impact of hair removal on surgical site infection rates: A prospective randomized noninferiority trial. J Am Coll Surg 2016;223(5):704–11.

50. Kurz A, Sessler DI, Lenhardt R. Perioperative normothermia to reduce the incidence of surgical-wound infection and shorten hospitalization. Study of wound infection and temperature group. N Engl J Med 1996;334(19):1209–15.

51. Seamon MJ, Wobb J, Gaughan JP, et al. The effects of intraoperative hypothermia on surgical site infection: an analysis of 524 trauma laparotomies. Ann Surg 2012;255(4):789–95.

52. Baucom RB, Phillips SE, Ehrenfeld JM, et al. Association of perioperative hypothermia during colectomy with surgical site infection. JAMA Surg 2015;150(6):570–5.

53. Rezapoor M, Tan TL, Maltenfort MG, et al. Incise draping reduces the rate of contamination of the surgical site during hip surgery: a prospective, randomized trial. J Arthroplasty 2018;33(6):1891–5.

54. Moores N, Rosenblatt S, Prabhu A, et al. Do iodine-impregnated adhesive surgical drapes reduce surgical site infections during open ventral hernia repair? A comparative analysis. Am Surg 2017;83(6):617–22.

55. Doorly M, Choi J, Floyd A, et al. Microbial sealants do not decrease surgical site infection for clean-contaminated colorectal procedures. Tech Coloproctol 2015;19(5):281–5.

56. Webster J, Alghamdi A. Use of plastic adhesive drapes during surgery for preventing surgical site infection. Cochrane Database Syst Rev 2015;2015(4): CD006353.
57. Bowater RJ, Stirling SA, Lilford RJ. Is antibiotic prophylaxis in surgery a generally effective intervention? Testing a generic hypothesis over a set of meta-analyses. Ann Surg 2009;249(4):551–6.
58. Bratzler DW, Dellinger EP, Olsen KM, et al. Clinical practice guidelines for antimicrobial prophylaxis in surgery. Surg Infect (Larchmt) 2013;14(1):73–156.
59. Deierhoi RJ, Dawes LG, Vick C, et al. Choice of intravenous antibiotic prophylaxis for colorectal surgery does matter. J Am Coll Surg 2013;217(5):763–9.
60. Weber WP, Marti WR, Zwahlen M, et al. The timing of surgical antimicrobial prophylaxis. Ann Surg 2008;247(6):918–26.
61. Weber WP, Mujagic E, Zwahlen M, et al. Timing of surgical antimicrobial prophylaxis: a phase 3 randomised controlled trial. Lancet Infect Dis 2017;17(6):605–14.
62. Classen DC, Evans RS, Pestotnik SL, et al. The timing of prophylactic administration of antibiotics and the risk of surgical-wound infection. N Engl J Med 1992; 326(5):281–6.
63. Berríos-Torres SI, Umscheid CA, Bratzler DW, et al, Healthcare Infection Control Practices Advisory Committee. Centers for disease control and prevention guideline for the prevention of surgical site infection, 2017. JAMA Surg 2017;152(8): 784–91. Erratum in: JAMA Surg. 2017 Aug 1;152(8):803. PMID: 28467526.

Challenging Surgical Dogma
Controversies in Diverticulitis

Aimal Khan, MD[a], Alexander T. Hawkins, MD, MPH[a],*

KEYWORDS

- Diverticulitis • Colorectal surgery • Antibiotics • Hartmann's • Colostomy

KEY POINTS

- Most patients with diverticular disease will remain asymptomatic throughout their life.
- Consumption of nuts, seeds, or popcorn does not increase the risk of diverticulitis in patients with diverticulosis.
- Only a small percentage (<20%) of patients with diverticulosis will develop diverticulitis.
- Selected patients with acute uncomplicated diverticulitis can be managed without antibiotics.
- When considering elective surgery for recurrent diverticulitis, every patient needs to be evaluated on a "case-by-case" basis as there is little evidence to support rigid treatment recommendations.

INTRODUCTION

Diverticulosis of the sigmoid colon is common in the developed world, affecting approximately 33% of persons older than 60 years.[1] Up to 15% of these patients will develop diverticulitis at some point in their lifetime. The incidence of diverticulitis has increased in the last decade,[2,3] accounting for nearly 300,000 US hospital admissions and $1.8 billion in annual direct medical costs.[4] With such a wide prevalence and diverse spectrum of clinical presentation, there are bound to be multiple controversies regarding disease management. Here the authors present six of the major points of contention in treatment of diverticular disease. First, the authors explore the still underdeveloped understanding of the natural history of disease. They then explore four crucial themes in the management of diverticulitis: the role of antibiotics in mild diverticulitis, when to operate on patients with acute diverticulitis, the role of laparoscopic lavage in the treatment of acute diverticulitis, and finally whether to perform a primary anastomosis (PA) in the acute setting. Finally, the authors try and determine which patients should undergo elective colectomy for recurrent disease. They identify

[a] Section of Colon & Rectal Surgery, Department of Surgery, Vanderbilt University Medical Center, 1161 21st Avenue South, Room D5203 MCN, Nashville, TN 37232, USA
* Corresponding author.
E-mail address: alex.hawkins@vumc.org

Surg Clin N Am 101 (2021) 967–980
https://doi.org/10.1016/j.suc.2021.05.024
0039-6109/21/© 2021 Elsevier Inc. All rights reserved.

surgical.theclinics.com

crucial studies to inform decision-making as well as identify knowledge gaps for future study. While by no means comprehensive, this article will serve to educate the reader on several important areas to consider when treating this ubiquitous disease.

NATURAL HISTORY OF DIVERTICULOSIS

Controversy regarding diverticulitis starts with our very fundamental understanding of the disease. Our knowledge of the pathophysiology and natural history of diverticular disease remains limited. The most widely accepted pathophysiologic mechanism of diverticulosis point the formation of colonic (pseudo)diverticulae as outpouchings of mucosa and submucosa in the inherently weak parts of the colon wall due to increased intraluminal pressure. The narrow diameter of sigmoid colon and excessive straining caused by altered bowel habits cause outward pressure leading to ballooning of mucosa and submucosa at points of entry of the vasa recta into the muscularis propria. Further understanding of the natural history is hampered by the lack of a working animal model for diverticular disease.

Various environmental and genetic factors have been implicated in the development of diverticular disease. Dietary fiber is by far the most studied factor, with several large prospective cohort studies showing benefit to fiber intake. The European Prospective Investigation into Cancer and Nutrition (EPIC)-Oxford study examined the eating habits of 47,033 subjects and observed that vegetarians had a 31% lower risk (risk ratio: 0.69, $P = .003$) of developing diverticular disease compared with meat eaters.[5] Similarly, the Nurses' Health Study found higher fiber intake to be protective against diverticulosis in women (odds ratio [OR]: 0.86, P value = .002).[6]

Despite historical recommendations to avoid nuts, seeds, and popcorn, there is no evidence that consumption of these items increases the risk of acute diverticulitis. The Health Professionals Follow-up Study prospective cohort study of 51,529 US men followed from 1986 to 2004 via self-administered questionnaires. The authors found inverse associations between nut and popcorn consumption and the risk of diverticulitis.[7]

Other studies have challenged this pivotal role of fiber by showing no protection against diverticular disease with the use of fiber.[8] Despite this, recommendations for fiber intake as primary prevention have been adopted by societies because of the little to no potential downside associated with increased fiber intake. The 2015 American Gastroenterological Association (AGA) Institute Guidelines on diverticulitis suggest a fiber-rich diet or fiber supplementation in patients with a history of acute diverticulitis.[9]

Several retrospective and observational studies have found smoking, obesity, decreased physical activity, and caffeine intake to be associated with diverticular disease.[10–13] The American Society of Colon and Rectal Surgeons (ASCRS) Clinical Practice Guidelines endorse tobacco cessation, reduced meat intake, physical activity, and weight loss as recommended interventions to potentially reduce the risk of diverticulitis.[14]

Over the last few years, increasing evidence has been pointing to the role of genetics in the development of diverticulosis. Both Swedish and Danish twin registries showed increased odds of development of diverticular disease among monozygotic twins compared with dizygotic twins.[15,16] In addition to twin registries, several inherited soft-tissue syndromes have been linked to increased risk of diverticular disease. Patient's with Ehlers-Danlos syndrome, Williams-Beuren syndrome, Marfan's syndrome, autosomal dominant polycystic kidney disease, and Coffin-Lowry syndrome are susceptible to development of diverticular disease.[17] Patients with a family history of diverticulosis have also been noted to develop diverticular disease at a younger age and are more susceptible to complicated recurrences than patients without a family history of the disease.[18] When taken together, the twin studies, connective tissues syndromes, and strong family association help establish compelling evidence of genetic influence on diverticulosis. Genetic association studies have identified several single-nucleotide polymorphisms in patients with diverticular disease, and more work continues to be carried out in this field.[19,20]

Despite the lack of working animal models, data from multiple small- and large-scale epidemiologic studies have helped chart the natural history of diverticular disease. It is well established that majority (80%–85%) of the patients with diverticulosis will remain asymptomatic for their whole life. Only 5% to 25% of patients will develop acute diverticulitis.[21,22] Of the patients who develop acute diverticulitis, only 20% to 40% will develop recurrent diverticulitis, and about 5% to 10% develop complicated diverticulitis (shock, free perforation, fistula, abscess, stricture, or obstruction).[23,24] The lifetime risk of bleeding in patients with diverticulosis range from 4% to 10%.[25,26] The risk of free perforation with feculent peritonitis is very small and almost exclusively occurs at the first episode of diverticulitis. Improvement in our understanding of the natural history of diverticular disease has challenged several decades old medical and surgical treatment dogmas, paving the way for more individualized approach to patients. **Fig. 1** represents the natural progression of sigmoid diverticular disease. The width of arrows has been sized proportional to the estimated number of patients in an individual disease state.

ROLE OF ANTIBIOTICS IN UNCOMPLICATED ACUTE DIVERTICULITIS

Before the last decade, antibiotics were considered the cornerstone of management for patients with acute uncomplicated diverticulitis. Since then, three prospective randomized controlled trials have challenged this treatment paradigm by showing similar outcomes in patients treated with and without antibiotics. This coincided with improvement in the understanding of the pathophysiologic progression from diverticulosis to diverticulitis. Diverticulitis as a primarily infectious process developing as a response to a microperforation has been replaced with primarily an inflammatory model where the inflamed segment of the colon can eventually lead a microperforation.

AVOD (Antibiotics in Acute Uncomplicated Diverticulitis RCT) was a multicenter randomized trial conducted in Sweden and Iceland in which patients with CT-scan-confirmed uncomplicated diverticulitis were randomized to be treated with or without antibiotics. The investigators found no difference in perforation or abscess formation (1.9% vs 1.0%, $P = .30$), median hospital stay (2.9 d vs 2.9 d, $P = .71$),

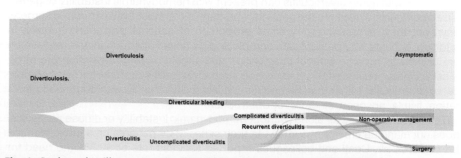

Fig. 1. Sankey plot illustrating the natural history of sigmoid diverticulosis.

or recurrent diverticulitis necessitating readmission to hospital (16%, $P = 881$) between the two groups.[27] On long-term follow up (median 11 years), these findings persisted with no difference in complications, recurrence rates, rate of surgery for diverticulitis, or findings of colorectal cancer. In addition, no difference was found in quality of life between these patients.[28] Similar results were noticed in the Dutch DIABLO (Diverticulitis: Antibiotics or Close Observation) trial where patients assigned to observation or antibiotic treatment strategies did not differ in their median time to recovery (primary end point), progression to complicated diverticulitis, recurrent diverticulitis, sigmoid resection, readmission, adverse events, or mortality.[29] Jaung and colleagues carried out a double-blind randomized trial where patients received a placebo or antibiotics for treatment of acute uncomplicated diverticulitis.[30] No significant difference was noted in their primary end point: length of hospital stay (40.0 h vs 45.8 h, $P = .2$) or other secondary endpoints (adverse events, readmission to the hospital within 1 wk, and readmission to the hospital within 30 d) between the two groups.[30]

In addition to these randomized trials, a multitude of retrospective studies, systematic reviews, and meta-analyses support the safety of managing patients with acute diverticulitis without antibiotics.[31–33] Despite these results, certain limitations of these studies can hinder the adoption of antibiotics-free approach. Almost universally, patients with compromised immune systems, severe diverticulitis, and extensive medical comorbidities were excluded from these trials. In addition, the lack of diverse patient populations may limit generalizability to the rest of the world. Despite these shortcomings, the 2020 ASCRS guidelines and 2021 AGA clinical practice guidelines now support the selective use of antibiotics for acute uncomplicated diverticulitis.[14,34] Further research is needed to identify the optimal duration and subset of patients that will benefit the most from an antibiotics-free approach. For now, the decision to pursue antibiotics-free approach in patients with acute diverticulitis needs be applied on a case-by-case basis.

WHEN TO OPERATE ON PATIENTS WITH ACUTE DIVERTICULITIS

The decision to operate on a patient with acute diverticulitis can be challenging. Fundamentally, surgery should only be undertaken when the risk of a patient's disease progression outweighs the risks associated with the surgery. In patients with diverticulitis, this is further complicated by the need for stoma (colostomy or diverting loop ileostomy [DLI]) and the wide variability in phenotypic presentations of acute diverticulitis. Despite these challenges, decisions grounded in safe surgical principles guided by the patient's physiologic state and disease progression can make this task less daunting.

Patients with acute diverticulitis can present with hemodynamic instability or generalized peritonitis. These are the patients who benefit the most from expedited surgery; however, they represent a very small proportion of patients presenting acutely. In addition, patients who present with complete large bowel obstruction and megacolon are unlikely to improve without intervention and should undergo resection promptly. Most patients present either as uncomplicated diverticulitis or other forms of complicated diverticulitis (other than hemodynamic instability), that is, with contained perforation, fistula, abscess, stricture, or obstruction.

The presence of free air alone (without hemodynamic instability or diffuse peritonitis) does not mandate emergent surgery. In their series of 39 patients presenting with extra digestive air, Costi and colleagues reported success rate of 92.3% (no need for surgery), morbidity of 23.1%, and no mortalities with their nonoperative approach.[35]

In general, most patients who have free air and/or free fluid, but localized pain and hemodynamic stability, can be managed nonoperatively with high success rates.

Most patients presenting with diverticulitis-related abscesses can be managed nonoperatively. However, CT- or ultrasound-guided drainage is usually warranted for abscesses >3 cm.[14] Patients presenting with inability to tolerate diet need to be categorized further. Patients whose symptoms are secondary to ileus can be managed conservatively. However, patients who have obstructive symptoms due to a diverticular stricture should be monitored closely. Some obstructions resolve as the inflammation decreases, but a low threshold for surgery should be used.

In summary, the decision to operate on a patient with diverticulitis in the acute setting should be individualized to each patient based on their physiologic parameters and response to conservative measures. Benefits of early surgical intervention should be juxtaposed with the significant morbidity associated with them. With increasing incidence of urgent surgery in patients with acute diverticulitis (7.1–10.2 per 1,000,000 between 1987 and 2012),[36] surgeons continue to play an integral role in the management of diverticulitis. Excellent understanding of patient's physiology and sound indications can ensure excellent outcomes for their patients.

ROLE OF LAPAROSCOPIC LAVAGE IN PERFORATED DIVERTICULITIS

Since its introduction in 1996 as an alternative to colectomy, laparoscopic lavage continues to be a source of significant scrutiny and debate. To date, three randomized controlled trials and several nonrandomized studies have assessed its efficacy in the management of patients with acute diverticulitis yielding mixed results (Table 1).

The Scandinavian diverticulitis (SCANDIV) and LOLA trial (Laparoscopic lavage (of the Ladies trial)), both published in 2015, failed to demonstrate superiority of laparoscopic lavage to sigmoid colectomy for acute diverticulitis. In the SCANDIV trial, the rate of severe postoperative complications (Clavien-Dindo score >IIIa) within 90 days was similar between laparoscopic lavage and sigmoid colectomy groups (30.7 vs 26.0, $P = .53$). In addition, patients who underwent laparoscopic lavage required reoperation at a higher rate than colectomy group (20.3% vs 5.7%, $P = .01$), and four participants had missed carcinomas in the lavage group.[38] The 5-year results of SCANDIV, published in 2020, showed no difference in severe complications (36% vs 35%, $P = .92$) and mortality (32% vs 25%, $P = .36$) between the two operative approaches.[45] The LOLA trial was terminated early after an interim analysis demonstrated a higher short-term adverse event rate in the laparoscopic lavage group than the colectomy group (39% vs 19%, $P = .04$). Simialr to SCANDIV, patients in the laparoscopic lavage group had higher rates of reoperation, although this finding was not statistically significant (20% vs 7%, $P = .12$).[37] Quality of life did not differ between laparoscopic lavage and colectomy groups in either trial. Similar to LOLA and SCANDIV, the DILALA (DIverticulitis – LAparoscopic LAvage versus resection for acute diverticulitis with peritonitis) trial, published in 2016, showed no difference in morbidity and short-term mortality between laparoscopic lavage and Hartman's groups (13.2% vs 17.1%, $P = .67$).[39] The operative time was found to be significantly shorter for the laparoscopic lavage group in all three trials.

Major limitations of these studies are their heterogeneity in selection criteria, primary outcomes, and the details of surgical technique (amount of fluid used and drain placed). All three of these studies excluded patients with Hinchey IV diverticulitis. Hinchey IV diverticulitis can be difficult to differentiate from Hinchey III diverticulitis on preoperative imaging, making preoperative planning difficult. In addition, the long-term results of SCANDIV also showed recurrence of diverticulitis was higher after

Table 1
Studies assessing the role of laparoscopic lavage in management of acute diverticulitis

Study, Publication Year	Study Design	No. of Patients	Primary Outcome	Major Findings
Randomized trials				
Vennix et al,[37] (LOLA) 2015	Randomized clinical trial (RCT)	90	Major morbidity and mortality within 12 mo	30-d adverse event rate Lavage group vs colectomy group (39% vs 19%, $P = .04$) 12-mo major morbidity or mortality Lavage group vs colectomy group (67% vs 60%, $P = .53$).
Schultz et al,[38] (SCANDIV) 2015	RCT	199	Severe postoperative complications (Clavien-Dindo score >IIIa) within 90 d	Severe postoperative complications within 90 d were similar between laparoscopic lavage and sigmoid colectomy (30.7% vs 26.0%, $P = .53$).
Angenete et al,[39] (DILALA) 2016	RCT	83	Reoperations within 12 mo postoperatively	No difference in morbidity and short-term mortality between laparoscopic lavage and Hartman's groups (13.2% vs 17.1%, $P = .67$)
Nonrandomized trials				
White et al,[40] 2010	Retrospective comparative analysis	78	Not specified	27 out 35 patients in lavage group recovered from initial peritonitis without resection. Of these 27 patients, 16 patients eventually underwent resection.
Franklin et al,[41] 2008	Retrospective case review	40	Not specified	Just over 50% of patients undergoing laparoscopic lavage underwent elective interval laparoscopic sigmoid colectomy during the mean follow-up period of 96 mo.
Karoui et al,[42] 2009	Prospective cohort matching with retrospective controls	59	Not specified	25/35 patients in peritoneal lavage group eventually underwent resection. Postoperative morbidity was similar between lavage and resection with anastomosis and DLI groups.

(continued on next page)

Table 1
(continued)

Study, Publication Year	Study Design	No. of Patients	Primary Outcome	Major Findings
Liang et al,[43] 2012	Retrospective comparative analysis	88	Not specified	Patients who underwent Hartmann's had significantly longer hospital stay than lavage (16.3 vs 6.7 d, *P* < .01) On the long-term follow-up, 44.7% of patients who underwent lavage had elective sigmoidectomy
Rogers et al,[44] 2012	Database review	427	Mortality	Patients selected for laparoscopic lavage had lower mortality (4.0% vs 10.4%, *P* < .001), complications (14.1% vs 25.0%, *P* < .001), and length of stay (10 d vs 20 d, *P* < .001) than those requiring resection.

laparoscopic lavage (21% vs 4%, *P* = .004), and 30% of the patients in the laparoscopic lavage group ultimately underwent a sigmoid resection.[45] Owing to these challenges, laparoscopic lavage has fallen out of favor with most surgeons, and its adoption remains low.[46] Ultimately, the 2020 ASCRS Clinical Practice Guidelines recommend against the use of laparoscopic lavage in patients with feculent peritonitis (Hinchey IV) and prefer colectomy over lavage in cases of purulent peritonitis (Hinchey III).[14]

PRIMARY ANASTOMOSIS VERSUS HARTMANN FOR PERFORATED DIVERTICULITIS

After source control and resection of inflamed bowel comes the question of reconstruction. In the 1980s, the 3-stage surgical procedure was replaced by the 2-stage procedure known as Hartmann's procedure (HP).[47] This procedure involved sigmoid colectomy with end descending colostomy and subsequent colostomy reversal with colorectal anastomosis weeks to months after patient recovery. While very useful in addressing the immediate issue at hand, reversal rates are low and associated with socioeconomic disparities.[48]

In recent years, several scientific reports have suggested that primary anastomosis (PA) with a DLI is a safe alternative to HP for selected complicated acute diverticulitis necessitating emergent or urgent operation. A 2012 Swiss study randomized 62 patients with acute left-sided colonic perforation (Hinchey III and IV) to HP (n = 30) and PA (with diverting ileostomy, n = 32), with a planned stoma reversal operation after 3 months in both groups.[49] Although the outcome after the initial colon resection did not show any significant differences (mortality 13% vs 9% and morbidity 67% vs 75% in HP vs PA), the stoma reversal rate after PA with diverting ileostomy was higher (90% vs 57%, *P* = .005) and serious complications (grades IIIb-IV: 0% vs 20%, *P* = .046), operating time (73 min vs 183 min, *P* < .001), hospital stay (6 d vs

9 d, P = .016), and in-hospital costs (US \$16,717 vs US \$24,014) were significantly reduced in the PA group.[49] The DIVERTI trial (Primary vs Secondary Anastomosis for Hinchey Stage III-IV Diverticulitis), published in 2017, randomized 102 patients. Morbidity for both resection and stoma reversal operations were comparable (39% in the HP arm vs 44% in the PA arm; P = .4233). Although the study observed no difference in mortality (HP: 7.7% vs PA: 4%, P = .42), 96% of PA patients and 65% of HP patients had a stoma reversal at 18 months (P = .0001). The LADIES trial (laparoscopic peritoneal lavage or resection for purulent peritonitis and Hartmann's procedure or resection with primary anastomosis for purulent or faecal peritonitis in perforated diverticulitis), published in 2019, enrolled 133 patients and randomly assigned them to HP (68 patients) or PA (65 patients).[50] Twelve-month stoma-free survival was significantly better for patients undergoing PA than for those undergoing HP (95% vs 72%; hazard ratio: 2.79; log-rank P < .0001). Gachabayov and colleagues performed a meta-analysis of 17 studies, including the randomized studies mentioned previously, and concluded that PA was associated with lower rates of organ space infection and stoma nonreversal rates.[51] Quality-of-life data obtained after undergoing emergency surgery for diverticulitis have observed worse quality of life after HP compared with patients who underwent resection with PA. This is mostly due to the presence of an end colostomy.[52]

Ultimately, national guidelines recommend that the decision to restore intestinal continuity and whether to perform proximal diversion in the setting of a PA should be individualized as the clinician considers the risks associated with anastomotic failure.[14] Some situations, including hemodynamic instability, acidosis, acute or chronic organ failure, and immunosuppression, may favor HP over a PA. In addition, certain older patients with poor bowel function and sphincter tone may be better served with an HP.

Despite emerging data supporting PA with a DLI, this approach is not widely used. An National Surgical Quality Improvement Program (NSQIP) study analyzed patients undergoing emergent colectomy for diverticulitis from 2012 to 2016 and found that only 7.6% underwent PA with DLI.[53] In multivariable analyses, compared with HP, PA with DLI was not associated with increased rates of mortality or morbidity. Further research is needed to identify and address barriers to PA with DLI.

ELECTIVE SURGERY FOR RECURRENT DIVERTICULITIS

The decision to pursue colectomy for recurrent diverticulitis is nuanced, and the threshold has changed greatly over the past 20 years. After a first episode of acute diverticulitis managed nonoperatively, it is estimated that 20% to 40% of individuals will experience a second episode, with the risk of recurrent diverticulitis peaking in the first 1 to 2 years of follow-up.[24]

Elective resection was previously recommended after 2 episodes of uncomplicated diverticulitis (or a single episode in young patients).[54] This practice was based on the idea that such patients demonstrated, by virtue of recurrence and age at onset, a more "virulent" syndrome at greater risk for recurrence. Thus, elective intervention was deemed necessary to prevent future complicated episodes, emergency operation, and/or colostomy. These assumptions have been essentially disproven over time.

Current ASCRS guidelines recommend that "the decision to recommend elective sigmoid colectomy after recovery from uncomplicated acute diverticulitis should be individualized."[14] In summary, the decision for elective surgery should not be made based on age, as the natural history of diverticulitis does not differ between young and old patients. There is also no specific number of attacks that should trigger surgery, as other factors such as attack severity, frequency, and impact on quality of life are more important than a specific number. Finally, elective surgery should not be performed to prevent a future hypothetical emergency, as patients with recurrent uncomplicated disease rarely progress to a free perforation and peritonitis.

As with any surgical procedure, the decision to proceed to the operating room is based on a calculus of potential risk and benefit to the patient. Several studies have revealed that there is minimal mortality benefit to elective surgery for diverticular disease.[55–57] Because of this, the choice for surgery should include input and preferences from the patients themselves, as they may opt for surgery if the frequency and severity of their episodes are sufficient to justify the burden of surgery.[58] Regrettably, there are data to suggest that the decision to proceed with elective colectomy may be due to hospital and market factors, rather than patient-level factors.[59]

Unfortunately, there is a paucity of data to aid in the decision-making process for colectomy in recurrent diverticular disease. The DIRECT trial (Surgery versus conservative management for recurrent and ongoing left-sided diverticulitis) was a multicenter randomized clinical trial from the Netherlands and compared conservative management (n = 56) to elective surgery (n = 53) in patients with either recurrent diverticulitis (≥3 episodes within 2 years) or persistent abdominal complaints (≥3 months) after a first episode of acute diverticulitis. Although the trial was terminated early because of poor recruitment, it reported a higher mean gastrointestinal quality of life (QoL) score (mean difference: 14.2, 95% confidence interval [CI]: 7.2–21.1, $P < .001$) in the surgery group.[60] In the 5-year follow-up study, the difference in QoL remained, and 46% of patients in the conservative management group ultimately crossed over to surgery because of severe ongoing complaints.[61] A recent Finnish trial randomized 72 patients (37 in the surgery group and 35 in the conservative treatment group) with recurrent diverticulitis.[62] The difference between gastrointestinal QoL scores at randomization and 6 months was a mean of 11.96 points higher in the surgery group than in the conservative treatment group (95% CI, 3.72–20.19; $P = .005$). There were 2 patients (5%) in the surgery group and 12 patients (31%) in the conservative treatment group who had new episodes of diverticulitis within 6 months. While these data suggest that colectomy may offer improved quality of life, there is still much to be learned about which particular subset of patients will benefit the most. Data from the ongoing PREDIC-DIV (PREDICtors for health-related quality of life after elective sigmoidectomy for DIVerticular disease) prospective observational study and the COSMID (Comparison of Surgery and Medicine on the Impact of Diverticulitis) trial should help illuminate the optimal treatment strategy to improve QoL in patients with recurrent diverticulitis.[63]

Patient who are immunosuppressed have a different risk profile of both observation and colectomy and require unique consideration. In terms of operative risk, a retrospective study of the NSQIP database compared 736 immunosuppressed patients with 21,980 immunocompetent patients undergoing elective colectomy for diverticulitis.[64] A multivariate regression analysis found that the groups had comparable mortality, but rates of major morbidity (OR: 1.46; 95% CI: 1.17–1.83) and wound dehiscence (OR: 2.69; 95% CI: 1.63–4.42) were significantly higher in the immunosuppressed group.

Several retrospective studies compare the risk of recurrent episodes between immunosuppressed and immunocompetent patients. A single-institution experience over a 14-year interval compared 107 immunosuppressed patients with 550 immunocompetent patients who had successful medical management of their first episode of diverticulitis with a mean follow-up duration of 81.6 months.[65] The rate of recurrent diverticulitis was similar in both groups (21.5% of immunosuppressed patients vs

20.5% of immunocompetent patients; $P = .82$). Although immunosuppressed patients who had a severe first episode (defined as abscess or perforation) were significantly more likely to have a recurrence or a complicated recurrence, the rate of requiring emergency surgery was comparable between the two groups. A similar study restricted to renal transplant patients also observed no difference in recurrence rates between the groups.[66] This stands in contrast to an older study that observed that a smaller group of "high-risk" patients (immunosuppression, chronic renal failure, and/ or collagen vascular disease) had a 5-fold higher risk of future diverticulitis with perforation.[67] Overall, this subset of patients need to be advised on the different risk profiles both for observation and surgery, with recommendations individualized. It is no longer recommended that elective colectomy be offered to immunocompromised patients after a single uncomplicated attack.

In summary, elective colectomy for recurrent diverticulitis remains a nuanced decision for both surgeons and patients. This area is ripe for future study, both in identification of patients who will benefit from surgery as well as improving the shared decision-making process. For now, patients and surgeons need to have a clear conversation about shared goals, as well as education as to the potential risk and benefits of colectomy.

CLINICS CARE POINTS

- Incidence of diverticulitis continues to increase across the globe.
- First episode of diverticulitis is usually the more virulent one.
- Colectomy is preferred over laparoscopic lavage in cases of purulent peritonitis.
- Decision for elective surgery in a patient needs to be made on a "case-by-case" basis in patient with recurrent diverticulitis.

DISCLOSURE

The authors have nothing to disclose.

REFERENCES

1. Everhart JE, Ruhl CE. Burden of digestive diseases in the United States part ii: lower gastrointestinal diseases. Gastroenterology 2009;136(3):741–54.
2. Etzioni DA, Mack TM, Beart RW, et al. Diverticulitis in the United States: 1998-2005: changing patterns of disease and treatment. Ann Surg 2009;249(2): 210–7.
3. Ricciardi R, Baxter NN, Read TE, et al. Is the decline in the surgical treatment for diverticulitis associated with an increase in complicated diverticulitis? Dis Colon Rectum 2009;52(9):1558–63.
4. Yen L, Davis KL, Hodhkins P, et al. Direct costs of diverticulitis in a US managed care population. Am J Pharm Benefits 2012;4(5):e118–29.
5. Crowe FL, Appleby PN, Allen NE, et al. Diet and risk of diverticular disease in Oxford cohort of European Prospective Investigation into Cancer and Nutrition (EPIC): prospective study of British vegetarians and non-vegetarians. BMJ 2011;343(jul19 4):d4131.
6. Ma W, Nguyen LH, Song M, et al. Intake of dietary fiber, fruits, and vegetables and risk of diverticulitis. Am J Gastroenterol 2019;114(9):1531–8.

7. Strate LL. Nut, corn, and popcorn consumption and the incidence of diverticular disease. JAMA 2008;300(8):907.
8. Peery AF, Barrett PR, Park D, et al. A high-fiber diet does not protect against asymptomatic diverticulosis. Gastroenterology 2012;142(2):266–72.e1.
9. Stollman N, Smalley W, Hirano I, et al. American gastroenterological association institute guideline on the management of acute diverticulitis. Gastroenterology 2015;149(7):1944–9.
10. Hjern F, Wolk A, Håkansson N. Smoking and the risk of diverticular disease in women. Br J Surg 2011;98(7):997–1002.
11. Hjern F, Wolk A, Håkansson N. Obesity, physical inactivity, and colonic diverticular disease requiring hospitalization in women: a prospective cohort study. Am J Gastroenterol 2012;107(2):296–302.
12. Strate LL, Liu YL, Aldoori WH, et al. Obesity increases the risks of diverticulitis and diverticular bleeding. Gastroenterology 2009;136(1):115–22.e1.
13. Cao Y, Strate LL, Keeley BR, et al. Meat intake and risk of diverticulitis among men. Gut 2018;67(3):466–72.
14. Hall J, Hardiman K, Lee S, et al. The American Society of colon and rectal surgeons clinical practice guidelines for the treatment of left-sided colonic diverticulitis. Dis Colon Rectum 2020;63(6):728–47.
15. Strate LL, Erichsen R, Baron JA, et al. Heritability and familial aggregation of diverticular disease: a population-based study of twins and siblings. Gastroenterology 2013;144(4):736–42.e1.
16. Granlund J, Svensson T, Olén O, et al. The genetic influence on diverticular disease - a twin study. Aliment Pharmacol Ther 2012. https://doi.org/10.1111/j.1365-2036.2012.05069.x.
17. Reichert MC, Lammert F. The genetic epidemiology of diverticulosis and diverticular disease: emerging evidence. United Eur Gastroenterol J 2015;3(5):409–18.
18. Almalki T, Garfinkle R, Kmiotek E, et al. Family history is associated with recurrent diverticulitis after an episode of diverticulitis managed nonoperatively. Dis Colon Rectum 2020;63(7):944–54.
19. Connelly TM, Berg AS, Hegarty JP, et al. The TNFSF15 gene single nucleotide polymorphism rs7848647 is associated with surgical diverticulitis. Ann Surg 2014;259(6):1132–7.
20. Maguire LH, Handelman SK, Du X, et al. Genome-wide association analyses identify 39 new susceptibility loci for diverticular disease. Nat Genet 2018; 50(10):1359–65.
21. Hughes LE. Postmortem survey of diverticular disease of the colon. II. The muscular abnormality of the sigmoid colon. Gut 1969;10(5):344–51.
22. Shahedi K, Fuller G, Bolus R, et al. Long-term risk of acute diverticulitis among patients with incidental diverticulosis found during colonoscopy. Clin Gastroenterol Hepatol 2013;11(12):1609–13.
23. Eglinton T, Nguyen T, Raniga S, et al. Patterns of recurrence in patients with acute diverticulitis. Br J Surg 2010;97(6):952–7.
24. Garfinkle R, Almalki T, Pelsser V, et al. Conditional risk of diverticulitis after non-operative management. Br J Surg 2020;107(13):1838–45.
25. Gennaro AR, Rosemond GP. Colonic diverticula and hemorrhage. Dis Colon Rectum 1973;16(5):409–15.
26. Niikura R, Nagata N, Shimbo T, et al. Natural history of bleeding risk in colonic diverticulosis patients: a long-term colonoscopy-based cohort study. Aliment Pharmacol Ther 2015;41(9):888–94.

27. Chabok A, Påhlman L, Hjern F, et al, for the AVOD Study Group. Randomized clinical trial of antibiotics in acute uncomplicated diverticulitis. Br J Surg 2012;99(4): 532–9.
28. Isacson D, Smedh K, Nikberg M, et al. Long-term follow-up of the AVOD randomized trial of antibiotic avoidance in uncomplicated diverticulitis. Br J Surg 2019; 106(11):1542–8.
29. Daniels L, Ünlü Ç, de Korte N, et al. Randomized clinical trial of observational *versus* antibiotic treatment for a first episode of CT-proven uncomplicated acute diverticulitis. Br J Surg 2016;104(1):52–61.
30. Jaung R, Nisbet S, Gosselink MP, et al. Antibiotics do not reduce length of hospital stay for uncomplicated diverticulitis in a pragmatic double-blind randomized trial. Clin Gastroenterol Hepatol 2021;19(3):503–10.e1.
31. van Dijk ST, Chabok A, Dijkgraaf MG, et al. Observational *versus* antibiotic treatment for uncomplicated diverticulitis: an individual-patient data meta-analysis. Br J Surg 2020;107(8):1062–9.
32. Emile SH, Elfeki H, Sakr A, et al. Management of acute uncomplicated diverticulitis without antibiotics: a systematic review, meta-analysis, and meta-regression of predictors of treatment failure. Tech Coloproctol 2018;22(7):499–509.
33. Moco D, Yeo H. Meta-analyses of current strategies to treat uncomplicated diverticulitis. Dis Colon Rectum 2019;62(3):371–8.
34. Peery AF, Shaukat A, Strate LL. AGA clinical practice update on medical management of colonic diverticulitis: expert review. Gastroenterology 2021;160(3): 906–11.e1.
35. Costi R, Cauchy F, Le Bian A, et al. Challenging a classic myth: pneumoperitoneum associated with acute diverticulitis is not an indication for open or laparoscopic emergency surgery in hemodynamically stable patients. A 10-year experience with a nonoperative treatment. Surg Endosc 2012;26(7):2061–71.
36. Simianu VV, Strate LL, Billingham RP, et al. The impact of elective colon resection on rates of emergency surgery for diverticulitis. Ann Surg 2016;263(1):123–9.
37. Vennix S, Musters GD, Mulder IM, et al. Laparoscopic peritoneal lavage or sigmoidectomy for perforated diverticulitis with purulent peritonitis: a multicentre, parallel-group, randomised, open-label trial. The Lancet 2015;386(10000): 1269–77.
38. Schultz JK, Yaqub S, Wallon C, et al. Laparoscopic lavage vs primary resection for acute perforated diverticulitis: The SCANDIV randomized clinical trial. JAMA 2015;314(13):1364.
39. Angenete E, Thornell A, Burcharth J, et al. Laparoscopic lavage is feasible and safe for the treatment of perforated diverticulitis with purulent peritonitis: the first results from the randomized controlled trial DILALA. Ann Surg 2016;263(1): 117–22.
40. White SI, Frenkiel B, Martin PJ. A ten-year audit of perforated sigmoid diverticulitis: highlighting the outcomes of laparoscopic lavage. Dis Colon Rectum 2010; 53(11):1537–41.
41. Franklin ME, Portillo G, Treviño JM, et al. Long-term experience with the laparoscopic approach to perforated diverticulitis plus generalized peritonitis. World J Surg 2008;32(7):1507–11.
42. Karoui M, Champault A, Pautrat K, et al. Laparoscopic peritoneal lavage or primary anastomosis with defunctioning stoma for hinchey 3 complicated diverticulitis: results of a comparative study. Dis Colon Rectum 2009;52(4):609–15.
43. Liang S, Russek K, Franklin ME. Damage control strategy for the management of perforated diverticulitis with generalized peritonitis: laparoscopic lavage and

drainage vs. laparoscopic Hartmann's procedure. Surg Endosc 2012;26(10):
2835–42.

44. Rogers AC, Collins D, O'Sullivan GC, et al. Laparoscopic lavage for perforated
diverticulitis: a population analysis. Dis Colon Rectum 2012;55(9):932–8.

45. Azhar N, Johanssen A, Sundström T, et al. Laparoscopic lavage vs primary
resection for acute perforated diverticulitis: long-term outcomes from the scandinavian diverticulitis (SCANDIV) randomized clinical trial. JAMA Surg 2021;
156(2):121.

46. O'Sullivan GC, Murphy D, O'Brien MG, et al. Laparoscopic management of
generalized peritonitis due to perforated colonic diverticula. Am J Surg 1996;
171(4):432–4.

47. Vermeulen J, Lange JF. Treatment of perforated diverticulitis with generalized
peritonitis: past, present, and future. World J Surg 2010;34(3):587–93.

48. Resio BJ, Jean R, Chiu AS, et al. Association of timing of colostomy reversal with
outcomes following hartmann procedure for diverticulitis. JAMA Surg 2019;
154(3):218–24.

49. Oberkofler CE, Rickenbacher A, Raptis DA, et al. A multicenter randomized clinical trial of primary anastomosis or Hartmann's procedure for perforated left
colonic diverticulitis with purulent or fecal peritonitis. Ann Surg 2012;256(5):
819–26 [discussion 826–7].

50. Lambrichts DPV, Vennix S, Musters GD, et al. Hartmann's procedure versus sigmoidectomy with primary anastomosis for perforated diverticulitis with purulent or
faecal peritonitis (LADIES): a multicentre, parallel-group, randomised, open-
label, superiority trial. Lancet Gastroenterol Hepatol 2019;4(8):599–610.

51. Gachabayov M, Oberkofler CE, Tuech JJ, et al. Resection with primary anastomosis vs nonrestorative resection for perforated diverticulitis with peritonitis: a
systematic review and meta-analysis. Colorectal Dis 2018;20(9):753–70.

52. Vermeulen J, Gosselink MP, Busschbach JJV, et al. Avoiding or reversing Hartmann's procedure provides improved quality of life after perforated diverticulitis.
J Gastrointest Surg 2010;14(4):651–7.

53. Lee JM, Bai P, Chang J, et al. Hartmann's procedure vs primary anastomosis with
diverting loop ileostomy for acute diverticulitis: nationwide analysis of 2,729 emergency surgery patients. J Am Coll Surg 2019;229(1):48–55.

54. Rafferty J, Shellito P, Hyman NH, et al, Standards Committee of American Society
of Colon and Rectal Surgeons. Practice parameters for sigmoid diverticulitis. Dis
Colon Rectum 2006;49(7):939–44.

55. Anaya DA, Flum DR. Risk of emergency colectomy and colostomy in patients with
diverticular disease. Arch Surg 2005;140(7):681–5.

56. Shaikh S, Krukowski ZH. Outcome of a conservative policy for managing acute
sigmoid diverticulitis. Br J Surg 2007;94(7):876–9.

57. Ritz J-P, Lehmann KS, Frericks B, et al. Outcome of patients with acute sigmoid
diverticulitis: multivariate analysis of risk factors for free perforation. Surgery
2011;149(5):606–13.

58. Regenbogen SE, Hardiman KM, Hendren S, et al. Surgery for diverticulitis in the
21st century: a systematic review. JAMA Surg 2014;149(3):292–303.

59. Hawkins AT, Samuels LR, Rothman R, et al. National variation in elective colon
resection for diverticular disease. Ann Surg 2020. https://doi.org/10.1097/SLA.
0000000000004236.

60. van de Wall BJM, Stam MAW, Draaisma WA, et al. Surgery versus conservative
management for recurrent and ongoing left-sided diverticulitis (DIRECT trial):

an open-label, multicentre, randomised controlled trial. Lancet Gastroenterol Hepatol 2017;2(1):13–22.

61. Bolkenstein HE, Consten ECJ, van der Palen J, et al. Long-term outcome of surgery versus conservative management for recurrent and ongoing complaints after an episode of diverticulitis: 5-year follow-up results of a multicenter randomized controlled trial (DIRECT-Trial). Ann Surg 2019;269(4):612–20.

62. Santos A, Mentula P, Pinta T, et al. Comparing laparoscopic elective sigmoid resection with conservative treatment in improving quality of life of patients with diverticulitis: the laparoscopic elective sigmoid resection following diverticulitis (LASER) randomized clinical trial. JAMA Surg 2021;156(2):129–36.

63. Sohn M, Agha A, Iesalnieks I, et al. PREDICtors for health-related quality of life after elective sigmoidectomy for DIVerticular disease: the PREDIC-DIV study protocol of a prospective multicentric transnational observational study. BMJ Open 2020;10(3):e034385.

64. Al-Khamis A, Abou Khalil J, Demian M, et al. Sigmoid colectomy for acute diverticulitis in immunosuppressed vs immunocompetent patients: outcomes from the ACS-NSQIP database. Dis Colon Rectum 2016;59(2):101–9.

65. Biondo S, Borao JL, Kreisler E, et al. Recurrence and virulence of colonic diverticulitis in immunocompromised patients. Am J Surg 2012;204(2):172–9.

66. Sugrue J, Lee J, Warner C, et al. Acute diverticulitis in renal transplant patients: should we treat them differently? Surgery 2018;163(4):857–65.

67. Klarenbeek BR, Samuels M, van der Wal MA, et al. Indications for elective sigmoid resection in diverticular disease. Ann Surg 2010;251(4):670–4.

Smoking, Obesity, and the Elective Operation

Sullivan A. Ayuso, MD, Jordan N. Robinson, MD, Paul D. Colavita, MD, B. Todd Heniford, MD*

KEYWORDS

- Smoking • Obesity • BMI • Complications • Preoperative • Preventative
- Prehabilitation

KEY POINTS

- Smoking and obesity increase the risk of postoperative complications, particularly wound and pulmonary complications.
- Smoking and obesity are modifiable risk factors, and their effects can be mitigated with smoking cessation 4 weeks before surgery and weight loss.
- Preoperative optimization should also focus on physical prehabilitation, glycemic control and medical management of other comorbidities.

INTRODUCTION

Smoking and obesity are two of the most prevalent public health issues facing society today. While the number of smokers has decreased in recent years, an estimated 15% of Americans are still active smokers.[1] In contrast, the number of people who are obese continues to rise as Americans are increasingly sedentary and have easy access to highly caloric, processed foods.[2] More than two-third of Americans are overweight or obese with nearly 40% falling in the obese category (**Table 1**).[3] It is projected that by 2030, over half of the adults in the United States will be obese.[4] Smoking and obesity both contribute to several health problems, including cardiovascular and pulmonary disease, and lead to a decreased lifespan.[5] Lifetime smokers have an associated reduction in life expectancy of more than 10 years.[6] When considered in combination, the detrimental effects of smoking and obesity tend to be additive with a 3- to 5-fold increased risk for all-cause mortality.[5]

Although smoking and obesity may be risk factors for a chronic disease, such as hypertension and coronary artery disease, they also serve as risk factors for acute

Gastrointestinal and Minimally Invasive Surgery, Department of Surgery, Carolinas Medical Center, Charlotte, NC 28204, USA
* Corresponding author. Gastrointestinal and Minimally Invasive Surgery, Department of Surgery, Carolinas Medical Center, 1025 Morehead Medical Drive Suite 300, Charlotte, NC 28204.
E-mail address: todd.heniford@gmail.com

Surg Clin N Am 101 (2021) 981–993
https://doi.org/10.1016/j.suc.2021.05.025
0039-6109/21/© 2021 Elsevier Inc. All rights reserved.

surgical.theclinics.com

Table 1
Centers for disease control BMI classification

Category	BMI (kg/m²)
Underweight	<18.5
Normal weight	18.5–24.9
Overweight	25.0–29.9
Class 1 obesity	30.0–34.9
Class 2 obesity	35.0–39.9
Class 3 obesity	>39.9

Table adapted from: 1. "Adult Body Mass Index." *Centers for Disease Control (CDC) and Prevention.* 2020.

problems in the perioperative period.[7,8] Smoking and obesity are risk factors that are potentially modifiable, and there is evidence to guide surgeons on the management of these patients in the perioperative period. The purpose of this article is to understand the impact of smoking and obesity on perioperative outcomes and identify ways to mitigate their associated risks. Moreover, other types of preoperative risk-modification will be discussed in an effort to provide a framework for surgeons to deliver personalized care that will improve patient outcomes.

CURRENT EVIDENCE—SMOKING

Pathologic changes in smokers are induced in multiple organ systems, including the cardiovascular, pulmonary, immune, and endocrine systems (**Table 2**).[9] The time to full organ system recovery when abstinent from smoking may range from 2 weeks to several months.[9] There are multiple pathophysiologic mechanisms by which smoking is believed to increase the risk for postoperative complications, in particular postoperative wound and pulmonary complications (PCs).[10,11] Smoking generates a stress response that leads to an increased presence of inflammatory mediators, vasoconstriction, and induction of tissue hypoxia.[12] Furthermore, there is an upregulation in fibroblasts that contributes to enhanced cellular adhesion and decreased collagen production.[9,13] The combination of hypoxia and the alteration in the cellular cytoskeleton create an environment for poor wound healing and increases the risk for wound-related complications, including surgical site infection (SSI).[12] The toxin production in cigarette smoke may also induce destruction of alveoli and impair gas exchange, which leads to increased risk of PCs. Patients may be at even greater risk for PC who have smoked for several years and are mechanically limited by obstructive lung disease.[14]

Large cohort studies and systematic reviews suggest that active smoking more than doubles the chance for developing a wound complication.[13,15–17] The wound complication that appears to be most affected by smoking is skin necrosis, which is due to peripheral vasoconstriction and subsequently poor perfusion of the skin.[15] In circumstances were there are large skin flaps, such as an abdominoplasty or open ventral hernia repair (VHR), the risk for wound complications is even higher.[18,19] Postoperative PC, including development of pneumonia and the need for reintubation, are 1.5 to 2 times more common in smokers.[13,20] Likewise, patients may be at an increased risk for cardiovascular disease in the perioperative period. Smoking is thought to enhance coagulopathy and decrease oxygen-carrying capacity, which can put patients at risk

Table 2
Systemic effects of smoking and diabetes

Smoking	System	Obesity
Atherosclerosis, ↑ sympathetic nervous system, ↑ RAAS activity Dx: HTN, HLD, CAD	Cardiovascular	↑ Sympathetic nervous system activity, ↑ RAAS activity, renal compression Dx: HTN, HLD, CAD
↑ Alveolar inflammation/destruction, reactive airway disease Dx: COPD, asthma	Pulmonary	↑ Mechanical stress, obesity hypoventilation, upper airway compression Dx: asthma, OSA
Vasoconstriction, poor perfusion Dx: delayed wound healing	Wound healing	Oxygen supply/demand mismatch Dx: delayed wound healing
B-cell destruction, inflammation Dx: diabetes	Endocrine	Insulin resistance, ↑ systemic inflammatory response Dx: diabetes
↑ Sympathetic nervous system activity, renal artery atherosclerosis Dx: ESRD	Renal	Renal compression, ↑ sympathetic nervous system activity Dx: Diabetic nephropathy, ESRD
Reflux, mesenteric artery atherosclerosis, ↑ dyslipidemia Dx: Barrett's esophagus, mesenteric ischemia	Gastrointestinal	Reflux, ↑ dyslipidemia Dx: Barrett's esophagus, NAFLD
Dyslipidemia, systemic hypertension Dx: stroke	Neurologic	Dyslipidemia, systemic hypertension Dx: stroke
N/A	Musculoskeletal	Mechanical stress Dx: Osteoarthritis

Abbreviations: CAD, coronary artery disease; ESRD, end-stage renal disease; HLD, hyperlipidemia; HTN, hypertension; NAFLD, nonalcoholic fatty liver disease; OSA, obstructive sleep apnea; RAAS, renin-angiotensin-aldosterone system.
aSmoking and obesity both predispose patients to cellular dysplasia and malignancy across systems.
Table adapted from: [1] "The Mortality Risk of Smoking and Obesity Combined." *Am J Prev Med.* 2006; and [2]. "Mechanisms, Pathophysiology, and Management of Obesity." *NEJM.* 2017.

for mortality-associated complications such as pulmonary embolism, stroke, and myocardial infarction.[7]

Although postoperative wound complications and cardioPCs are most common, there are other specific situations worth mentioning. For instance, for patients who undergo an intestinal anastomosis, smoking increases the risk for an anastomotic leak.[21] A recent study of patients undergoing left colon resection found that anastomotic leak rate was increased over three-fold (17% vs 5%, $P = .01$) in smokers.[21] In addition to anastomotic leak, patients who smoke and undergo gastric bypass surgery are at an added risk for the development of marginal ulcers, which predispose patients to anastomotic stricture and perforation.[22] Because of the multiplicity of risk factors in this patient population, smoking cessation requirements for patients should be more stringent.[22]

A meta-analysis by Sorenson examined four randomized controlled trials that evaluated the timing of smoking cessation relative to date of surgery.[23] In these four trials, smoking cessation took place anywhere from two to 8 weeks before operation.[24,25] The study that required smoking abstinence just 2 weeks before elective colorectal surgery did not reduce the risk of wound complications or other complications within 30 days of surgery.[25] The other three studies, which included both general surgery and orthopedic surgery patients, required smoking cessation at least 4 weeks before surgery.[24,26,27] Each of these studies showed a significant decrease in overall short-term complications. However, two of these three randomized trials did not show a decrease in wound complications.[23] These trials were limited primarily by the small number of patients that they were able to enroll and, therefore, may have been affected by type II error. Nevertheless, it is now generally recommended that smoking cessation occurs at least 4 weeks before elective surgery.[28] In an elegant, prospective, volunteer study of nonsmoking patients versus smokers versus abstinent smokers with and without nicotine patches with small, peri-sacral incisions performed and followed up for 4 to 12 weeks, a significant, 6-fold decrease in wound complications was noted in nonsmokers. Abstinence for 4 weeks resulted in outcomes being equal to those of nonsmokers, and the use of nicotine patches did not reduce the positive outcomes of stopping smoking.

Other studies, however, demonstrate that former smokers, while at decreased risk compared with active smokers, are still at increased risks in comparison to patients who have never smoked.[13,23] In the largest retrospective review of patients designated as "former smokers," Hawn and colleagues demonstrated that patients who had any history of smoking demonstrated an increased risk of postoperative pneumonia, SSI, and mortality.[13] Furthermore, the relationship between pack years and postoperative complication appears dose-dependent; patients who have a pack-year history that is greater than 20 years are at greatest risk for postoperative complications.[13] The results of this study were further substantiated by the frequently sited meta-analysis by Sorensen. In this meta-analysis, it was concluded that former smokers had a one-third higher incidence of wound healing complications than nonsmokers.[23]

Preoperative smoking cessation intervention programs take on a variety of forms. For example, programs may use pharmacologic interventions, such as nicotine replacement or buproprion, in addition to counseling by nurses or physicians.[24] A Cochrane review of interventions for preoperative smoking cessation recommended that behavioral interventions, such as weekly counseling session, along with nicotine replacement therapy may be the optimal elements of a smoking intervention program.[29] The use of other pharmacologic agents, such as varenicline, did not affect early abstinence rates but did improve smoking cessation rates when patients were followed up for 1 year postoperatively.[30] The Cochrane review also concluded that intervention programs were more effective if they began four to 8 weeks before surgery.[29]

CURRENT EVIDENCE—OBESITY

Excess adiposity in obese patients leads to pathophysiologic changes on a multi-system level (see **Table 2**). Adiposity leads to low-grade systemic inflammation, a heightened sympathetic response, and insulin resistance.[31] It is important to note that these obesity-induced systemic changes appear more pronounced with central adiposity than with peripheral adiposity (**Fig. 1**). Central adipocytes produce several chemokines (eg, leptin) and cytokines (eg, interleukins, tumor necrosis factor) that generate a profound systemic inflammatory response that contributes to chronic disease states such metabolic syndrome.[32] The presence of increased fat can also alter the pharmokinetics of drugs administered in the perioperative period, with Body Mass Indices (BMI) greater than 40 kg/m^2 altering bioavailability.[33]

Obesity may also make an operation more technically challenging. Even before the beginning of the operation, patients who are obese have more challenging airways, which increases the difficulty of intubation.[31] Intraoperatively, obesity can decrease visualization in open and minimally invasive surgery (MIS) cases making it harder to perform key technical steps in an operation. Excess adiposity can make retraction difficult, and surgeons may find themselves operating in small and narrow spaces. In MIS cases, obese patients also require a higher rate of conversion to open surgery.[34] Despite this, it is thought that the benefits of MIS, such as a reduction in wound complications and decreased length of stay, may be particularly beneficial in the obese patient population and help to lessen other surgical risks.[35]

The relationship between obesity and increased postoperative wound complications is also well-established.[36–38] A strong contributing factor includes decreased oxygen tension in the tissues as a result of a mismatch of oxygen supply and demand.[39] A review of colorectal surgery patients demonstrates that obese patients are 50%

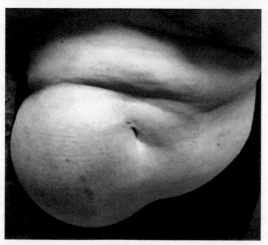

Fig. 1. An obese patient with a ventral hernia. Before operation, the patient was required to lose weight through a ketogenic diet and daily exercise. Referral to a bariatric surgeon was also considered before scheduling surgery.

more likely than patients with normal BMI to develop a postoperative SSI[39] Another study by Gupta and colleagues using National Surgical Quality Improvement Program (NSQIP) data reviewed elective general surgery cases over a 5-year period and stratified patients by BMI.[40] In this study, the authors found that there was a graduated escalation in risk for wound complications that occurred with increased BMI, and patients in the "super super obese" (BMI ≥ 60) category had nearly double the risk of SSI compared with normal BMI patients. The study by Gupta and colleagues was one of the first studies to stratify patients into subcategories with BMIs ≥40.[40]

Studies in abdominal wall reconstruction have demonstrated much the same. Increases in obesity stepwise increase the incidence of wound complications and the need for reoperation and can triple the incidence of hernia repair failure.[41] Indeed, long-term (2–5 years) recurrence rates have been reported to be as high as 50%.[42] In one report of 850 MIS VHRs, the recurrence rate was four times higher for patients with a BMI of 40 or greater versus that of those with normal weight.[43] A BMI of less than 40 is typically targeted for patients undergoing VHR at this institution, but similar to many academic centers, there is no true barrier to surgery according to BMI.[44] Indeed, the authors have shown that for each point of BMI increase beyond 26 kg/m^2, there is a 1.08 times increase in wound complications.[44] This leads one to consider a push to decrease BMI in any patient who is overweight or obese.

Obese patients are at a higher risk for intraoperative PCs and failed extubation after surgery.[32] Once successfully extubated, obesity further predisposes patients to hypoventilation and atelectasis, which may result in PC, including the need for reintubation.[45] Patients who are obese and/or have a history of obstructive sleep apnea may benefit from the use of noninvasive positive pressure techniques, such as continuous positive airway pressure, or supplemental oxygen while they are in the hospital.[46] Early ambulation is particularly important in this population because it can help prevent atelectasis and deep vein thrombosis, which have an increased incidence in obese patients.[45]

A decreased body weight of even 5% to 10% has been associated with decreased risk for associated PC.[45] However, BMI alone may not be the only consideration driving postoperative PC. Schlosser and colleagues used 3-D volumetric analysis to analyze computed tomography scans of the abdomen and pelvis and found that the volume and location of adiposity (eg, extra-abdominally in a hernia sac) also play a role in the likelihood of PC.[47] Furthermore, obese patients who have pre-existing respiratory conditions, such as asthma or chronic obstructive pulmonary disorder (COPD), are at the highest risk for developing postoperative PC.[47] While there is no universal target BMI for performing an elective operation, there have been studies performed that have attempted to answer this question. An example includes national data from NSQIP which evaluated patients who underwent open VHR over a 14-year period. It concluded that patients who are morbidly obese (BMI ≥40) were nearly three times as likely to develop postoperative complications as patients in the normal weight group.[48]

In a similar vein to smoking cessation programs, the approach to optimizing patient weight before elective surgery is heterogeneous. The combination of a low-calorie, low-carbohydrate diet and daily physical activity is the mainstay for weight loss before surgery.[31] A comprehensive program with high-intensity behavioral counseling can result in mean weight loss that ranges from 5% to 8%.[49] The use of medications for weight loss, such as the phentermine, which is the sympathomimetic that is most commonly prescribed, are generally not part of perioperative routines. The utilization of new medications has been limited by the concerns for long-term safety, in particular, in regard to long-term cardiovascular side effects.[31]

While obesity, especially morbid obesity, is generally recognized as a risk factor before major surgical operations, the data are not unanimous as it is with smoking. Notably, the landmark article by Dindo and colleagues published in *The Lancet* in 2003 noted that obesity was not predictive for the development of postoperative complications in Swiss patients undergoing general surgery procedures.[36] In this study, patients with BMI above 30 kg/m^2 were grouped and compared with those patients with BMI less than 30 kg/m^2. The results of this study indicated that there were no differences in in-hospital postoperative complications between obese and nonobese patients. Since this study, there have been other publications, such as that by Mullen and colleagues, which examine rates of mortality in obese patients undergoing nonbariatric general surgery.[37] In this study, which used NSQIP data, the authors found that patients who were overweight (BMI: 25.1–30 kg/m^2) or moderately obese (BMI: 35.1–40.0 kg/m^2) actually had a lower rate of mortality after surgery.[37] While these study outcomes are uncommon, they do add to confusion on the topic.

DISCUSSION

Smoking and obesity are two commonly encountered risk factors in patients undergoing elective surgery. A smoking history of any kind places a patient at increased for a myriad of postoperative complications, most notably wound and PCs. Effective interventions for smoking cessation include behavioral counseling and nicotine replacement therapy and should begin at least 4 weeks before surgery.[29] Similarly, obesity increases rates of postoperative complications and may enhance the technical difficulty of the operation being performed. Unlike for smoking, there is no specific BMI that is used to mitigate risk; however, a BMI less than 40 kg/m^2 has been associated with a decreased risk of SSI and other specific postoperative complications, such as hernia recurrence. Surgical prehabilitation with targeted lifestyle modification through diet and exercise can lead to weight loss that may lessen risk for postoperative complications.

The perioperative period can be the ideal time for a lifestyle intervention.[50] For example, studies suggest that 80% of smokers who seek medical care have the desire to quit and that the perioperative period may be the best time to do so.[51,52] Although it may be considered outside of the "traditional" purview of the surgeon, a recognition of the importance of smoking cessation can have a major impact on patient outcomes. By conveying the risks of smoking (and similarly, obesity) that are specific to surgery, it may provide patients with tangible evidence that motivates them to quit. The goal of perioperative smoking cessation need not necessarily target long-term cessation or be maintained by counseling with the surgeon. Evidence suggests that smoking cessation programs that emphasize temporary abstinence from smoking around the time of surgery result in sustainable quit-rates over time.[52,53]

It may be difficult to tell whether or not a patient has quit smoking. There are several tests that can be used by providers to reliably tell if a patient has quit smoking. At this institution, chronic smokers routinely undergo cotinine testing and are not offered surgery if they are currently smoking. A cotinine test evaluates the level of cotinine in a patient's urine and has a high sensitivity and specificity, which have both been reported to be greater than 90%.[54]

For patients who are former smokers, there are other ways to help diminish associated complications. For example, in high-risk patient populations, the use of negative pressure wound therapy has been shown to reduce the development of postoperative SSI.[55] Other means of improving patient outcomes in the perioperative period include early ambulation, the use of incentive spirometry, and continuation of home medications, such as inhaled steroids, for pre-existing pulmonary conditions such as asthma and COPD.[56]

For an obese patient, referral to a bariatric surgeon is an option if the risks of complications from obesity present a greater risk to the patient than nonoperative management. Referral to a bariatric surgeon is considered at this institution when a patient is morbidly obese and is going to undergo VHR.[57] Often a gastric sleeve can be performed laparoscopically despite the presence of a ventral hernia. In general, bariatric procedures are safe with an overall postoperative complication rate of around 5%.[58] Bariatric surgery can result in sustained weight loss of greater than 20% compared with patients' presurgery weight.[59] Not only is bariatric surgery a safe way to drastically decrease obesity but also it can improve and even eliminate hyperglycemia, hypertension, and obstructive sleep apnea, which add to perioperative risk.[59,60] Another option that may be considered in patients with excessive central adiposity who are undergoing elective open abdominal operations, in particular, open VHR, is a concurrent panniculectomy. A panniculectomy, which may require the expertise of a plastic surgeon, frequently helps with operative exposure and can decrease the strain on repair and has an acceptable wound complication rate.[61,62]

The "obesity paradox," which refers to the potential protective effect of nonmorbid obesity, should be further evaluated. There are several published studies, such as a study by Mullen and colleagues, that suggest improved outcomes for patients who are overweight and have mild to moderate obesity.[37] These studies primarily focus specifically on mortality, and mortality alone does not adequately convey the degree of perioperative risk conferred by obesity.[63] In the article by Mullen and colleagues, which asserted that overweight and moderately obese patients have improved postoperative mortality, it was still concluded that there was an increased wound morbidity with increasing BMI.[37] Also, this article used information from a national database to evaluate short-term outcomes, and longer term complication were not characterized. The use of BMI as the lone marker for obesity is problematic because it does adequately describe the amount of adiposity or muscle mass that a patient possesses. The message being conveyed by "obesity paradox" studies needs careful evaluation as the long-term effects of obesity are without question deleterious for patients.

There are other modifiable preoperative factors to consider that have a substantial impact on patient outcomes and should be addressed in conjunction with smoking and diabetes. Patients who have uncontrolled diabetes are at a higher risk for the development of postoperative wound complications and delayed wound healing.[44] It is standard practice at this institution to target a hemoglobin A1c level of less than 7.2 before surgery.[38] Prospective data at this institution have shown that an A1c of 7.2 serves as a cutoff for increased wound morbidity in patients undergoing VHR.[44] Even in "smaller" outpatient cases, such as repair of umbilical hernias, uncontrolled diabetes carries an increased risk for developing postoperative wound complications.[14] Postoperative glycemic control is similarly important for reducing wound morbidity. Generally, a blood sugar below 200 mg/dL is targeted postoperatively in hospital with care taken to avoid hypoglycemia.[64]

Prehabilitation programs are gaining widespread popularity, particularly in the fields of colorectal surgery, surgical oncology, and abdominal wall reconstruction.[65–67] Although there is little standardization among prehabilitation programs, there are certain elements that are common, which include a focus on nutrition, physical activity, and psychosocial counseling.[68] Liang and colleagues published results from a randomized-controlled trial suggesting that participation in a structured prehabilitation program decreases 30-day complication and hernia recurrence rates in patients undergoing VHR.[42] In patients undergoing an operation for colorectal cancer, randomization into a trimodal prehabilitation program was found to increase disease-free survival by over 20% in patients with stage 3 cancer.[66]

Using a multidisciplinary approach to optimize patients should be encouraged to provide comprehensive care for patients. This approach is particularly useful when surgeons have limited time to discuss the nonsurgical parts of a patient's care. In the surgical clinic at this institution, geriatricians are routinely consulted for patients older than 65 years to assess frailty, which is predictive of discharge to an institutional care facility, and help with perioperative medication management.[69] Routine completion of a comprehensive geriatric assessment improves health outcomes in geriatric patients and is cost-effective.[70] Specialists from other disciplines, such as endocrinology, nutrition, and bariatrics, are also used to address specific needs of patients. The goal of a perioperative management strategy is to personalize care in a way that improves patient outcomes.

SUMMARY

Nearly one in five Americans is a smoker, and two out of every five Americans are obese. Both smoking and obesity increase the risk of postoperative complications, particularly wound and PCs. The relationship of smoking and obesity appears to be dose-dependent with patients who have greater pack-histories and higher BMIs having the greatest risk of complications. While smoking and obesity do increase perioperative risk, they are potentially modifiable. Smoking cessation 4 weeks before surgery and weight loss through diet and exercise before surgery can improve outcomes. Other factors, such as diabetes, frailty, and additional medical comorbidities should be optimized to ensure the best outcomes for patients.

CLINICS CARE POINTS

- Smoking and obesity are commonly encountered risk factors in patients who are undergoing elective surgery.
- Smoking places patients at risk for postoperative complications, particularly wound and pulmonary complications.
- Preoperative smoking cessation should take place at least *4 weeks* before the scheduled operation.
- Smoking cessation intervention programs should include behavioral counseling and nicotine replacement therapy.
- Obesity can make an operation more technically challenging and place a patient at a risk for a variety of perioperative complications.
- While there is no cutoff BMI that is used before scheduling a surgery, a BMI of 40 kg/m^2 is associated with a higher rate of surgical site infection and other important outcomes, such as hernia recurrence.
- Lifestyle modification through a combination of low-calorie, low-carbohydrate diet and daily exercise is considered first line for weight loss before elective surgery.
- Other means of preoperative optimization are important to consider and include glycemic control for diabetic patients and physical optimization of patients through structured prehabilitation programs.
- Preoperative optimization of patients should be individualized to maximize outcomes in the postoperative period.

REFERENCES

1. Petro CC, Haskins IN, Tastaldi L, et al. Does active smoking really matter before ventral hernia repair? An AHSQC analysis. Surgery 2019;165(2):406–11.
2. Chooi YC, Ding C, Magkos F. The epidemiology of obesity. Metabolism 2019; 92:6–10.
3. Sifferlin A. More than two thirds of americans are overweight or obese | Time. Time 2015.
4. Finkelstein EA, Khavjou OA, Thompson H, et al. Obesity and severe obesity forecasts through 2030. Am J Prev Med 2012;42(6):563–70.
5. Freedman DM, Sigurdson AJ, Rajaraman P, et al. The Mortality Risk of Smoking and Obesity Combined. Am J Prev Med 2006;31(5):355–62.
6. Centers for Disease Control. Fast Facts | Fact Sheets | Smoking & Tobacco Use | CDC. Available at: https://www.cdc.gov/tobacco/data_statistics/fact_sheets/fast_facts/index.htm. Accessed March 24, 2021.
7. Khullar D, Maa J. The impact of smoking on surgical outcomes. J Am Coll Surg 2012;418–26.
8. Quante M, Dietrich A, Elkhal A, et al. Obesity-related immune responses and their impact on surgical outcomes. Int J Obes 2015;877–83.
9. Tønnesen H, Nielsen PR, Lauritzen JB, et al. Smoking and alcohol intervention before surgery: evidence for best practice. Br J Anaesth 2009;102(3):297–306.
10. Davies OJ, Husain T, Stephens RCM. Postoperative pulmonary complications following non-cardiothoracic surgery. BJA Educ 2017;17(9):295–300.
11. Sereysky J, Parsikia A, Stone ME, et al. Predictive factors for the development of surgical site infection in adults undergoing initial open inguinal hernia repair. Hernia 2020;24(1):173–8.
12. Sorensen LT, Karlsmark T, Gottrup F. Abstinence from smoking reduces incisional wound infection. Ann Surg 2003;238(1):1–5.
13. Hawn MT, Houston TK, Campagna EJ, et al. The attributable risk of smoking on surgical complications. Ann Surg 2011;254(6):914–20.
14. Henriksen NA, Bisgaard T, Helgstrand F. Smoking and obesity are associated with increased readmission after elective repair of small primary ventral hernias: a nationwide database study. Surg 2020;168(3):527–31.
15. Sørensen LT. Wound healing and infection in surgery. Ann Surg 2012;255(6): 1069–79.
16. DeLancey JO, Blay E, Hewitt DB, et al. The effect of smoking on 30-day outcomes in elective hernia repair. Am J Surg 2018;216(3):471–4.
17. Novitsky YW, Porter JR, Rucho ZC, et al. Open preperitoneal retrofascial mesh repair for multiply recurrent ventral incisional hernias. J Am Coll Surg 2006; 203(3):283–9.
18. Cox TC, Blair LJ, Huntington CR, et al. The cost of preventable comorbidities on wound complications in open ventral hernia repair. J Surg Res 2016;206(1): 214–22.
19. Theocharidis V, Katsaros I, Sgouromallis E, et al. Current evidence on the role of smoking in plastic surgery elective procedures: a systematic review and meta-analysis. J Plast Reconstr Aesthet Surg 2018;624–36.
20. Mills E, Eyawo O, Lockhart I, et al. Smoking cessation reduces postoperative complications: a systematic review and meta-analysis. Am J Med 2011;124(2): 144–54.
21. Baucom RB, Poulose BK, Herline AJ, et al. Smoking as dominant risk factor for anastomotic leak after left colon resection. Am J Surg 2015;210(1):1–5.

22. Chow A, Neville A, Kolozsvari N. Smoking in bariatric surgery: a systematic review. Surg Endosc 2020;1–20.

23. Sørensen LT. Wound healing and infection in surgery: the clinical impact of smoking and smoking cessation: a systematic review and meta-analysis. Arch Surg 2012;373–83.

24. Møller AM, Villebro N, Pedersen T, et al. Effect of preoperative smoking intervention on postoperative complications: a randomised clinical trial. Lancet 2002; 359(9301):114–7.

25. Sorensen LT, Jorgensen T. Short-term pre-operative smoking cessation intervention does not affect postoperative complications in colorectal surgery: a randomized clinical trial. Color Dis 2003;5(4):347–52.

26. Lindström D, Azodi OS, Wladis A, et al. Effects of a perioperative smoking cessation intervention on postoperative complications. Ann Surg 2008;248(5):739–45.

27. Sørensen LT, Hemmingsen U, Jørgensen T. Strategies of smoking cessation intervention before hernia surgery - effect on perioperative smoking behavior. Hernia 2007;11(4):327–33.

28. Surgeons AC of. Quit Smoking Before Your Operation.

29. Thomsen T, Villebro N, Møller AM. Interventions for preoperative smoking cessation. Cochrane Database Syst Rev 2014. https://doi.org/10.1002/14651858. CD002294.pub4.

30. Wong J, Abrishami A, Yang Y, et al. A perioperative smoking cessation intervention with varenicline: a double-blind, randomized, placebo-controlled trial. Anesthesiology 2012;117(4):755–64.

31. Heymsfield SB, Wadden TA. Mechanisms, pathophysiology, and management of obesity. N Engl J Med 2017;376(3):254–66.

32. Carron M, Safaee Fakhr B, Ieppariello G, et al. Perioperative care of the obese patient. Br J Surg 2020;107(2):e39–55.

33. Smit C, De Hoogd S, Brüggemann RJM, et al. Obesity and drug pharmacology: a review of the influence of obesity on pharmacokinetic and pharmacodynamic parameters. Expert Opin Drug Metab Toxicol 2018;275–85.

34. Moghadamyeghaneh Z, Masoomi H, Mills SD, et al. Outcomes of conversion of laparoscopic colorectal surgery to open surgery. J Soc Laparoendosc Surg 2015;18(4). https://doi.org/10.4293/JSLS.2014.00230.

35. Scheib SA, Tanner E, Green IC, et al. Laparoscopy in the morbidly obese: physiologic considerations and surgical techniques to optimize success. J Minim Invasive Gynecol 2014;182–95.

36. Dindo D, Muller MK, Weber M, et al. Obesity in general elective surgery. Lancet 2003;361(9374):2032–5.

37. Mullen JT, Moorman DW, Davenport DL. The obesity paradox: body mass index and outcomes in patients undergoing nonbariatric general surgery. Ann Surg 2009;250(1):166–72.

38. Heniford BT, Ross SW, Wormer BA, et al. Preperitoneal ventral hernia repair: a decade long prospective observational study with analysis of 1023 patient outcomes. Ann Surg 2020;271(2):364–74.

39. Gurunathan U, Ramsay S, Mitrić G, et al. Association between obesity and wound infection following colorectal surgery: systematic review and meta-analysis. J Gastrointest Surg 2017;21(10):1700–12.

40. Gupta M, Dugan A, Chacon E, et al. Detailed perioperative risk among patients with extreme obesity undergoing nonbariatric general surgery. Surg 2020; 168(3):462–70.

41. Desai KA, Razavi SA, Hart AM, et al. The effect of BMI on outcomes following complex abdominal wall reconstructions. Ann Plast Surg 2016;76:S295–7.
42. Liang MK, Bernardi K, Holihan JL, et al. Modifying risks in ventral hernia patients with prehabilitation: a randomized controlled trial. Ann Surg 2018;268(4):674–80.
43. Heniford BT, Park A, Ramshaw BJ, et al. Laparoscopic repair of ventral hernias: nine years' experience with 850 consecutive hernias. Ann Surg 2003;238: 391–400.
44. Augenstein VA, Colavita PD, Wormer BA, et al. CeDAR: carolinas equation for determining associated risks. J Am Coll Surg 2015;221(4):S65–6.
45. Taylor A, DeBoard Z, Gauvin JM. Prevention of postoperative pulmonary complications. Surg Clin North Am 2015;237–54.
46. Carron M, Zarantonello F, Ieppariello G, et al. Obesity and perioperative noninvasive ventilation in bariatric surgery. Minerva Chir 2017;248–64.
47. Schlosser KA, Maloney SR, Prasad T, et al. Too big to breathe: predictors of respiratory failure and insufficiency after open ventral hernia repair. Surg Endosc 2020;34(9):4131–9.
48. Pernar LIM, Pernar CH, Dieffenbach BV, et al. What is the BMI threshold for open ventral hernia repair? Surg Endosc 2017;31(3):1311–7.
49. Apovian CM, Aronne L, Rubino D, et al. A randomized, phase 3 trial of naltrexone SR/bupropion SR on weight and obesity-related risk factors (COR-II). Obesity 2013;21(5):935–43.
50. Prestwich A, Moore S, Kotze A, et al. How can smoking cessation be induced before surgery? A systematic review and meta-analysis of behavior change techniques and other intervention characteristics. Front Psychol 2017;8:915.
51. Lebrun-Harris LA, Fiore MC, Tomoyasu N, et al. Cigarette smoking, desire to quit, and tobacco-related counseling among patients at adult health centers. Am J Public Health 2015;105(1):180–8.
52. Saxony J, Cowling L, Catchpole L, et al. Evaluation of a smoking cessation service in elective surgery. J Surg Res 2017;212:33–41.
53. Lee SM, Landry J, Jones PM, et al. Long-term quit rates after a perioperative smoking cessation randomized controlled trial. Anesth Analg 2015;120(3):582–7.
54. Achilihu H, Feng J, Wang L, et al. Tobacco use classification by inexpensive urinary cotinine immunoassay test strips. J Anal Toxicol 2019;43(2):149–53.
55. Javed AA, Teinor J, Wright M, et al. Negative pressure wound therapy for surgical-site infections: a randomized trial. Ann Surg 2019;269(6):1034–40.
56. Moore JA, Conway DH, Thomas N, et al. Impact of a peri-operative quality improvement programme on postoperative pulmonary complications. Anaesthesia 2017;72(3):317–27.
57. Newcomb WL, Polhill JL, Chen AY, et al. Staged hernia repair preceded by gastric bypass for the treatment of morbidly obese patients with complex ventral hernias. Hernia 2008;12(5):465–9.
58. Birkmeyer JD, Finks JF, O'Reilly A, et al. Surgical Skill and Complication Rates after Bariatric Surgery. N Engl J Med 2013;369(15):1434–42.
59. Schauer PR, Bhatt DL, Kirwan JP, et al. Bariatric surgery versus intensive medical therapy for diabetes — 5-year outcomes. N Engl J Med 2017;376(7):641–51.
60. Auclair A, Biertho L, Marceau S, et al. Bariatric surgery-induced resolution of hypertension and obstructive sleep apnea: impact of modulation of body fat, ectopic fat, autonomic nervous activity, inflammatory and adipokine profiles. Obes Surg 2017;27(12):3156–64.
61. Shubinets V, Fox JP, Tecce MG, et al. Concurrent panniculectomy in the obese ventral hernia patient: assessment of short-term complications, hernia

recurrence, and healthcare utilization. J Plast Reconstr Aesthet Surg 2017;70(6): 759–67.

62. Elhage SA, Marturano MN, Deerenberg EB, et al. Impact of panniculectomy in complex abdominal wall reconstruction: a propensity matched analysis in 624 patients. Surg Endosc 2020. https://doi.org/10.1007/s00464-020-08011-7.

63. Donini LM, Pinto A, Giusti AM, et al. Obesity or BMI paradox? Beneath the tip of the iceberg. Front Nutr 2020;7:53.

64. Sathya B, Davis R, Taveira T, et al. Intensity of peri-operative glycemic control and postoperative outcomes in patients with diabetes: a meta-analysis. Diabetes Res Clin Pract 2013;102(1):8–15.

65. Siegal SR, Orenstein S. A pilot trial of prehabilitation for sarcopenic patients undergoing complex ventral hernia repairs. n.d.

66. Trépanier M, Minnella EM, Paradis T, et al. Improved disease-free survival after prehabilitation for colorectal cancer surgery. Ann Surg 2019;270(3):493–501.

67. Barberan-Garcia A, Ubré M, Roca J, et al. Personalised prehabilitation in high-risk patients undergoing elective major abdominal surgery : a randomized blinded controlled trial. Ann Surg 2018;267(1):50–6.

68. Baimas-George M, Watson M, Elhage S, et al. Prehabilitation in frail surgical patients: a systematic review. World J Surg 2020;3668–78.

69. Robinson TN, Wallace JI, Wu DS, et al. Accumulated frailty characteristics predict postoperative discharge institutionalization in the geriatric patient. J Am Coll Surg 2011;213(1):37–42.

70. Eamer G, Saravana-Bawan B, van der Westhuizen B, et al. Economic evaluations of comprehensive geriatric assessment in surgical patients: a systematic review. J Surg Res 2017;218:9–17.

Dissecting the Perioperative Care Bundle

Kyle G. Cologne, MD*, Christine Hsieh, MD

KEYWORDS

- Enhanced recovery after surgery (ERAS) • Enhanced recovery protocols (ERP)
- Fast-track surgery

KEY POINTS

- Enhanced recovery after surgery (ERAS) has been shown to be safe and effective, improving outcomes and decreasing length of stay after major abdominal surgery.
- Individual components of ERAS bundles have varying levels of supporting literature, and it is often difficult to dissect out their true contributions.
- Nonnarcotic agents to assist with pain control are integral to the success of an ERAS pathway.

INTRODUCTION

Enhanced recovery after surgery (ERAS) protocols are comprehensive perioperative care pathways designed to mitigate the physiologic stressors associated with surgery and, in turn, improve clinical outcomes.[1] Also referred to as enhanced recovery protocols or previously "fast-track" surgery, these programs combine the multidisciplinary efforts of those involved in a patient's journey through surgery to create a "bundle" of interventions that are purportedly more effective than the sum of the individual parts.[2] A robust body of literature supports adoption of such programs, touting diminished perioperative morbidity, reduced postop complications, and overall improved clinical outcomes (including a reduced length of stay without corresponding increase in readmission rates).[3–5] There are also resultant cost savings associated with these programs.[6] Given that implementing ERAS protocols requires significant time, effort, and institutional change,[7,8] there are ongoing efforts to study the components of these perioperative care bundles to assess their efficacy as stand-alone interventions and the degree with which they contribute to improved outcomes within the context of a care bundle. This manuscript examines some of the critical components, describes some areas where the science is weak (but dogma may be strong), and provides some of the evidence (or lack thereof) behind components of a standard ERAS protocol.

Division of Colon and Rectal Surgery, Department of Surgery, Keck School of Medicine of the University of Southern California, 1441 Eastlake Avenue, Suite 7418, Los Angeles, CA 90033, USA
* Corresponding author.
E-mail address: kyle.cologne@med.usc.edu

Surg Clin N Am 101 (2021) 995–1006
https://doi.org/10.1016/j.suc.2021.05.026
0039-6109/21/© 2021 Elsevier Inc. All rights reserved.

surgical.theclinics.com

WHAT IS ENHANCED RECOVERY AFTER SURGERY AND HOW DOES IT WORK?

In the 1990s, the Danish surgeon Dr Henrik Kehlet postulated that the surgical stress response induced widespread physiologic changes that increased demand on various organ systems, thereby increasing the risk of postoperative morbidity.[9] Subsequent research expanded on this idea and examined the various biological cascade systems and metabolic pathways involved in maintaining homeostasis.[2] From here, various points of intervention were identified, and this ultimately led to the development of protocols meant to ameliorate the adverse effects of surgical stress in hopes of producing improved clinical outcomes.[10–12]

The first enhanced recovery protocols focused specifically on the care of the patient undergoing colon resection in the early 2000s.[13,14] Since then, ERAS protocols have been developed and fine-tuned by numerous academic and professional societies, with adaptations made for specific surgical specialties and institutions.[2,15–17] Although some individual components differ, ERAS protocols are generally organized into 3 interlinked sections: preoperative, intraoperative, and postoperative (**Fig. 1**). Several professional societies have also published guidelines or clinical practice guidelines detailing these most common components.[18]

Preoperative care generally focuses on optimization of existing medical comorbidities and nutritional status. Counseling patients about recovery milestones and discharge criteria is strongly recommended, as is education about particular aspects of recovery, such as stoma care.[18] Advising patients to stop smoking cigarettes or drinking alcohol is commonly recommended,[19] and even brief periods of smoking cessation can have beneficial effects on recovery of pulmonary function. It is estimated that smoking increases the cost of postoperative care by just more than $300 in the initial 3 months following surgery, so smoking cessation efforts are worthwhile.[20]

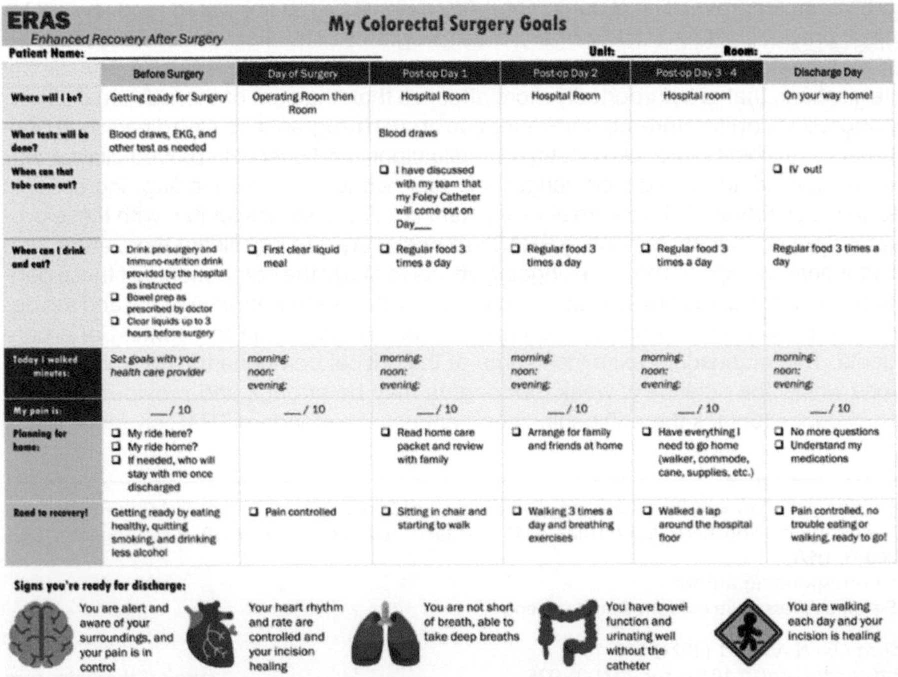

ERAS
Enhanced Recovery After Surgery

My Colorectal Surgery Goals

Patient Name: _____ Unit: _____ Room: _____

	Before Surgery	Day of Surgery	Post-op Day 1	Post-op Day 2	Post-op Day 3 - 4	Discharge Day
Where will I be?	Getting ready for Surgery	Operating Room then Room	Hospital Room	Hospital Room	Hospital room	On your way home!
What tests will be done?	Blood draws, EKG, and other test as needed		Blood draws			
When can that tube come out?			❏ I have discussed with my team that my Foley Catheter will come out on Day___			❏ IV out!
When can I drink and eat?	❏ Drink pre-surgery and immuno-nutrition drink provided by the hospital as instructed ❏ Bowel prep as prescribed by doctor ❏ Clear liquids up to 3 hours before surgery	❏ First clear liquid meal	❏ Regular food 3 times a day	❏ Regular food 3 times a day	❏ Regular food 3 times a day	Regular food 3 times a day
Today I walked ___ minutes:	Set goals with your health care provider	morning: noon: evening:	morning: noon: evening:	morning: noon: evening:	morning: noon: evening:	morning: noon: evening:
My pain is:	___ / 10	___ / 10	___ / 10	___ / 10	___ / 10	___ / 10
Planning for home:	❏ My ride here? ❏ My ride home? ❏ If needed, who will stay with me once discharged		❏ Read home care packet and review with family	❏ Arrange for family and friends at home	❏ Have everything I need to go home (walker, commode, cane, supplies, etc.)	❏ No more questions ❏ Understand my medications
Road to recovery!	Getting ready by eating healthy, quitting smoking, and drinking less alcohol	❏ Pain controlled	❏ Sitting in chair and starting to walk	❏ Walking 3 times a day and breathing exercises	❏ Walked a lap around the hospital floor	❏ Pain controlled, no trouble eating or walking, ready to go!

Signs you're ready for discharge:

You are alert and aware of your surroundings, and your pain is in control

Your heart rhythm and rate are controlled and your incision is healing

You are not short of breath, able to take deep breaths

You have bowel function and urinating well without the catheter

You are walking each day and your incision is healing

Fig. 1. Example of ERAS pathway at tertiary care medical center

Malnourished patients may be provided with an oral nutritional supplement to be taken starting 7 to 10 days before surgery,[14] as this has been one of the biggest risk factors for complications.[21] The traditional "NPO past midnight" recommendation has fallen out of favor, with most protocols allowing ingestion of clear liquids up to 2 hours before surgery, in accordance with recent American Society of Anesthesiologists practice guidelines,[22] which reduces physiologic stress and actually results in a decreased risk of aspiration compared with old NPO after midnight practices. Those deemed at-risk for postoperative nausea or vomiting can be identified at this juncture and flagged to receive prophylactic medications. Similarly, prehabilitation programs such as a 6-minute walk regimen are most beneficial when implemented before surgery, so patients come in to surgery more prepared to deal with the physiologic stresses of surgery.[23] These "prehabilitation" efforts are gaining traction, and the evidence is mounting that addressing correctable risk factors before surgery can significantly improve outcomes. Therefore, prehabilitation programs are increasingly integrated into enhanced recovery bundles. Such programs make intuitive sense and consider preoperative conditioning for surgery as analogous to training for a marathon race.

Intraoperative protocols aim to dampen the body's response to surgical stress. Efforts such as multimodal analgesia and judicious administration of intravenous fluids fall into this category, as do minimally invasive surgical approaches. Surgical "dogma" involving intraabdominal drains and nasogastric tubes have been called into question for years,[24] and routine use of both these types of tubes is increasingly discouraged.[18,19] Restrictive versus goal-directed fluid strategies have been debated. Both seem to be more beneficial versus more liberal strategy. However, it is possible to give too little fluid. Particularly with colorectal surgery, where patients may take a bowel prep and become dehydrated, keeping patients euvolemic during surgery can be a challenge. The best method for this remains uncertain.[25] As there are increased costs associated with various monitoring technologies (such as noninvasive stroke volume variation), each institution should assess their own outcomes, including rates of postoperative renal insufficiency, oliguria, and need for bolus fluid infusion and the like postoperatively to determine an appropriate protocol.

Postoperative management in ERAS protocols entails continuation of measures started in the preop or intraop setting, plus early resumption of presurgical activities, that is, early mobilization and oral intake. Considerable variation abounds regarding optimal postoperative regimens for nausea, pain relief, and prevention of ileus, except to unequivocally recommend minimizing of opiate medications. What seems to be an overarching theme is that although the exact medications may not matter, an overall opioid-sparing approach using multimodal nonnarcotic medications is key. Consideration can also be given to add alvimopan (Entereg), a mu-opioid receptor blocker, which has been shown independently to reduce ileus and facilitate return of bowel function after intestinal resection.[26] Its inclusion in ERAS protocols is inconsistently recommended due to only modest benefit in minimally invasive surgery, if at all,[27] but still may have a role in open surgery. Other strategies such as "sham" feeding with sugar-free chewing gum have been widely studied and favorably received,[28] but as alvimopan, may not reach protocol status.

OUTCOMES

ERAS protocols are designed to tackle several factors that prolong a patient's recuperation period after surgery. Interestingly, no single item included in ERAS protocols can be identified as the major contributor to reduction of perioperative morbidity or mortality[29]; this is inherent in the way these protocols were developed—as multimodal care "bundles," which generate cumulative benefit from those interventions that when taken individually, produce only marginal gains,[30] and this creates significant difficulty when trying to define the extent to which each intervention contributes to patient outcomes and explains why there continues to be so much variation in ERAS protocols.

Nevertheless, multiple studies have shown that for patients in ERAS care pathways, there is an overall decrease in perioperative complications, hospital length of stay, and time to return of preoperative quality of life.[4,5] Assessment of patient quality of life and satisfaction scores has found that ERAS care has no negative impact on the patient's subjective feelings of satisfaction and readiness for discharge and in fact shows that patients may suffer less fatigue and resume usual activities sooner.[31]

As a result, the success of ERAS in producing favorable outcomes is now tied to compliance with all aspects of the protocol, and this requires buy-in from all parties involved in a patient's care, from surgeons to anesthesiologists, nurses to physical therapists, practice administrators to physician extenders, and physicians-in-training.[32] Therefore, it follows that better compliance with ERAS protocols should lead to better outcomes, and this has been suggested in numerous studies examining short-term and long-term outcomes.[33–35] Barriers to implementation have been described as all the "Buts": but my patients are sicker, but my patients are not appropriate for this, but my partners will never comply with this, and so forth. Across multiple disciplines and age ranges, ERAS protocols are shown to be effective. With increased compliance comes decreased overall complication rate. The incidence of severe complications resulting in reoperation or intensive care unit admission decreases, and mortality rates improve.[36]

Embedded within the various ERAS protocols is a recommendation for minimally invasive surgical approaches, when expertise is available.[18] In analyzing outcomes related to implementation of ERAS protocols, there remains a significant challenge when considering the broad variability in surgical technique and intraoperative conditions. Nonetheless, some studies associate laparoscopic surgery with improved short-term outcomes such as length of stay, readmission, and 30-day mortality, with the caveat that other components of the fast-track protocol could have influenced these outcomes[37] or that the measured outcomes improve as compliance with the entire ERAS care bundle increases.

CONTROVERSIAL COMPONENTS OF TYPICAL ENHANCED RECOVERY AFTER SURGERY BUNDLES

Although mounting evidence supports adaptation of ERAS protocols, the individual components of these protocols are under increasing scrutiny not just for their beneficial contributions but also for any associated adverse effects. Areas of controversy include the usage of nonsteroidal antiinflammatory drugs (NSAIDs) due to their association with anastomotic leak, gabapentanoid administration in the elderly patient, prophylactic placement of thoracic epidural catheters for pain management, mechanical bowel preparation, early ambulation, and sham feeding.

Nonsteroidal Antiinflammatory Drugs and Anastomotic Leak

Several studies suggest caution when administering NSAIDs in patients undergoing intestinal surgery due to the potential increase in risk of anastomotic leak; however, the quality of these studies is poor.[38–42] Most of these are small, retrospective studies, and the question remains unanswered. Analysis of the data suggests that the evidence is mixed—although there does seem to be molecule and class-specific effect, the potential risk of leak is lowest with cyclooxygenase-2 (COX-2) inhibitors.

A 2011 review of 3 observational studies (n = 33,246 patients) looked more specifically at the data. The investigators reviewed data acquired before, during, and after withdrawal of NSAID use and determined that leak rates varied from 3% to 4% with COX-2 inhibitors to 15% to 20% with nonspecific formulations (eg, diclofenac).[38] In 2012, a retrospective analysis of 795 patients receiving NSAIDs (either selective, nonselective, both, or none) also showed an increased risk of anastomotic leak: 13.2% versus 7.6% (odds ratio [OR] 1.84).[39] However, a more recent meta-analysis published in 2014 showed the leak effect may in fact be limited to emergent surgery.[40] In addition, a propensity-matched study using the Michigan Surgical Quality Collaborative database (with more than 4000 patients included) showed no difference in leak rates but a higher rate of sepsis.[41] Finally, a propensity-matched cohort of 173 hospitals in the United Kingdom (with more than 1000 patients receiving perioperative NSAIDs) demonstrated no difference in either acute kidney injury (adjusted OR [aOR] 0.8 [0.63–1.00, $P = .057$]) or anastomotic leak (aOR 0.85 [0.58–1.21, $P = .382$]).[42] Smaller studies arrive at similar conclusions, suggesting a nonsignificant increase in leak rates or a higher leak rate with nonselective agents, but all with bias.[43,44]

Gabapentanoids and the Elderly Patient

Although the data for gabapentanoids as a part of a multimodal regimen is so far quite sparse, there is gathering evidence that usage of these does have opioid-sparing effects. The data for gabapentanoids as part of a multimodal regimen are the least robust; however, the evidence is mounting that it does have opioid-sparing effects.[45–49] A known side effect of the medication is somnolence or drowsiness, and this is most pronounced in the elderly. For this reason, it should be used with caution in this population. Of note, these effects seem to be dose dependent and more prominent when gabapentin is administered at 300 mg 3 times per day (TID). Many newer protocols that involve multiple phases of care will include a smaller preoperative dose of 100 mg TID, then escalate to 300 mg TID postoperative in an effort to reduce side effects.

Epidural Analgesia

Minimizing the use of opioids is a central tenet of ERAS, and indeed, early iterations of ERAS protocols included routine use of epidural analgesia.[11,12] However, there are many potential problems with epidurals. They require a highly specialized team not only to place the catheters safely (which can be a time-consuming process) but also to manage issues, such as hypotension or urinary retention, that arise postoperatively. As a result, there is ongoing debate about the merits of epidural anesthesia, balanced with potential adverse effects, including also the systems-related issues that arise when trying to implement these in a comprehensive ERAS protocol.[50–52] The suggestion that up to one-third of catheters are nonfunctional[53] requires investigation into alternative methods that may be more effective. Modern regional nerve blocks such as transversus abdominus plane, quadratus lumborum, or erector spinae blocks are excellent alternatives and may even be more effective than epidurals in head-to-head comparison[54] with shorter lengths of stay. The reasons for this are unclear, but when used with a robust multimodal pain regimen, the length of stay seen even in larger, open surgical cases is much shorter compared with previous eras. In general, epidural analgesia has a limited role in the protocols for laparoscopic cases.

AREAS OF FURTHER STUDY

The number of studies demonstrating the advantages of ERAS pathway care for surgical patients continues to grow. The original concept of bundled care creating positive outcomes that are amplified beyond the sum of the individual components holds firm. However, these care pathways must be continuously examined for areas of improvement, omission, and addition, concurrent with developments in each of the treatment phases. Advances in pain management, surgical practice, and pharmacology, plus improvements in the systems delivering care to patients slated for surgery, will all require careful evaluation and vetting before incorporation into a protocol where every component counts, albeit to varying and sometimes inscrutable degrees.

Bowel Preparation

The practice of bowel preparation in anticipation of colon surgery has fluctuated significantly over the past several years. Usage of mechanical bowel preparation, either with or without antibiotic agents, is highly variable in the United States as well as Europe. In recent years, increasing data highlight several interesting features, namely, that oral antibiotic agents alone may have a more significant impact than using only a mechanical preparation[55] but that combining the 2 routes may be most beneficial for the patient.[56,57] Both oral antibiotics and mechanical preparation are recommended strongly in recent clinical practice guidelines for colorectal surgery[18,58] in the United States; however, this is not always the case. Although some studies conclude that bowel preparation may be safely omitted,[59] there are other reasons why it may be required. Laparoscopic manipulation of a colon full of stool is difficult. Furthermore, if intraoperative colonoscopy is necessary to localize a lesion that cannot otherwise be identified, mechanical bowel preparation is required.

Early Postoperative Ambulation

Early ambulation is often touted as a routine part of enhanced recovery, due to the widely accepted idea that doing so will reduce or ward off postoperative ileus and promote faster return of bowel function. Although widely practiced, early ambulation has not been demonstrated to have any effect on postoperative bowel function. There are, of course, many other benefits to early ambulation, including reduced risk of thromboembolism, reduced pulmonary complications, and a faster return to normal activity. In addition, this often adds to the patient's overall sense of well-being. The effects of postoperative early ambulation in combination with a well-defined prehabilitation program has been studied, and research in this area is ongoing.[60]

Postoperative "Sham" Feeding

Sham feeding with chewing gum has been suggested as a way to significantly reduce ileus rates after gastrointestinal surgery. The theory was that the mastication motion would trick the body into thinking that it was eating and thus improve intestinal mobility. Some also feel that the hexitols in the sugar-free gum act as laxatives. Chewing gum has been shown to be safe to administer, but reality is that in a typical enhanced recovery program, where early feeding is implemented, the addition of chewing gum may have little additional effect. In one meta-analysis, this was a 30-minute improvement in time to first bowel movement and 31 minutes to first flatus.[61]

In general, chewing gum is a safe and simple component of the ERAS bundle, but its contribution is perhaps not as crucial as other steps such as limiting opioid intake. Because it will not harm the patient,[62] and may in fact have some benefit,[63] it remains present in most mature ERAS bundles.

PROMISING ADDITIONS TO ENHANCED RECOVERY AFTER SURGERY PROTOCOLS

Further iterations of ERAS protocols will potentially make use of ileus-reducing medications. Two such medications have been prescribed for years in selected cases: alvimopan and methylnaltrexone.

Alvimopan is a mu-receptor antagonist that has shown reduced rates of postoperative ileus, with faster return of bowel function and shorter hospital stay.[64–68] The effect is most pronounced after open surgery. Cost, which can be upward of $170 per pill, remains the main drawback of using this medication. However, in several analyses, mean hospital costs were reduced when using alvimopan: overall by $2,021[64] or broken down into savings of $2345 overall, $1382 laparoscopic, and $3218 for open surgery[65] owing to the reduced length of stay from ileus.

Because of the up-front expense of alvimopan, other pharmacologic alternatives have been investigated. Most of these are employed for off-label use and include prokinetics and some antibiotics. Other agents such as propranolol[69] and neostigmine[70] have been used to treat ileus; however, robust clinical data showing benefit are lacking.

Methylnaltrexone deserves special mention. Although it also is a mu-opioid receptor antagonist that was Food and Drug Administration approved in April 2008, it is indicated for treatment of opioid-induced constipation, particularly in the palliative care setting. Two phase 3 trials for ileus prevention did not demonstrate any significant reduction in time to recovery of gastrointestinal function.[71]

SUMMARY

Ongoing examination of the individual components of ERAS protocols may be inherently complicated by the nature of how these care bundles are proposed to work. The efficacy and contribution of each component to the patient's overall well-being may be vague and difficult to quantify in relation to each other. However, as ERAS protocols gain traction across disciplines and health systems, ongoing examination of the various elements of the protocols and their utility in varying contexts will be necessary in order to continue improving patient outcomes, quality of comprehensive surgical care, and ultimately health care costs.

CLINICS CARE POINTS

- The traditional NPO after midnight has been supplanted by clear liquids until 2-3 hours prior to surgery.
- Minimally invasive approaches should be utilized whenever possible to enhance recovery.
- It remains controversial if NSAIDS contribute to anastomotic leak.
- Gabapentanoids should be avoided/minimized in the elderly due to the risk of somnolence.
- Oral antibiotics with (or without) mechanical bowel preparation is recommended to reduce SSI.
- Regional nerve blocks and/or epidurals can serve as adjuncts to a multimodal regimen, if used effectively.
- Ileus reducing medications such as Alvimopan have potential benefit, which must be weighed against the cost.

DISCLOSURE

The authors have nothing to disclose.

REFERENCES

1. Lau CSM, Chamberlain RS. Enhanced recovery after surgery programs improve patient outcomes and recovery: a meta-analysis. World J Surg 2017;41:899–913.
2. Ljungqvist O, Scott M, Fearon KC. Enhanced recovery after surgery: a review. JAMA Surg 2017;152(3):292–8.
3. Ban KA, Berian JR, Ko CY. Does implementation of Enhanced Recovery after Surgery (ERAS) protocols in colorectal surgery improve patient outcomes? Clin Colon Rectal Surg 2019;32:109–13.
4. Greco M, Capretti G, Beretta L, et al. Enhanced recovery program in colorectal surgery: a meta-analysis of randomized controlled trials. World J Surg 2014;38: 1531–41.
5. Varadhan KK, Neal KR, Dejong CH, et al. The Enhanced Recovery After Surgery (ERAS) pathway for patients undergoing major elective open colorectal surgery: a meta-analysis of randomized controlled trials. Clin Nutr 2010;29(4):434–40.
6. Joliat GR, Ljungqvist O, Wasylak T, et al. Beyond surgery: clinical and economic impact of enhanced recovery after surgery programs. BMC Health Serv Res 2018;18(1):1008.
7. Cavallaro P, Bordeianou L. Implementation of an ERAS pathway in colorectal surgery. Clin Colon Rectal Surg 2019;32:102–8.
8. Geltzeiler CB, Rotramel A, Wilson C, et al. Prospective study of colorectal enhanced recovery after surgery in a community hospital. JAMA Surg 2014; 149(9):955–61.
9. Kehlet H. Multimodal approach to control postoperative pathophysiology and rehabilitation. Br J Anaesth 1997;78:606–17.
10. Engelman RM, Rousou JA, Flack JE III, et al. Fast-track recovery of the coronary bypass patient. Ann Thorac Surg 1994;58(6):1742–6.
11. Bardram L, Funch-Jensen P, Jensen P, et al. Recovery after laparoscopic colonic surgery with epidural analgesia, and early oral nutrition and mobilisation. Lancet 1995;345(8952):763–4.
12. Kehlet H, Mogensen T. Hospital stay of 2 days after open sigmoidectomy with a multimodal rehabilitation programme. Br J Surg 1999;86(2):227–30.
13. Fearon KC, Ljungqvist O, Von Meyenfeldt M, et al. Enhanced recovery after surgery: a consensus review of clinical care for patients undergoing colonic resection. Clin Nutr 2005;24:466–77.
14. Wind J, Polle SW, Fung K, et al. Laparoscopy and/or fast track multimodal management versus standard care (LAFA) study group. Enhanced recovery after surgery (ERAS) group. Br J Surg 2006;93(7):800–9.
15. Arumainayagam N, McGrath J, Jefferson KP, et al. Introduction of an enhanced recovery protocol for radical cystectomy. BJU Int 2008;101(6):698–701.
16. Cerantola Y, Valerio M, Persson B, et al. Guidelines for perioperative care after radical cystectomy for bladder cancer: enhanced recovery after surgery (ERAS®) society recommendations. Clin Nutr 2013;32(6):879–87.
17. Gotlib Conn L, Rotstein OD, Greco E, et al. Enhanced recovery after vascular surgery: protocol for a systematic review. Syst Rev 2012;2(1):52.
18. Carmichael JC, Keller DS, Baldini G, et al. Clinical practice guidelines for enhanced recovery after colon and rectal surgery from the American Society of Colon and Rectal Surgeons and Society of American Gastrointestinal and Endoscopic Surgeons. Dis Colon Rectum 2017;60(8):761–84.

19. Gustafsson UO, Scott MJ, Hubner M, et al. Guidelines for perioperative care in elective colorectal surgery: enhanced recovery after surgery (ERAS®) society recommendations: 2018. World J Surg 2019;43:659–95.

20. Gaskill CE, Kling CE, Varghese TK. Financial benefit of a smoking cessation program prior to elective colorectal surgery. J Surg Res 2017;215:183–9.

21. Williams DGA, Molinger J, Wischmeyer PE. The malnourished surgery patient: a silent epidemic in perioperative outcomes? Curr Opin Anaesthesiol 2019;32(3): 405–11.

22. Practice guidelines for preoperative fasting and the use of pharmacologic agents to reduce the risk of pulmonary aspiration: application to healthy patients undergoing elective procedures: an updated report by the American Society of Anesthesiologists Task Force on preoperative fasting and the use of pharmacologic agents to reduce the risk of pulmonary aspiration. Anesthesiology 2017;126: 376–93.

23. Mayo NE, Feldman L, Scott S, et al. Impact of preoperative change in physical function on postoperative recovery: an argument supporting prehabilitation for colorectal surgery. Surgery 2011;150(3):505–14.

24. Nelson R, Edwards S, Tse B. Prophylactic nasogastric decompression after abdominal surgery. Cochrane Database Syst Rev 2007;3:CD004929.

25. Minto G, Scott MJ, Miller TE. Monitoring needs and goal-directed fluid therapy within an enhanced recovery program. Anesthesiol Clin 2015;33(1):35–49.

26. Al-Mazrou AM, Baser O, Kiran RP. Alvimopan, regardless of ileus risk, significantly impacts ileus, length of stay, and readmission after intestinal surgery. J Gastrointest Surg 2018;22:2104–16.

27. Barletta JF, Asgeirsson T, El-Badawi KI, et al. Introduction of alvimopan into an enhanced recovery protocol for colectomy offers benefit in open but not laparoscopic colectomy. J Laparoendosc Adv Surg Tech 2011;21:887–91.

28. Roslan F, Kushairi A, Cappuyns L, et al. The impact of sham feeding with chewing gum on postoperative ileus following colorectal surgery: a meta-analysis of randomised controlled trials. J Gastrointest Surg 2020;24:2643–53.

29. Greer NL, Gunnar WP, Dahm P, et al. Enhanced recovery protocols for adults undergoing colorectal surgery: a systematic review and meta-analysis. Dis Colon Rectum 2018;61(9):1108–18.

30. MacFie J. Enhanced recovery after surgery is obsolete. Dis Colon Rectum 2016; 59(10):1002–3.

31. Li D, Jensen CC. Patient satisfaction and quality of life with enhanced recovery protocols. Clin Colon Rectal Surg 2019;32(2):138–44.

32. Stone AB, Leeds IL, Efron J, et al. Enhanced recovery after surgery pathways and resident physicians: barrier or opportunity? Dis Colon Rectum 2016;59(10): 1000–1.

33. Gustafsson UO, Hausel J, Thorell A, et al. Adherence to the enhanced recovery after surgery protocol and outcomes after colorectal cancer surgery. Arch Surg 2011;146(5):571–7.

34. ERAS Compliance Group. The impact of enhanced recovery protocol compliance on elective colorectal cancer resection. Ann Surg 2015;261(6):1153–9.

35. Pisarska M, Torbicz G, Gajewska N, et al. Compliance with the ERAS protocol and 3-year survival after laparoscopic surgery for non-metastatic colorectal cancer. World J Surg 2019;43:2552–60.

36. Gustafsson UO, Oppelstrup H, Thorell A, et al. Adherence to the ERAS protocol is associated with 5-year survival after colorectal cancer surgery: a retrospective cohort study. World J Surg 2016;40:1741–7.

37. Zhao JH, Sun JX, Huang XZ, et al. Meta-analysis of the laparoscopic versus open colorectal surgery within fast track surgery. Int J Colorectal Dis 2016;31(3): 613–22.

38. Rushfeldt CF, Sveinbjørnsson B, Søreide K, et al. Risk of anastomotic leakage with use of NSAIDs after gastrointestinal surgery. Int J Colorectal Dis 2011; 26(12):1501–9.

39. Gorissen KJ, Benning D, Berghmans T, et al. Risk of anastomotic leakage with non-steroidal anti-inflammatory drugs in colorectal surgery. Br J Surg 2012; 99(5):721–7.

40. Hakkarainen TW, Steele SR, Bastaworous A, et al. Nonsteroidal anti-inflammatory drugs and the risk for anastomotic failure: a report from Washington State's Surgical Care and Outcomes Assessment Program (SCOAP). JAMA Surg 2015; 150(3):223–8.

41. Paulasir S, Kaoutzanis C, Welch KB, et al. Nonsteroidal anti-inflammatory drugs: do they increase the risk of anastomotic leaks following colorectal operations? Dis Colon Rectum 2015;58(9):870–7.

42. STARsurg Collaborative. Perioperative nonsteroidal anti-inflammatory drugs (NSAID) administration and acute kidney injury (AKI) in major gastrointestinal surgery: a prospective, multicenter, propensity matched cohort study. Ann Surg 2020. https://doi.org/10.1097/SLA.0000000000004314.

43. Bhangu A, Singh P, Fitzgerald JE, et al. Postoperative nonsteroidal anti-inflammatory drugs and risk of anastomotic leak: meta-analysis of clinical and experimental studies. World J Surg 2014;38(9):2247–57.

44. Hawkins AT, McEvoy MD, Wanderer JP, et al. Ketorolac use and anastomotic leak in elective colorectal surgery: a detailed analysis. Dis Colon Rectum 2018;61(12): 1426–34.

45. Dauri M, Faria S, Gatti A, et al. Gabapentin and pregabalin for the acute postoperative pain management. A systematic-narrative review of the recent clinical evidences. Curr Drug Targets 2009;10(8):716–33.

46. Ho KY, Gan TJ, Habib AS. Gabapentin and postoperative pain – a systematic review of randomized controlled trials. Pain 2006;126(1–3):91–101.

47. Zhang J, Ho KY, Wang Y. Efficacy of pregabalin in acute postoperative pain: a meta-analysis. Br J Anaesth 2011;106(4):454–62.

48. Dahl JB, Mathiesen O, Kehlet H. An expert opinion on postoperative pain management, with special reference to new developments. Expert Opin Pharmacother 2010;11(15):2459–70.

49. Moore RA, Straube S, Wiffen PJ, et al. Pregabalin for acute and chronic pain in adults. Cochrane Database Syst Rev 2009;(3):CD007076.

50. Rosen DR, Wolfe RC, Damle A, et al. Thoracic epidural analgesia: does it enhance recovery? Dis Colon Rectum 2018;61(12):1403–9.

51. Hill AG. Epidurals and colorectal surgery: have they had their day? Dis Colon Rectum 2018;61(12):1342–3.

52. Marecik SJ, Borsuk DJ, Studniarek A, et al. Epidurals preclude ultra-fast discharges after colorectal resections. Dis Colon Rectum 2019;62(7):e405.

53. Saclarides TJ. Current choices – good or bad – for the proactive management of postoperative ileus: a surgeon's view. J Perianesth Nurs 2006;21(2A Suppl): S7–15.

54. Warren JA, Carbonell AM, Jones LK, et al. Length of stay and opioid dose requirement with transversus abdominis plane block vs epidural analgesia for ventral hernia repair. J Am Coll Surg 2019;228(4):680–6.

55. Atkinson SJ, Swenson BR, Hanseman DJ, et al. In the absence of a mechanical bowel prep, does the addition of pre-operative oral antibiotics to parental antibiotics decrease the incidence of surgical site infection after elective segmental colectomy? Surg Infect 2015;16(6):728–32.

56. Klinger AL, Green H, Monlezun DJ, et al. The role of bowel preparation in colorectal surgery: results of the 2012-2015 ACS-NSQIP data. Ann Surg 2019; 269(4):671–7.

57. Kiran RP, Murray AC, Chiuzan C, et al. Combined preoperative mechanical bowel preparation with oral antibiotics significantly reduces surgical site infection, anastomotic leak, and ileus after colorectal surgery. Ann Surg 2015;262(3):416–25.

58. Migaly J, Bafford AC, Francone TD, et al. Clinical Practice Guidelines Committee of the American Society of Colon and Rectal Surgeons. The American Society of Colon and Rectal Surgeons clinical practice cuidelines for the use of bowel preparation in elective colon and rectal surgery. Dis Colon Rectum 2019;62(1):3–8.

59. Zmora O, Mahajna A, Bar-Zakai B, et al. Is mechanical bowel preparation mandatory for left-sided colonic anastomosis? Results of a prospective randomized trial. Tech Coloproctol 2006;10(2):131–5.

60. Zutshi M, Delaney CP, Senagore AJ, et al. Shorter hospital stay associated with fasttrack postoperative care pathways and laparoscopic intestinal resection are not associated with increased physical activity. Colorectal Dis 2004;6(6):477–80.

61. Ho YM, Smith SR, Pockney P, et al. A meta-analysis on the effect of sham feeding following colectomy: should gum chewing be included in enhanced recovery after surgery protocols? Dis Colon Rectum 2014;57(1):115–26.

62. Matros E, Rocha F, Zinner M, et al. Does gum chewing ameliorate postoperative ileus? Results of a prospective, randomized, placebo-controlled trial. J Am Coll Surg 2006;202(5):773–8.

63. Schuster R, Grewal N, Greaney GC, et al. Gum chewing reduces ileus after elective open sigmoid colectomy. Arch Surg 2006;141(2):174–6.

64. Kelley SR, Wolff BG, Lovely JK, et al. Fast-track pathway for minimally invasive colorectal surgery with and without alvimopan (Entereg)™: which is more cost-effective? Am Surg 2013;79(6):630–3.

65. Delaney CP, Craver C, Gibbons MM, et al. Evaluation of clinical outcomes with alvimopan in clinical practice: a national matched-cohort study in patients undergoing bowel resection. Ann Surg 2012;255(4):731–8.

66. Wolff BG, Michelassi F, Gerkin TM, et al, Alvimopan Postoperative Ileus Study Group. Alvimopan, a novel, peripherally acting mu opioid antagonist: results of a multicenter, randomized, double-blind, placebo-controlled, phase III trial of major abdominal surgery and postoperative ileus. Ann Surg 2004;240(4):728–34 [discussion 734-5].

67. Delaney CP, Weese JL, Hyman NH, et al, Alvimopan Postoperative Ileus Study Group. Phase III trial of alvimopan, a novel, peripherally acting, mu opioid antagonist, for postoperative ileus after major abdominal surgery. Dis Colon Rectum 2005;48(6):1114–25 [discussion 1125-6]; [author reply 1127-9].

68. Ludwig K, Enker WE, Delaney CP, et al. Gastrointestinal tract recovery in patients undergoing bowel resection: results of a randomized trial of alvimopan and placebo with a standardized accelerated postoperative care pathway. Arch Surg 2008;143(11):1098–105.

69. Hallerbäck B, Carlsen E, Carlsson K, et al. Beta-adrenoceptor blockade in the treatment of postoperative adynamic ileus. Scand J Gastroenterol 1987;22(2): 149–55.

70. Neostigmine bromide/neostigmine methylsulfate. In: McEvoy GK, editor. American hospital formulary service drug information 2007. Bethesda, MD: American Society of Health-System Pharmacists; 2007. p. 1245–7.

71. Yu CS, Chun HK, Stambler N, et al. Safety and efficacy of methylnaltrexone in shortening the duration of postoperative ileus following segmental colectomy: results of two randomized, placebo-controlled phase 3 trials. Dis Colon Rectum 2011;54(5):570–8.

Controversies in Abdominal Wall Reconstruction

Kevin F. Baier, MD[a], Michael J. Rosen, MD[b],*

KEYWORDS

- Ventral hernia repair • Abdominal wall reconstruction • Robotic hernia repair
- Hernia mesh • Prophylactic mesh

KEY POINTS

- There is a growing need for standardization of outcome reporting in hernia surgery.
- The role for prophylactic stoma mesh is not as clear as once thought.
- No clear benefit for use of biologic and synthetic absorbable mesh has been demonstrated, but prospective studies comparing them with synthetic mesh are lacking.
- Robotic intraperitoneal onlay mesh (IPOM) has not demonstrated clinically measurable benefits compared with laparoscopic IPOM but shows promise in more complex ventral hernia repair and abdominal wall reconstruction.

INTRODUCTION

Hernia operations are among the most commonly performed procedures by general surgeons. Despite their frequency, there are several controversies surrounding hernia repair. With the development of new prosthetics and surgical approaches, decision making for hernia care has become increasingly complex. There remain many controversial topics in hernia surgery that require further understanding and improved research capability. This article examines some of the key controversies, including outcome reporting, mesh selection, robotics, and prophylactic stoma mesh reinforcement, and explores the current literature pertaining to these areas of controversy.

A CALL FOR STANDARDIZATION OF OUTCOMES REPORTING IN HERNIA SURGERY

In understanding and communicating the technical aspects of an operation and most importantly comparing the ultimate outcome of these procedures, surgeons need a common language with which to report these details. Surgeons at a minimum always should explain the location of the mesh and the manipulation, or release, of various

[a] Cleveland Clinic Foundation, 9500 Euclid Avenue, Building A-100, Cleveland, OH 44195, USA;
[b] Center for Abdominal Core Health, Cleveland Clinic Foundation, 9500 Euclid Avenue, Building A-100, Cleveland, OH 44195, USA
* Corresponding author.
E-mail address: rosenm@ccf.org

Surg Clin N Am 101 (2021) 1007–1022
https://doi.org/10.1016/j.suc.2021.08.002
0039-6109/21/© 2021 Elsevier Inc. All rights reserved.

components of the abdominal wall. It is common for various names or acronyms to be given to these different procedures (**Table 1**). To avoid confusion, it is best to describe exactly what was done to the abdominal wall accurately and precisely and where the mesh was placed. See **Fig. 1** for a depiction of the EuraHS description of mesh positions during ventral hernia repair (VHR).[1] With the continuing advancement of minimally invasive surgical (MIS) repairs, many of these procedures now are attempted utilizing laparoscopic or robotic approaches but the tenets of the procedures and their descriptors should remain constant.

Despite the prevalence of hernia disease and the frequency of repair, there is significant heterogeneity in the reporting of postoperative outcomes. Although multiple outcomes are relevant in hernia surgery, for the purposes of this article, the focus is on wound morbidity, hernia recurrence, and patient-reported outcomes (PROs).

Wound Morbidity

There are several different standardized definitions for reporting wound events that have been put forth by the Centers for Disease Control and Prevention, the American College of Surgeons National Surgery Quality Improvement Program, the Ventral Hernia Working Group, and the Clavien-Dindo classification system. In an article by Haskins and colleagues,[2] researchers found that of the top 50 cited articles in VHR, 18% used 1 or more standardized definitions for reporting postoperative wound events, 28% used study-specific definitions, and 54% of articles listed wound event types without including a formal definition for postoperative wound events. This variability contributes to the difficulty of interpreting the current hernia literature and comparing outcomes across studies. The investigators proposed standardizing the reporting of ventral hernia–related wound events to 3 categories: surgical site infection (SSI), surgical site occurrence (SSO), and SSO requiring procedural intervention (SSOPI). See **Table 2** for definitions and examples of each.

Although most surgeons are familiar with the terms SSO and SSI, SSOPI allows surgeons to better capture and describe the clinically significant SSIs and SSOs. Because the majority of hernia surgery involves the use of prosthetic material, the need to portray the safety of various surgical techniques and prosthetics in relation to the severity of associated wound events accurately is paramount.

Patient-reported Outcomes

Hernia surgeons historically have defined success with 1 measure: hernia recurrence. Because the health care system grapples with defining quality of care, there has been a movement from clinician reported outcomes to PROs. Validated measures, like the National Institutes of Health Patient-Reported Outcomes Measurement Information System (PROMIS) pain scale, have been developed to help clinicians understand the evolution of pain from the preoperative period, throughout recovery, and long after repair.[3] Similarly, disease-specific tools were developed to assess the impact of hernia disease on patients' quality of life, including the Hernia-related Quality-of-Life Survey (HERQLES)[4] and Carolinas Comfort Scale.[5] These PRO tools are beginning to shed light on the long-lasting impacts of hernia repair from the patient perspective. As understanding of pain and the functional impact of hernia repair continues to evolve, definitions of "success" and "failure" will become more nuanced than simply recurrence or no recurrence, and PROs will become a more important factor in the shared clinical decision making between surgeons and patients.

Table 1
Common abbreviations in ventral hernia repair

Abbreviation	Definition	Mesh Location
IPOM	Intraperitoneal onlay mesh	Intraperitoneal
TAPP	Transabdominal preperitoneal	Preperitoneal
TEP	Totally extraperitoneal	Preperitoneal
eTEP	Endoscopic totally extraperitoneal	Retromuscular/preperitoneal
Rives-Stoppa	Open retrorectus repair	Retromuscular
TAR	Transversus abdominus release	Retromuscular
ACS	Anterior component separation	Onlay, retromuscular, preperitoneal, or intraperitoneal

Hernia Recurrence

Although the utility of PROs in hernia repair is likely to grow in the coming years, hernia recurrence will remain a core outcome worthy of close tracking and reporting. With socialized health care systems in Europe, it is possible to use claims data to identify recurrences that require reoperation, which is meaningful but likely an underestimate of the incidence of hernia recurrence. The US health care system often is limited by long-term follow-up and, with a lack of socialized health care, this process cannot be utilized for the majority of the population. On the other hand, this means that most studies in the United States utilize clinical or radiographic assessment. Although more sensitive, these methods typically require an in-person visit. In an article by Baucom and colleagues,[6] the investigators developed the Ventral Hernia Recurrence Inventory in an effort to understand if PROs could detect long-term hernia recurrence reliably. Patient were asked if they felt or saw a bulge and if they had any pain at their hernia site. They found that a patient-reported bulge was 85% sensitive and 81% specific in detecting hernia recurrence. Patients who answered no to both questions had a 0% chance of hernia recurrence. Although this measure is likely to over-predict the true incidence of hernia recurrence, it can be administered without an in-person visit and can be used to focus a surgeon's attention on patients who merit clinical or radiographic evaluation and help surgeons to better estimate the true incidence of long-term hernia recurrence. It is important for the hernia community to agree on standards of reporting for recurrence so that studies can be fairly compared in the future.

THE PERFECT MESH

There is no perfect mesh, at least not yet. Moreover, it is likely that most meshes perform reasonably well with appropriate surgical technique and the perfect mesh not perform well if placed inappropriately. It is important, however, to understand basic mesh constructs to guide in appropriate mesh selection for any given scenario. In general, mesh types can be divided into 3 broad categories: permanent synthetic, synthetic absorbable, and biologic. It generally is accepted that synthetic mesh is appropriate for all clean cases and significantly reduces the risk of hernia recurrence.[7] Synthetic mesh can be divided further into lightweight (LW) (<40 g/m^2), medium weight (MW) ($40–75$ g/m^2), and heavy weight (HW) (>75 g/m^2). The trend toward increased hernia recurrence with LW mesh[8,9]; favorable bacterial clearance in monofilament, uncoated, polypropylene, and polyester mesh[10]; and report of favorable rates of infection, mesh removal, and hernia recurrence with MW mesh in clean-contaminated and contaminated VHRs reported by Carbonell and colleagues[11] have led to the

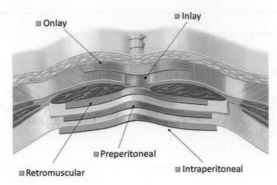

Fig. 1. Potential layers in the abdominal wall to place mesh.

widespread adoption of MW mesh for clean VHRs and abdominal wall reconstruction. No prospective study has compared MW to HW mesh in clean or contaminated VHR directly. Despite the findings of Carbonell and colleagues, the use of permanent synthetic mesh in clean-contaminated or contaminated hernia repair remains controversial and has heavily influenced the growing number of synthetic absorbable and biologic products on the market.

Biologic Mesh

One of the first prospective evaluations of biologic mesh in contaminated fields was published in 2012. The RICH trial[12] is a prospective, multicenter, single-arm study examining the outcomes associated with use of non–cross-linked porcine dermis, Strattice (LifeCell Corporation, Branchburg, New Jersey), in 80 contaminated VHRs greater than 9 cm^2, with an average hernia width of 16 cm. With 75% follow-up, the 2-year hernia recurrence was 28%. Primary closure of the fascia was not achieved in 19% of cases despite 65% of patients undergoing anterior component separation. It now is known that biologic and synthetic absorbable mesh should not be used as definitive repair when bridging the fascial defect due to the unacceptably high rates of recurrence.[13] The high rate of hernia recurrence in bridging repairs limits the ability to extrapolate from this study to other series with complete fascial closure and speaks more to surgical technique than choice of mesh.

To date, only 2 randomized controlled trials (RCTs) have compared biologic mesh to synthetic mesh. Olavarria and colleagues[14] undertook a single-center pilot RCT comparing retromuscular biologic (porcine acellular dermal matrix) to synthetic (MW, macroporous polypropylene) mesh in 87 patients with a median hernia width of 6 cm and 81.4% follow-up at 1 year. They reported no benefit to biologic mesh, with an increased trend toward major complication, SSI, wound dehiscence, readmission, and recurrence associated with biologic mesh without meeting statistical significance. Another recent larger multicenter trial from Europe, the LAPSIS trial,[15] compared biologic, Surgisis Gold (Cook Medical, Bloomington, Indiana) to synthetic mesh in open (retromuscular) repairs and laparoscopic (bridging intraperitoneal onlay mesh [IPOM]) repairs. This study has several significant design limitations, notably the use of a biologic mesh for bridging laparoscopic repairs and lack of standardization of the comparative laparoscopic synthetic mesh (barrier-coated polypropylene or expanded polytetrafluoroethylene at the surgeon's discretion). If only the open, retromuscular repairs are examined, 127 patients in total, biologic mesh had a reported recurrence rate of 13.6% whereas the reported recurrence rate with synthetic mesh

Table 2
Definitions and examples of surgical site infection, surgical site occurrence, and surgical site occurrence requiring procedural intervention[2]

	Surgical Site Infection	Surgical Site Occurrence	Surgical Site Occurrence Requiring Procedural Intervention
Definition	An infection that occurs in the part of the body where the surgery took place and is defined based further on the compartment involved	Includes any SSI as well as any of the examples below	Any SSO that requires a procedural intervention
Examples	Superficial	Wound cellulitis	Wound opening
	Deep	Skin/soft tissue ischemia or necrosis	Wound débridement
	Organ space	Nonhealing incisional wound	Suture excision
		mucocutaneous anastomotic disruption	Percutaneous drainage
		Fascial disruption	Partial mesh removal
		Enterocutaneous fistula	Complete mesh removal
		Exposed mesh	
		Hematoma	
		Seroma	
		Wound serous drainage	
		Chronic sinus drainage	

was 9.8%. Although these numbers were reported, no direct subgroup analysis between open repairs was performed making the statistical significance uncertain.

Long-acting Resorbable Mesh

There are no RCTs comparing long-acting resorbable (LAR) synthetic mesh to permanent synthetic mesh to date. The feasibility of use for LARs has been demonstrated in several studies. In a prospective, multicenter study, The COBRA trial[16] examined the outcomes associated with placement of Gore Bio-A (W. L. Gore and Associates, Flagstaff, Arizona) in the retromuscular (90%) or intraperitoneal (10%) position in 104 patients undergoing clean contaminated or contaminated open VHR. Bio-A takes approximately 6 months to break down completely. The average hernia width was 9 cm, and more than two-thirds of patients required component separation, either anterior (20%) or posterior (48%), and fascial closure was achieved in 100% of patients. With 84% follow-up at 2 years, the hernia recurrence rate was 17%. Although the complexity of cases addressed in this study is a major strength, the inclusion of parastomal hernias (PSHs) (21% of patients) and lack of control arm or randomization make it difficult to compare the outcomes to other types of mesh.

Phasix mesh (C.R. Bard, Warwick, Rhode Island) is a naturally derived monofilament poly-4-hydroxybutyrate polymer produced by *Escherichia coli* K12 bacteria and takes approximately 18 months to fully break down.[17] In a study by Roth and colleagues,[18] Phasix mesh was used in 120 patients undergoing open, clean VHR repair with defects greater than 10 cm. Fascial closure was achieved in 94% of cases, component separation was utilized in 44% of cases, the mesh was placed in the retrorectus position in 73%, and the onlay position in 27% of cases. The incidence of SSI was 9.3%. With 79% follow-up at 18 months, the recurrence rate was 9% and with 67.8% follow-up at 3 years, hernia recurrence increased to 17.9%. The lack of control for comparison and the fact that all hernia repairs were clean cases make it difficult to compare the outcomes from this study with the RICH and COBRA trials. There is no large prospective evaluation of Tigr Matrix (Novus Scientific, Uppsala, Sweden) in VHR, another LAR that takes approximately 36 months to fully break down.[17] A systematic review of biologic and absorbable synthetic mesh use in VHR found no role for the routine use of biologic or synthetic absorbable mesh in any ventral hernia patient population, including contaminated fields, bridging situations, PSH repair, or hernia prevention.[19]

Briefly, the role for rapid-absorbing synthetic mesh, namely Vicryl mesh (Ethicon, Somerville, New Jersey), particularly in the setting of staged approach to abdominal wall reconstruction remains a viable option. When primary closure cannot be achieved but a patient would benefit from delayed reconstruction in order to allow for better preoperative optimization or to minimize the risk of postoperative mesh infection, Vicryl mesh is a relatively cheap alternative to LARs and can be used as an inlay in order to bridge a fascial defect.[20] The concern for fistula formation in the presence of Vicryl mesh certainly is warranted; however, the incidence does not appear as high as once thought, with both small RCTs and systematic reviews finding the incidence to be 5% among patients undergoing temporary abdominal closure with Vicryl mesh.[21,22] Rapid-absorbing synthetic mesh provides surgeons with 1 additional tool when tackling complex cases involving heavy contamination, the excision of prior infected mesh, or intolerance of anesthesia.

Summary

Only 2 RCTs have compared biologic mesh to synthetic mesh and neither has demonstrated any advantage to biologic mesh. There are no RCTs comparing LAR mesh to synthetic mesh, and the prospective data available do not suggest a significant advantage over synthetic mesh. At this point, the role for biologic and LAR mesh remains uncertain but its routine use cannot be recommended at this time.

ROBOTIC VENTRAL HERNIA REPAIR

Laparoscopic IPOM (lapIPOM) first was described in 1993 and marked the beginning for minimally invasive hernia repair.[23] The adaptation of IPOM to the robotic IPOM (rIPOM) platform first was described in 2003 by Ballantyne and colleagues,[24] and, since that time, the number and complexity of operations performed for VHR on the robotic platform have grown exponentially. The quality of the literature identifying the indications and benefits of various robotic approaches, however, remains limited. The current state of the literature and understanding of the robotic platform for VHR to date are discussed.

Robotic Intraperitoneal Onlay Mesh Repair

One of the first large scale studies to systematically evaluate the robotic approach for IPOM was a propensity score analysis of 631 patients undergoing either rIPOM or lapIPOM from the Abdominal Core Health Quality Collaborative (ACHQC), a national hernia registry.[25] The investigators found that rIPOM reduced length of stay (LOS) (1 day vs 0 days, respectively; $P < .001$), reduced the incidence of SSO (14% vs 5%, respectively; $P = .001$) without any difference in SSOPI (0% vs 1%, respectively; $P = 1$), and was associated with increased operative times. Although the exact mechanism for this reduction in LOS was not clear, this work prompted 2 subsequent RCTs to determine if a reduction in pain potentially was a mechanism for these favorable results.

The first RCT to compare rIPOM to lapIPOM was published by Olavarria and colleagues,[26] included 124 patients, and measured LOS as its primary outcome, including both postoperative days and readmissions. The average body mass index (BMI) was 32 kg/m^2, and 88% of hernia defects were less than 4 cm in width. After randomization, the patient demographics and hernia characteristics were similar between the 2 groups, with the minor exception that there were more incisional hernias in the rIPOM group than in the lapIPOM group (88% vs 73%, respectively) and more recurrent hernias in the lapIPOM group than in the rIPOM group (12% vs 25%, respectively); no P values were reported. A MW, barrier-coated polypropylene mesh with a minimum mesh overlap of 5 cm on all sides relative to the hernia defect was utilized in both groups. In the lapIPOM group, fascial defects were closed with 0 polydioxanone sutures and the mesh was fixated with transfascial sutures (permanent vs absorbable not specified) and a circumferential double crown of permanent tacks. In the rIPOM group, fascial defects were closed with a locking barbed 0 polydioxanone suture and the mesh was secured with circumferential running locking barbed 2-0 polydioxanone sutures. At 90 days, the investigators found no difference in LOS (0 vs 0, respectively; P = .82), recurrence (0 vs 0, respectively; P = 1.0), or PROs, including AW-QOL score or interquartile ratio pain scores. Operative times were significantly longer rIPOM group compared with lapIPOM (141 vs 77 minutes, respectively; P < .001) and rIPOM was significantly more expensive ($15,865 vs $12,955, respectively; P = .004) One unique strength to this study is a ramp-up period prior to the start of the study in which the 3 participating surgeons at 2 centers performed 50 standardized cases per site in order to optimize the workflow and decrease any potential learning curve effect. The group recently published their 1-year outcomes, with 91% of patients completing 1-year follow-up, finding no difference in hernia recurrence between rIPOM and lapIPOM (7% vs 9%, respectively; P = .576), and no difference in PROs; however, they did find a significant increase in patients undergoing reoperation in the lapIPOM group (0 vs 9%, respectively; P = .020).[27] The 5 reoperations included 2 seroma excisions, 1 incision and drainage of an abdominal wall abscess, 1 diagnostic laparoscopy with removal of a tack for chronic pain, and 1 patient who presented for repair of a hernia recurrence. The increase in reoperation rate is interesting but difficult to draw conclusions from, because the study was not powered to detect a difference in reoperations after repair. The investigators estimate 476 patients would be required to adequately power a study to detect a true difference.

The second RCT, by Petro and colleagues,[28] included 75 patients and measured postoperative pain with an 11-point numerical rating scale (NRS-11) as its primary outcome. The investigators chose pain instead of LOS due to the referral pattern of their institution and the number of patients traveling from afar that could confound LOS as the primary outcome. After randomization, the 2 arms were comparable in demographics and hernia characteristics with the exception that the rIPOM group had a higher median BMI (35 vs 31, respectively; P = .02). At 30 days, postoperatively, there was no difference in NRS-11 scores, LOS, recurrence, or postoperative complications as well as no difference in PROs, including the PROMIS 3a pain score and HerQLes score at 30 days. Similar to the findings by Olavarria and colleagues,[26] rIPOM was associated with increased cost, largely driven by increased operative time. Neither study included the capital costs associated with purchase of the laparoscopic or robotic equipment or the associated maintenance costs of the equipment in their cost analyses. This study only reports short-term outcomes and the long-term follow-up will be important in understanding if one approach demonstrates a benefit over time. There was a relatively high rate of conversion to open, 7% overall, with 3 patients in each arm. That said, there were no missed enterotomies or unplanned reoperations so this could be considered appropriate surgical judgment. The investigators did not include these conversions to open in their analysis in order to isolate the comparison of the 2 minimally invasive techniques, and this diversion from intention-to-treat analysis could be considered a weakness. Another criticism of this study is the potential effect of learning curve on outcomes because 1 of the 2 surgeons was in their first year of practice. A comparison between the 2 surgeons involved showed no difference in operative times over the course of the study, and the average operative times for the 2 operations are comparable to those reported in the study by Olavarria and colleagues,[26] 146 minutes versus 141 minutes for rIPOM and 94 minutes versus 77 minutes for lapIPOM.

To date, although the rIPOM allows for precise suturing of the fascial defect and transabdominal circumferential suture fixation, there appear to be no measurable improvements in PROS or early hernia recurrence. Larger RCTs and continued long-term follow-up re necessary to understand the role of the robot in minimally invasive IPOM VHR.

Robotic Endoscopic Total Extraperitoneal

After the total extraperitoneal (TEP) approach was described for the management on inguinal hernias, Belyansky and colleagues[29] described adapting the approach to laparoscopic VHR in a retrospective series of 79 patients and then robotically in a retrospective review of 37 patients.[30] This approach is now known as an endoscopic TEP (eTEP) and provides the opportunity for retromuscular mesh placement, theoretically decreasing the risk of complications associated with intraperitoneal mesh, and allowing for the use of cheaper, uncoated mesh, that is known to perform better in cases of contamination.[10] The robotic series reported by Belyansky and colleagues[29] included patients with a mean age of 54, mean BMI of 35.5, and mean American society of Anesthesiology (ASA) of 2.4 with no intraoperative complications and 2 patients developing postoperative SSOPIs, both seromas requiring percutaneous drainage. In this study, 29 patients underwent eTEP, with an average hernia defect size of 5.9 cm, LOS of 0.3 days, and operative time of 141 minutes whereas 8 patients underwent eTEP in combination with transversus abdominus release (TAR) for an average hernia defect size of 11.3 cm, LOS of 2.1 days, and average operative time of 240 minutes. Only 30-day outcomes are reported. This study demonstrates the feasibility of the approach but lacks long-term follow-up and a comparison arm.

The first retrospective case-control study to evaluate laparoscopic eTEP to lapIPOM (with midline closure) was published in 2021 by Bellido Luque and colleagues.[31] In this study, patients 39 patients who underwent lapIPOM were compared with 40 patients who underwent laparoscopic eTEP. There were no significant differences in the patient demographics or hernia characteristics between the 2 groups. All hernias were less than 8 cm in width, with the average defect measuring 5.2 cm in the lapIPOM group and 4.6 cm in the eTEP group. No patients with incarcerated or strangulated hernias were included. The investigators reported an increased operative time in the eTEP group (106 minutes vs 61 minutes, respectively; $P < .05$) and a decreased LOS (1.3 days vs 1.8 days, respectively; $P < .05$). Using the EuraHS quality-of-life scale, which assesses pain, activity restriction, and cosmetic discomfort, the investigators found no difference in baseline pain, activity restriction, or cosmetic discomfort but found decreased pain at 1 day, 7 days, and 30 days postoperatively in the eTEP group as well as decreased activity restrictions and cosmetic discomfort at 30 days and 180 days postoperatively. Only 1 recurrence was identified in the lapIPOM group and none in the eTEP, group with average follow-up of 28.3 months and 15.9 months, respectively. Because this is a retrospective case-control study with relatively small sample size, it is prone to selection bias but offers insight into the potential benefits of the eTEP approach. Larger retrospective studies utilizing propensity score matching to limit bias, and, ultimately, prospective RCTS are required to further evaluate laparoscopic eTEP and robotic eTEP.

Robotic Transversus Abdominus Release

Laparoscopic TAR first esd described in 2016 by Belyansky and colleagues,[32] and, soon after, its adaptation to the robotic platform was described by Warren and colleagues.[33] Multiple retrospective studies have demonstrated a decreased LOS, on average 2 days to 3 days, associated with robotic TAR compared with its open counterpart.[33–36] The largest of these retrospective reviews was published by Carbonell and colleagues,[37] in 2018, and examined 1205 patients undergoing retromuscular VHR, and, after 2:1 propensity score matching, compared 111 patients who underwent robotic retromuscular VHR (rRVHR) to 222 patients who underwent open retromuscular VHR. A TAR was utilized in 85% of robotic repairs and 83% of open repairs, with a majority of hernias between 4 cm and 10 cm. The investigators found a reduced LOS for rRVHR compared with open retromuscular VHR (2 days vs 3 days, respectively; $P < .001$) and no difference in 30-day readmissions or SSIs. There was an increased rate of SSO associated with rRVHR (32% vs 14%, respectively; $P < .001$), largely consisting of seromas that did not require intervention. The operative times were longer in the rRVHR group (45% vs 12% of cases requiring >240 minutes, respectively; $P < .001$). One of the major findings of this trial is after appropriate statistical matching, the actual defect sizes were fairly small; thus, the difference in LOS was only 1 day, unlike many other trials comparing more complex open abdominal wall reconstruction to less complex robotic repairs. These studies suggest, however, a potential clinical benefit to robotic abdominal wall reconstruction but, due to their retrospective nature, are at risk for selection bias and prospective trials still are required to truly understand the advantages of robotic retromuscular hernia repairs.

The Cost of Robotic Ventral Hernia Repair

The cost of care associated with the robotic platform is an important consideration in value-based health care delivery. As discussed previously, 2 RCTs have found the robotic platform to add time and cost without clinically measurable benefit compared with laparoscopy for IPOM VHRs.[26,28] The IPOM technique is relatively straightforward and many investigators argue that the benefit to the robot is more significant in complex hernia repair. The potential for the robotic platform to result in cost savings exists when the costs associated with increased operative time and capital cost of equipment are exceed by the cost savings associated with decreased LOS or some other improved clinical outcome. The retrospective literature to date suggests that this may be possible in patients with larger defects requiring TAR. A study by Belyansky and colleagues[38] retrospectively reviewed the costs associated with open TAR versus MIS TAR. The investigators included 104 consecutive patients undergoing open abdominal wall reconstruction, 57 open abdominal wall reconstructions and 47 MIS abdominal wall reconstructions, consisting of 38 laparoscopic and 9 robotic repairs. There was no difference in age, BMI, or ASA between the 2 groups; however, the open abdominal wall reconstruction group had larger hernia defects (293.2 cm^2 vs 206 cm^2, respectively; $P < .01$). They found that MIS abdominal wall reconstruction was associated with similar operative times compared with open AWR (232 minutes vs 234 minutes, respectively; $P = .92$), decreased LOS (1.4 days vs 5.3 days, respectively; $P < .01$), and decreased hospital cost ($12,295 vs $20,924, respectively; $P < .01$). The capital expense or depreciation of laparoscopic and robotic equipment was not measured. The benefits of decreased LOS on the cost of hernia care are clear; however, the retrospective nature of this study puts it at risk for selection bias, and, with only 9 patients undergoing repair utilizing the robotic platform, it cannot be generalized to all robotic abdominal wall reconstructions.

Summary

As surgeons continue to evaluate the robot in VHR and new robotic platforms become available, the economic impact of robotic-assisted VHR will become clearer. Ultimately, the role of robotic hernia surgery likely will be defined by its effect on the value equation, where improvements in outcomes that matter to patients will need to exceed the cost associated with this technology.

PROPHYLACTIC STOMA MESH
Introduction

PSHs are a frequent occurrence after ostomy creation. The incidence of PSH varies widely in the literature, from 2% to 28% after end ileostomy creation to 4% to 48% after end colostomy creation.[39] PSH often occur within the first 2 years after creation of an ostomy but can occur any time.[40] The recurrence rate after repair of PSH is similarly high and variable, with reports as high as 69% for suture repair and 6.9% to 17% for mesh repair.[41] These characteristics of PSHs led lead many surgeons to shift their focus from hernia repair to hernia prevention, igniting the ongoing debate over the use of prophylactic stoma mesh.

The use of prophylactic mesh at the time of stoma creation first was reported by Bayer and colleagues[42] in 1986. The RCT comparing the use of prophylactic synthetic mesh to conventional ostomy creation was published by Jänes and colleagues[43] and included 54 patients. In it, all procedures were performed via midline laparotomy. The retrorectus space was developed by releasing the posterior sheath from the midline and dissecting laterally. A macroporous, LW polypropylene mesh was placed in the retrorectus position and the stoma was brought through cruciate incisions that were aligned in the posterior sheath, mesh, and anterior sheath. Two absorbable sutures were used to fixate the lateral corners of the mesh and the medial corners were incorporated into the midline fascial closure. The investigators found the clinical incidence of PSH at 1 year to be 50% in controls and 4% in the prophylactic mesh group ($P = .00$). This study inspired a series of small trials over the next decade, most with similarly favorable results, finding prophylactic mesh decreased the rate of PSH formation with no increase in wound morbidity.[44–47] The exception to this was a study published in 2015 by Vierimaa and colleagues[48] that found laparoscopic keyhole IPOM mesh at the time of end colostomy creation was associated with a decrease in unblinded clinical incidence of PSH at 12 months (37.5% vs 14.7%, respectively; $P = .049$), but no difference in radiographic PSH (53.1% vs 51.4%, respectively; $P = 1.00$). This study demonstrates the importance of blinded evaluation and correlation with radiographic evaluation.

Current Evidence

The Dutch PREVENT trial[49] was published in 2016, included 150 patients, and found a reduced incidence in clinical PSH from 24.2% in controls to 4.5% in the prophylactic mesh group at 1 year (P = .0011), with no difference in SSIs, 25% versus 21%, respectively. In this study, a 10-cm × 15-cm LW polypropylene mesh was placed in the retromuscular position using the surgical technique, as described by Jänes and colleagues,[43] with the exception that the entire medial border of the mesh was incorporated into the midline closure. Following randomization, the preoperative demographics between the 2 arms were similar, including age (63), sex (60% male), BMI (26), indication for surgery (malignancy in 87% of patients), and clinical risk factors for hernia formation, including history of aneurysm, prior hernias, diabetes, and immunosuppression. Tobacco use was not assessed. One of the biggest limitations of this trial, and several others from Europe, is the fairly low BMI of participants compared with many series in the United States, questioning the results and the applicability to American patients. Clinical assessment of PSH was not blinded and cross-sectional imaging was used only to confirm clinical assessment. This study was the largest to date, generating enthusiasm for the technique but was soon followed by another larger RCT with contradictory conclusions.

Soon to follow, the STOMAMESH trial,[50] published in 2019 and including 211 patients, found the rate of clinical PSH at 1 year to be 30% in controls and 29% in the prophylactic mesh group (P = .866), with similar findings on radiographic assessment (34% vs 32%, respectively; P = .748) and no difference in SSI (22% versus 21%, respectively). Aside from using a smaller 10-cm × 10-cm piece of LW polypropylene mesh, the surgical technique was identical between the 2 studies. Preoperative patient demographics were similar between the 2 groups and similar to those in the PREVENT trial, including age (69), sex (68% male), BMI (26), indication for surgery (malignancy in 91% of patients), and tobacco use (8% of patients). Clinical and radiographic assessments both were blinded. The contradictory conclusions reached by these studies requires surgeons to dissect the factors that may contribute to and influence their findings.

With similar patient demographics, surgical technique, mesh selection, and location of the mesh, a possible explanation for the difference between the 2 trials is the unblinded clinical assessment in the PREVENT trial and lack of routine CT assessment for comparison. Additionally, all operations in the PREVENT trial were performed at teaching hospitals and university centers. The operations in the STOMAMESH trial were performed at a mix of university hospitals, regional hospitals, and county hospitals. Although a prerequisite for colorectal surgeon participation was an annual volume of greater than 100 major surgical procedures, the increased operative times reported in the STOMAMESH trial compared with the PREVENT trial, 287 versus 156 minutes for controls and 323 minutes versus 182 minutes for the mesh group, respectively, may indicate the limited reproducibility of the results generated by highly specialized centers. Additionally, the results of these studies can be applied only to elective colostomy formation because the PREVENT trial excluded emergent operations and the STOMAMESH trial included only 1 patient who underwent emergent colostomy creation. Importantly, no mesh-related complications were identified in either study and no mesh had to be removed.

A Cochrane review published in 2018 that examined the results of 10 RCTs, including the STOMAMESH trial, amounting to 844 patients and found the risk of PSH hernia was less in participants who received prophylactic mesh (relative risk [RR] 0.53; 95% CI, 0.43–0.66).[51] In absolute numbers, the investigators found the rate of PSH to be 22% in the prophylactic mesh group and 41% in controls; however, in conclusion, the investigators noted that the "Confidence in [their] estimate [was] low due to large degree of clinical heterogeneity and variability in follow-up duration and technique of parastomal hernia detection." The 2019 European Hernia Society

Guidelines followed with the "strong" recommendation for routine use of prophylactic mesh at the time of permanent colostomy creation based on "Low"-quality evidence,[52] a seemingly contradictory position likely based on the results of Cochrane review and other and prior systematic reviews.[53,54]

Since that time, the GRECCAR 7 trial,[55] a double-blinded RCT published in 2021 and including 200 patients, found no difference in the clinical or radiographic incidence of PSH at 2 years between the control arm and prophylactic mesh group (28% vs 31%, respectively; $P = .77$, and 34% vs 22%, respectively; $P = .17$) and no difference in stoma-related complications (32% versus 38%, respectively) and no mesh infections reported. Although the indications for surgery and patient demographics of this study appear similar to those in both the PREVENT and STOMAMESH trials, there are a few notable differences in methodology. In this trial, the retrorectus space was developed bluntly and the mesh delivered through the aperture of the ostomy with no fixation, a technique that could increase the difficulty of achieving a flat, fully unfurled mesh in the retrorectus space. Patients undergoing laparoscopic and open cases were included in this trial, introducing a new surgical variable; 40 patients were lost to follow-up due to death from progression of disease and only 135 patients completed the 2-year follow-up. This loss to follow-up puts the study at risk for type II error because the study design required 177 patients to obtain 80% power. The rate of PSH was higher in centers contributing greater than 20 patients to the trial (hazard ratio 2.835; $P<.001$). The source of this difference is unclear and there was no difference in rate of PSH when comparing the 2 groups by surgeons performing less than 2 procedures, 2 to 7 procedures, or greater than 7 procedures, but it may reflect the difficulty of standardization of practice across various institutions and care settings. These factors increase the difficulty of comparison between this trial and the 2 aforementioned trials.

In addition to synthetic mesh, the prophylactic use of biologic mesh in the retrorectus space was evaluated in an RCT by Fleshman and colleagues.[56] The researchers included 113 patients undergoing laparoscopic and open permanent end ileostomy or colostomy creation and randomized patients to no mesh or insertion of a 6-cm × 6-cm or 8-cm × 8-cm porcine-derived acellular dermal matrix in the retromuscular position delivered through the ostomy aperture, similar in fashion to the GRECCAR 7 trial. By blinded clinical assessment at 2 years postoperatively, the researchers found the incidence of PSH between the control and mesh groups to be similar (13.2% vs 12.2%, respectively; RR 0.85; 95% CI, 0.42–1.72). CT evaluation was not performed routinely and was obtained only if there was clinical suspicion for PSH. One major limitation of this trial was the higher than anticipated enrollment of end ileostomies and the lower-than-expected rate or PSHs in the control arm. The rate of PSH after end ileostomy creation is known to be lower than after end colostomy creation and compared with the aforementioned studies, in which malignancy was the indication for surgery in approximately 90% of cases, malignancy accounted for only 47% of the operations in this study whereas inflammatory bowel disease accounted for 34% along with a variety of other benign conditions that accounted for the rest. These differences likely explain the lower incidence of PSH hernia reported in this study compared with aforementioned studies of synthetic mesh.

Summary

At this point in time, the jury still is out on the use of prophylactic mesh at the time of permanent ostomy creation, and the benefits may not be as strong as once thought. Taking into consideration that most of these patients have numerous comorbidities, wound contamination by definition, and that understanding of the benefits and limitations of various prosthetics as well as their location in the abdominal wall continues to evolve, the authors still do not advocate for the routine use of prophylactic stoma mesh at this time.

SUMMARY

Understanding of abdominal core health and the nuances to hernia care continue to evolve. Despite that hernia operations are some of the most common operations performed by general surgeons, much of the controversy around mesh, operative approach, and technologic adjuncts centers on the paucity of high-quality data and RCTs. It is time that surgeons begin to make data collection a priority in order to provide patients with the best possible care.

DISCLOSURE

K.F. Baier has nothing to disclose. M.J. Rosen is the ACHQC Medical Director, with salary support and research grants paid to his institution by Intuitive Surgical and Pacira.

REFERENCES

1. Muysoms F, Campanelli G, Champault GG, et al. EuraHS: the development of an international online platform for registration and outcome measurement of ventral abdominal wall Hernia repair. Hernia 2012;16(3):239–50.
2. Haskins IN, Horne CM, Krpata DM, et al. A call for standardization of wound events reporting following ventral hernia repair. Hernia 2018;22(5):729–36.
3. Broderick J, DeWit EM, Rothrock N, et al. Advances in patient reported outcomes: the NIH PROMIS(®) measures. EGEMS (Wash DC) 2013;1(1):1015.
4. Krpata DM, Schmotzer BJ, Flocke S, et al. Design and initial implementation of HerQLes: A hernia-related quality-of-life survey to assess abdominal wall function. J Am Coll Surg 2012;215(5):635–42.
5. Heniford BT, Lincourt AE, Walters AL, et al. Carolinas comfort scale as a measure of hernia repair quality of life. Ann Surg 2018;267(1):171–6.
6. Baucom RB, Ousley J, Feurer ID, et al. Patient reported outcomes after incisional hernia repair—establishing the ventral hernia recurrence inventory. Am J Surg 2016;212(1):81–8.
7. Luijendijk RW, Hop WCJ, van den Tol MP, et al. A comparison of suture repair with mesh repair for incisional hernia. N Engl J Med 2000;343(6):392–8.
8. Conze J, Kingsnorth AN, Flament JB, et al. Randomized clinical trial comparing lightweight composite mesh with polyester or polypropylene mesh for incisional hernia repair. Br J Surg 2005;92(12):1488–93.
9. Burgmans JPJ, Voorbrood CEH, Simmermacher RKJ, et al. Long-term results of a randomized double-blinded prospective trial of a lightweight (ultrapro) versus a heavyweight mesh (prolene) in laparoscopic total extraperitoneal inguinal hernia repair (TULP-trial). Ann Surg 2016;263(5):862–6.
10. Blatnik JA, Krpata DM, Jacobs MR, et al. In vivo analysis of the morphologic characteristics of synthetic mesh to resist MRSA adherence. J Gastrointest Surg 2012;16(11):2139–44.
11. Carbonell AM, Criss CN, Cobb WS, et al. Outcomes of synthetic mesh in contaminated ventral hernia repairs. J Am Coll Surg 2013;217(6):991–8.

12. Itani KMF, Rosen M, Vargo D, et al. Prospective study of single-stage repair of contaminated hernias using a biologic porcine tissue matrix: the RICH study. Surgery 2012;152(3):498–505.

13. Albino FP, Patel KM, Nahabedian MY, et al. Does mesh location matter in abdominal wall reconstruction? A systematic review of the literature and a summary of recommendations. Plast Reconstr Surg 2013;132(5):1295–304.

14. Olavarria OA, Bernardi K, Dhanani NH, et al. Synthetic versus biologic mesh for complex open ventral hernia repair: a pilot randomized controlled trial. Surg Infect (Larchmt) 2020. https://doi.org/10.1089/sur.2020.166.

15. Miserez M, Lefering R, Famiglietti F, et al. Synthetic versus biological mesh in laparoscopic and open ventral hernia repair (LAPSIS): results of a multinational, randomized, controlled, and double-blind trial. Ann Surg 2021;273(1):57–65.

16. Rosen MJ, Bauer JJ, Harmaty M, et al. Multicenter, prospective, longitudinal study of the recurrence, surgical site infection, and quality of life after contaminated ventral hernia repair using biosynthetic absorbable mesh: the COBRA study. Ann Surg 2017;265(1):205–11.

17. Petro CC, Rosen MJ. A current review of long-acting resorbable meshes in abdominal wall reconstruction. Plast Reconstr Surg 2018;142(3S):84S–91S.

18. Roth JS, Anthone GJ, Selzer DJ, et al. Prospective, multicenter study of P4HB (Phasix™) mesh for hernia repair in cohort at risk for complications: 3-year follow-up. Ann Med Surg (Lond) 2020;61:1–7.

19. Köckerling F, Alam NN, Antoniou SA, et al. What is the evidence for the use of biologic or biosynthetic meshes in abdominal wall reconstruction? Hernia 2018;22(2):249–69.

20. Petro CC, Rosen MJ. Fight or flight: the role of staged approaches to complex abdominal wall reconstruction. Plast Reconstr Surg 2018;142(3S):38S–44S.

21. Bee TK, Croce MA, Magnotti LJ, et al. Temporary abdominal closure techniques: a prospective randomized trial comparing polyglactin 910 mesh and vacuum-assisted closure. J Trauma 2008;65(2):337–42.

22. Boele Van Hensbroek P, Wind J, Dijkgraaf MGW, et al. Temporary closure of the open abdomen: a systematic review on delayed primary fascial closure in patients with an open abdomen. World J Surg 2009;33(2):199–207.

23. LeBlanc KA, Booth WV. Laparoscopic repair of incisional abdominal hernias using expanded polytetrafluoroethylene: preliminary findings. Surg Laparosc Endosc 1993;3(1):39–41.

24. Ballantyne GH, Hourmont K, Wasielewski A. Telerobotic laparoscopic repair of incisional ventral hernias using intraperitoneal prosthetic mesh. JSLS 2003;7(1):7–14.

25. Prabhu AS, Dickens EO, Copper CM, et al. Laparoscopic vs robotic intraperitoneal mesh repair for incisional hernia: an americas hernia society quality collaborative analysis. J Am Coll Surg 2017;225(2):285–93.

26. Olavarria OA, Bernardi K, Shah SK, et al. Robotic versus laparoscopic ventral hernia repair: Multicenter, blinded randomized controlled trial. BMJ 2020;370:m2457.

27. Dhanani NH, Olavarria OA, Holihan JL, et al. Robotic versus laparoscopic ventral hernia repair: one-year results from a prospective, multicenter, blinded randomized controlled trial. Ann Surg 2021. https://doi.org/10.1097/SLA.0000000000004795.

28. Petro CC, Zolin S, Krpata D, et al. Patient-reported outcomes of robotic vs laparoscopic ventral hernia repair with intraperitoneal Mesh: the PROVE-IT randomized clinical trial. JAMA Surg 2021;156(1):22–9.

29. Belyansky I, Daes J, Radu VG, et al. A novel approach using the enhanced-view totally extraperitoneal (eTEP) technique for laparoscopic retromuscular hernia repair. Surg Endosc 2018;32(3):1525–32.

30. Belyansky I, Reza Zahiri H, Sanford Z, et al. Early operative outcomes of endoscopic (eTEP access) robotic-assisted retromuscular abdominal wall hernia repair. Hernia 2018;22(5):837–47.

31. Bellido Luque J, Gomez Rosado JC, Bellido Luque A, et al. Endoscopic retromuscular technique (eTEP) vs conventional laparoscopic ventral or incisional hernia repair with defect closure (IPOM +) for midline hernias. A case–control study. Hernia 2021. https://doi.org/10.1007/s10029-021-02373-0.

32. Belyansky I, Zahiri HR, Park A. Laparoscopic transversus abdominis release, a novel minimally invasive approach to complex abdominal wall reconstruction. Surg Innov 2016;23(2):134–41.

33. Warren JA, Cobb WS, Ewing JA, et al. Standard laparoscopic versus robotic retromuscular ventral hernia repair. Surg Endosc 2017;31(1):324–32.

34. Martin-del-Campo LA, Weltz AS, Belyansky I, et al. Comparative analysis of perioperative outcomes of robotic versus open transversus abdominis release. Surg Endosc 2018;32(2):840–5.

35. Abdu R, Vasyluk A, Reddy N, et al. Hybrid robotic transversus abdominis release versus open: propensity-matched analysis of 30-day outcomes. Hernia 2020. https://doi.org/10.1007/s10029-020-02249-9.

36. Bittner JG, Alrefai S, Vy M, et al. Comparative analysis of open and robotic transversus abdominis release for ventral hernia repair. Surg Endosc 2018;32(2): 727–34.

37. Carbonell AM, Warren JA, Prabhu AS, et al. Reducing length of stay using a robotic-assisted approach for retromuscular ventral hernia repair: a comparative analysis from the americas hernia society quality collaborative. Ann Surg 2018; 267:210–7.

38. Belyansky I, Weltz AS, Sibia US, et al. The trend toward minimally invasive complex abdominal wall reconstruction: is it worth it? Surg Endosc 2018;32(4): 1701–7.

39. Carne PWG, Robertson GM, Frizelle FA. Parastomal hernia. Br J Surg 2003;90(7): 784–93.

40. Glasgow SC, Dharmarajan S. Parastomal hernia: avoidance and treatment in the 21st century. Clin Colon Rectal Surg 2016. https://doi.org/10.1055/s-0036-1584506.

41. Hansson BME, Slater NJ, Van Der Velden AS, et al. Surgical techniques for parastomal hernia repair: a systematic review of the literature. Ann Surg 2012;255(4): 685–95.

42. Bayer I, Kyzer S, Chaimoff C. A new approach to primary strenthening of colostomy with Marlex mesh to prevent paracolostomy hernia. Surg Gynecol Obstet 1986;163(6):579–80.

43. Jänes A, Cengiz Y, Israelsson LA. Preventing parastomal hernia with a prosthetic mesh: a randomized study. Arch Surg 2004;139(12):1356–8.

44. Serra-Aracil X, Bombardo-Junca J, Moreno-Matias J, et al. Randomized, controlled, prospective trial of the use of a mesh to prevent parastomal hernia. Ann Surg 2009;249(4):583–7.

45. Lambrecht JR, Larsen SG, Reiertsen O, et al. Prophylactic mesh at end-colostomy construction reduces parastomal hernia rate: a randomized trial. Color Dis 2015;17(10):O191–7.

46. López-Cano M, Lozoya-Trujillo R, Quiroga S, et al. Use of a prosthetic mesh to prevent parastomal hernia during laparoscopic abdominoperineal resection: a randomized controlled trial. Hernia 2012;16(6):661–7.

47. López-Cano M, Serra-Aracil X, Mora L, et al. Preventing parastomal hernia using a modified sugarbaker technique with composite mesh during laparoscopic: abdominoperineal resection a randomized controlled trial. Ann Surg 2016;264(6): 923–8.

48. Vierimaa M, Klintrup K, Biancari F, et al. Prospective, randomized study on the use of a prosthetic mesh for prevention of parastomal hernia of permanent colostomy. Dis Colon Rectum 2015;58(10):943–9.

49. Brandsma H-T, Hansson BME, Aufenacker TJ, et al. Prophylactic mesh placement during formation of an end-colostomy reduces the rate of parastomal hernia. Ann Surg 2017;265(4):663–9.

50. Odensten C, Strigård K, Rutegård J, et al. Use of prophylactic mesh when creating a colostomy does not prevent parastomal hernia: a randomized controlled trial - STOMAMESH. Ann Surg 2019;269(3):427–31.

51. Jones HG, Rees M, Aboumarzouk OM, et al. Prosthetic mesh placement for the prevention of parastomal herniation. Cochrane Database Syst Rev 2018;2018(7): CD008905.

52. Antoniou SA, Agresta F, Garcia Alamino JM, et al. European hernia Society guidelines on prevention and treatment of parastomal hernias. Hernia 2018;22(1): 183–98.

53. Wang S, Wang W, Zhu B, et al. Efficacy of prophylactic mesh in end-colostomy construction: a systematic review and meta-analysis of randomized controlled trials. World J Surg 2016;40(10):2528–36.

54. López-Cano M, Brandsma HT, Bury K, et al. Prophylactic mesh to prevent parastomal hernia after end colostomy: a meta-analysis and trial sequential analysis. Hernia 2017;21(2):177–89.

55. Prudhomme M, Rullier E, Lakkis Z, et al. End colostomy with or without mesh to prevent a parastomal hernia (GRECCAR 7). Ann Surg 2021. https://doi.org/10.1097/sla.0000000000004371.

56. Fleshman JW, Beck DE, Hyman N, et al. A prospective, multicenter, randomized, controlled study of non-cross-linked porcine acellular dermal matrix fascial sublay for parastomal reinforcement in patients undergoing surgery for permanent abdominal wall ostomies. Dis Colon Rectum 2014;57:623–31.

Modern Management of the Appendix: So Many Options

CPT Samuel Grasso, DO, LTC Avery Walker, MD*

KEYWORDS

- Appendicitis • Nonoperative management • Operative management • Antibiotics
- Modern

KEY POINTS

- All uncomplicated cases of appendicitis, including those with a fecalith, should undergo operative management.
- Complicated cases of appendicitis (abscess, mass, phlegmon) should have an interval appendectomy performed.
- All appendicitis patients older than 40 years should have surveillance endoscopy performed to rule out neoplasm.

INTRODUCTION

Acute appendicitis continues to be the most common abdominal surgical emergency in the world with a lifetime risk of 8.6% in men and 6.9% in women.[1] Surgical excision has historically been the cornerstone of management for the past 120 years, with the appropriate transition from open exposures to minimally invasive techniques over the last several decades.[2] Recent investigations, motivated by optimizing resource utilization, have reexamined operative management (OM) in the setting of acute appendicitis. These efforts force the modern surgeon to be familiar with different treatment approaches and surveillance options to best treat their patients while minimizing unnecessary risk and health care expenditures.

Ruling out a Complicated Case

If the patient does not have a periappendiceal mass, phlegmon, perforation, or abscess, their case of acute appendicitis is referred to as "uncomplicated." These cases are also known as "simple" or "nonperforated." Most cases (80%–87%) present this way.[3] This delineation between uncomplicated and complicated appendicitis has been found to be extremely important in management.

Department of General Surgery, William Beaumont Army Medical Center, 5005 N Piedras Street, El Paso, TX 79920, USA
* Corresponding author.
E-mail address: avery.s.walker.mil@mail.mil

Surg Clin N Am 101 (2021) 1023–1031
https://doi.org/10.1016/j.suc.2021.08.003
0039-6109/21/Published by Elsevier Inc.

In the United States, computed tomography (CT) scans seem ubiquitous in the acute care setting, and most surgeons will get to benefit from this cross-sectional anatomy. Without a CT scan, one must rely on clinical history and physical examination to determine risk of a complicated case. Obstruction, hemodynamic instability, peritonitis, and duration of symptoms greater than 24 hours can all serve as indicators of a complicated case.[4]

New research has also examined the neutrophil-to-lymphocyte ratio (NLR) as a predictor of complicated versus uncomplicated disease. A systematic review in 2020 looked at 8914 patients in 17 different studies, revealing that NLR can predict both diagnosis and severity of appendicitis[5]: NLR greater than 4.7 is an independent predictor of appendicitis, whereas an NLR greater than 8.8 is an independent predictor of complicated appendicitis. Use of this relatively novel and inexpensive calculation can assist the surgeon in determining if the operating room or surgical ward is the appropriate next step for the patient.

UNCOMPLICATED APPENDICITIS
Nonoperative Management

To date, numerous studies have examined the nonoperative management (NOM) of uncomplicated appendicitis. The Appendicitis Acute (APPAC) trial was a multicenter, open-label, noninferiority randomized clinical trial. It was conducted from 2009 to 2012 in Finland, randomizing 530 patients to either open appendectomy or NOM with antibiotics. The NOM arm performed well overall, with only 27.3% of patients requiring appendectomy within 12 months of randomization (21% during the index hospitalization and 79% after a readmission). This study had a high impact on the medical community and is heavily referenced to validate NOM with more than 495 citations,[6] but it should be stressed that the study did not meet its prespecified noninferiority margin for NOM. The long-term quality of life (QoL) scores were similar between NOM and OM; however, they were lower in those who originally underwent NOM but had to convert to OM for recurrence.[7,8]

The Comparison of the Outcomes of antibiotic Drugs and Appendectomy (CODA) Collaborative conducted a larger and more recent trial across 25 medical centers in the United States.[9] The investigators enrolled 1552 patients with uncomplicated appendicitis from 2016 to 2020, randomizing them to either appendectomy or NOM with 10 days of antibiotics. Ninety-six percent of the surgical arm underwent laparoscopic appendectomy. Forty-seven percent of patients in the NOM arm did not require hospital admission. At 90 days, 29% of the NOM had undergone appendectomy (41% of patients with an appendicolith and 25% of those without). Using 30-day QoL scores as the primary outcome, this study demonstrated that antibiotics were noninferior to appendectomy.

Of note, NOM of uncomplicated appendicitis has been repeatedly found to be more cost-effective than OM in both pediatric and adult populations.[10,11] One paper reported a $10,000 difference between approaches initially. Five-year follow-up of the APPAC trial group demonstrated persistent significant cost savings associated with NOM.[12]

Antibiotic Selection

Antibiotic selection depends on patient risk factors, patient allergies, severity of infection, local antibiogram, and surgeon preference. The obvious target is appendiceal/colonic flora (gram-negative aerobes and anaerobes).

All patients (NOM and OM) should be given antibiotics. OM patients should be given single-dose preoperative antibiotics within the 60-minute preincision "window" for surgical prophylaxis.[13] The investigators prefer a combination of ceftriaxone and metronidazole per our local antibiogram.

In the APPAC trial, patients in the NOM arm were given intravenous (IV) ertapenem (1 g/d) for 3 days followed by 7 days of oral (PO) levofloxacin (500 mg/d) and metronidazole (500 mg/TID). The CODA trial included a minimum of 24 hours of IV antibiotics (most commonly being ertapenem, cefoxitin, or cefazolin/metronidazole) followed by PO antibiotics (ciprofloxacin/metronidazole or cefdinir/metronidazole) for a total of 10 days.

Efficacy of Nonoperative Management

Besides the aforementioned APPAC and CODA trials, numerous other trials have examined the efficacy of NOM. When compared with surgery, NOM has demonstrated reduced overall symptoms of appendicitis,[9,14] reduced leukocyte count,[15] lower risk of peritonitis,[16] similar or lower pain scores,[15,16] and fewer days of missed work for patient or caregiver.[9] There was no difference in overall health at 30 days compared with OM.[9]

Considering these favorable outcomes, the largest hindrance to widespread adoption of NOM is the high risk of recurrent appendicitis. Because of this, a significant percentage of these patients will ultimately go on to require appendectomy, even if NOM was initially successful (**Table 1**).

The Fecalith's Impact on Decision-Making

The presence of a fecalith (also known as appendicolith, coprolith, or appendiceal calculi) on imaging in an otherwise uncomplicated case of appendicitis may influence the surgeon to avoid NOM. Rate of fecaliths found in appendectomy specimens vary largely in the literature (1%–51%), but the best estimate is that about 15% of patients will have a fecalith.[18,19] Fecaliths are associated with higher rates of complicated appendicitis.[20]

Patients in the APPAC trial with a fecalith were designated as "complicated" and excluded from the study. The CODA trial included patients with fecaliths, and as mentioned earlier, they were associated with a significantly higher rate of failure of NOM. They were also associated with a higher rate of complications.[9] The higher incidence of NOM failure with fecaliths has also been demonstrated in pediatric patients.[21]

Decision-Making for Uncomplicated Appendicitis

For adult and pediatric patients in the developed world, most uncomplicated cases should still undergo appendectomy. Although more expensive, surgical management is more effective as definitive care without an increased risk of complications.[22,23] This recommendation aligns with that of the American College of Surgeons, Society of

Table 1		
Appendicitis recurrence after nonoperative management		
Time Frame	Risk of Recurrence	Data
Within initial admission	10%	Becker et al.[17]
Within 90 d	29%	CODA trial[9]
Within 1 y	27.3%	APPAC trial[6]
Within 5 y	39.1%	APPAC trial[7]

American Gastrointestinal and Endoscopic Surgeons, European Association of Endoscopic Surgery, and World Society of Emergency Surgery.[24,25] However, there are always patient and disease factors that make surgery particularly difficult or undesirable for certain individuals, and the recent literature suggests that a nonoperative approach to appendicitis is safe in these select patients.

COMPLICATED APPENDICITIS

For patients with complicated appendicitis, including free perforation, periappendiceal mass, phlegmon, or abscess, management is variable. Of the approximately 300,000 appendectomies performed annually in the United States, 25% of them are for complicated appendicitis.[26] Patients with generalized peritonitis due to free perforation in the abdominal cavity need to undergo preoperative resuscitation (crystalloid, antibiotics, and vasopressor support) before emergency appendectomy to achieve source control. However, most patients with complicated disease have more localized sepsis and do not require emergent surgery. Instead, mos of these patients should not undergo immediate surgery, as it is associated with high rates of complications, extended resections, and conversions to open surgery.[27–31] Immediate surgery for complicated appendicitis is also associated with high rates of postoperative abscess and fistula.[30]

NOM of complicated appendicitis includes crystalloid resuscitation, intravenous antibiotics, and percutaneous drainage of any abscesses that develop. Image-guided percutaneous drainage of abscesses as needed leads to decreased risk of complications and shorter hospital stay.[28] With NOM, more than 80% of complicated appendicitis patients will not need an immediate appendectomy.[31]

Interval Appendectomy

Patients with resolved complicated appendicitis have historically undergone elective interval appendectomy 6 to 8 weeks after resolution of symptoms; this was due to 2 concerns: cecal or appendiceal neoplasm masquerading as appendicitis (see later discussion) and recurrent appendicitis. Of note, the appendiceal lumen is often obliterated by the index infection, so recurrence rates are not as high as one might expect. Although it certainly varies by age and extent of follow-up, a 2016 meta-analysis reported an overall 12.4% rate of recurrent appendicitis.[32]

Recent investigation into the cost-effectiveness of performing interval appendectomies on all patients has shown significantly increased costs on hospital systems without persistent benefits for all patients.[32] One study ultimately recommended a cost-benefit risk-reduction break-even point of 34 years old (ie, patients younger than 34 years should have an interval appendectomy performed from a cost perspective).[33]

Appendiceal Neoplasm

Appendiceal neoplasms are a common finding on final pathology report after appendectomy. They are sometimes the source of luminal obstruction, and other times they are found incidentally. The likelihood of finding a neoplasm in complicated appendicitis is significantly higher than in uncomplicated cases (12.6% vs 1.2%).[34,35] The risk of a neoplasm also strongly correlates with age (**Table 2**).

An important study to evaluate the risk of appendiceal neoplasms was the Peri-Appendicitis Acuta (periAPPAC) trial, published in 2019 by the same group that conducted the APPAC trial.[38] This trial focused on patients aged 18 to 60 years who had an appendiceal abscess that was successfully treated with antibiotics and percutaneous drainage. These patients underwent colonoscopy to exclude a cecal tumor

Table 2 Appendiceal neoplasms based on the age of the patient	
Age Group	Risk of Harboring Neoplasm in Complicated Appendicitis[36,37]
Younger than 30 years	0%
Between 30 and 50 years old	11%
Older than 50 years	16%

and were then randomized to either interval appendectomy or continued NOM with and abdominal MRI ordered at 3 months.

The periAPPAC trial had a planned enrollment of 120 patients, but the trial was prematurely terminated after an interim analysis of the first 60 patients demonstrated an unexpectedly high rate of appendiceal neoplasm (17%). Patients initially randomized to the observation arm were then offered appendectomy, and this led to a 20% overall rate of neoplasm. The neoplasm rate was 35% for patients older than 40 years.

Based on the available data regarding both recurrent appendicitis and neoplasm, the investigators recommend interval appendectomy on all patients who are healthy enough to undergo surgery. The authors' justification depends on the patient's age; if younger than 34 years, the patient should undergo interval appendectomy from a hospital cost perspective. If older than 40 years, the patient should undergo interval appendectomy (after colonoscopy, see later discussion) from a neoplasm risk-reduction perspective. The authors find it more pragmatic from a systems-based approach to recommend interval appendectomy for all patients than to exclude those aged 35 to 39 years.

Colonoscopy after Appendicitis

As discussed earlier, complicated appendicitis is linked with underlying neoplasm in a significant number of patients. In addition, uncomplicated appendicitis has also been linked with right-sided colonic neoplasm, albeit at a much lower rate than complicated cases.[39] For patients older than 40 years who experience appendicitis, the risk of colon cancer is higher than the general public, with odds ratios as high as 38.5.[40] Unfortunately, because of the acute care context to appendicitis and lack of durable follow-up for many patients, 60% to 80% of patients do not undergo surveillance endoscopy within 3 years of appendicitis.[39,41]

Based on the available evidence, the investigators recommend that postappendicitis colonoscopy should be performed in all patients older than 40 years to rule out right-sided colonic neoplasms.

SURGICAL APPROACH

When surgery is to be performed (uncomplicated, complicated, or interval cases of appendicitis), the authors recommend for a laparoscopic approach. Assuming surgeon familiarity and institutional capability, the minimally invasive laparoscopic exposure has been well studied and proved to be superior over doing the case open.[42] It has resulted in lower wound infections, less postoperative pain, less postoperative adhesions,[43] and a shorter length-of-stay. It also has advantages in the obese, elderly, and those in whom the diagnosis is not clear. Initial concerns about increased risk

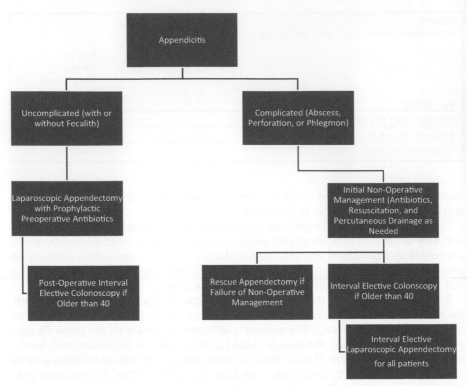

Fig. 1. Recommended algorithm for treating appendicitis.

of postoperative intraabdominal abscess and longer operative times[42] are decreasing.[44] It is suspected that this is due to increasing surgeon familiarity and improving technology.

SUMMARY

Appendicitis is extremely common, and the immediate and long-term management must take into consideration several patient and disease factors. In uncomplicated cases of appendicitis, NOM is safe and cost-effective, but it is associated with high rates of recurrence, and so patients should be appropriately counseled, and appropriate follow-up should be arranged. For those with complicated diverticulitis, most will not receive appendectomy at the index hospitalization. Interval colonoscopy is appropriate for patients 40 years and older. This algorithmic approach to appendicitis can be found in **Figure 1**. Until more data emerges, the safest decision is to offer interval appendectomy in all patients, regardless of age.

DISCLOSURE

The authors have nothing to disclose.

REFERENCES

1. Körner H, Söndenaa K, Söreide JA, et al. Incidence of acute nonperforated and perforated appendicitis: age-specific and sex-specific analysis. World J Surg 1997;21(3):313–7.

2. Baird DL, Simillis C, Kontovounisios C, et al. Acute appendicitis. BMJ 2017;357: j1703.
3. Andersson RE, Hugander A, Thulin AJ. Diagnostic accuracy and perforation rate in appendicitis: association with age and sex of the patient and with appendicectomy rate. Eur J surg 1992;158(1):37–41.
4. Temple CL, Huchcroft SA, Temple WJ. The natural history of appendicitis in adults. A prospective study. Ann Surg 1995;221(3):278.
5. Hajibandeh S, Hajibandeh S, Hobbs N, et al. Neutrophil-to-lymphocyte ratio predicts acute appendicitis and distinguishes between complicated and uncomplicated appendicitis: A systematic review and meta-analysis. Am J Surg 2020; 219(1):154–63.
6. Salminen P, Paajanen H, Rautio T, et al. Antibiotic therapy vs appendectomy for treatment of uncomplicated acute appendicitis: the APPAC randomized clinical trial. JAMA 2015;313(23):2340–8.
7. Salminen P, Tuominen R, Paajanen H, et al. Five-year follow-up of antibiotic therapy for uncomplicated acute appendicitis in the APPAC randomized clinical trial. JAMA 2018;320(12):1259–65.
8. Sippola S, Haijanen J, Viinikainen L, et al. Quality of life and patient satisfaction at 7-year follow-up of antibiotic therapy vs appendectomy for uncomplicated acute appendicitis: a secondary analysis of a randomized clinical trial. JAMA Surg 2020;155(4):283–9.
9. CODA Collaborative. A randomized trial comparing antibiotics with appendectomy for appendicitis. N Engl J Med 2020;383(20):1907–19.
10. Wu JX, Sacks GD, Dawes AJ, et al. The cost-effectiveness of nonoperative management versus laparoscopic appendectomy for the treatment of acute, uncomplicated appendicitis in children. J Pediatr Surg 2017;52(7):1135–40.
11. Wu JX, Dawes AJ, Sacks GD, et al. Cost effectiveness of nonoperative management versus laparoscopic appendectomy for acute uncomplicated appendicitis. Surgery 2015;158(3):712–21.
12. Haijanen J, Sippola S, Tuominen R, et al. Cost analysis of antibiotic therapy versus appendectomy for treatment of uncomplicated acute appendicitis: 5-year results of the APPAC randomized clinical trial. PLoS One 2019;14(7): e0220202.
13. Bratzler DW, Houck PM. Antimicrobial prophylaxis for surgery: an advisory statement from the National Surgical Infection Prevention Project. Clin Infect Dis 2004; 38:1706–15.
14. Hansson J, Körner U, Khorram-Manesh A, et al. Randomized clinical trial of antibiotic therapy versus appendicectomy as primary treatment of acute appendicitis in unselected patients. Br J Surg 2009;96(5):473–81.
15. Eriksson S, Granström L. Randomized controlled trial of appendicectomy versus antibiotic therapy for acute appendicitis. Br J Surg 1995;82(2):166–9.
16. Vons C, Barry C, Maitre S, et al. Amoxicillin plus clavulanic acid versus appendicectomy for treatment of acute uncomplicated appendicitis: an open-label, non-inferiority, randomised controlled trial. Lancet 2011;377(9777):1573–9.
17. Becker P, Fichtner-Feigl S, Schilling D. Clinical management of appendicitis. Visc Med 2018;34(6):453–8.
18. Ramdass MJ, Sing QY, Milne D, et al. Association between the appendix and the fecalith in adults. Can J Surg 2015;58(1):10.
19. Nitecki S, Karmeli R, Sarr MG. Appendiceal calculi and fecaliths as indications for appendectomy. Surg Gynecol Obstet 1990;171(3):185–8.

20. Singh JP, Mariadason JG. Role of the faecolith in modern-day appendicitis. Ann R Coll Surg Engl 2013;95(1):48–51.
21. Huang L, Yin Y, Yang L, et al. Comparison of antibiotic therapy and appendectomy for acute uncomplicated appendicitis in children: a meta-analysis. JAMA Pediatr 2017;171(5):426–34.
22. Prechal D, Damirov F, Grilli M, et al. Antibiotic therapy for acute uncomplicated appendicitis: a systematic review and meta-analysis. Int J Colorectal Dis 2019; 34(6):963–71.
23. Podda M, Gerardi C, Cillara N, et al. Antibiotic treatment and appendectomy for uncomplicated acute appendicitis in adults and children: a systematic review and meta-analysis. Ann Surg 2019;270(6):1028–40.
24. Gorter RR, Eker HH, Gorter-Stam MA, et al. Diagnosis and management of acute appendicitis. EAES consensus development conference 2015. Surg Endosc 2016;30(11):4668–90.
25. Sartelli M, Chichom-Mefire A, Labricciosa FM, et al. The management of intra-abdominal infections from a global perspective: 2017 WSES guidelines for management of intra-abdominal infections. World J Emerg Surg 2017;12(1):1–34.
26. Perez KS, Allen SR. Complicated appendicitis and considerations for interval appendectomy. JAAPA 2018;31(9):35–41.
27. Simillis C, Symeonides P, Shorthouse AJ, et al. A meta-analysis comparing conservative treatment versus acute appendectomy for complicated appendicitis (abscess or phlegmon). Surgery 2010;147(6):818–29.
28. Brown CV, Abrishami M, Muller M, et al. Appendiceal abscess: immediate operation or percutaneous drainage? Am Surg 2003;69(10):829.
29. Cheng Y, Xiong X, Lu J, et al. Early versus delayed appendicectomy for appendiceal phlegmon or abscess. Cochrane Database Syst Rev 2017;(6):CD011670.
30. Mentula P, Sammalkorpi H, Leppäniemi A. Laparoscopic surgery or conservative treatment for appendiceal abscess in adults? A randomized controlled trial. Ann Surg 2015;262(2):237–42.
31. Fagenholz PJ, Peev MP, Thabet A, et al. Abscess due to perforated appendicitis: factors associated with successful percutaneous drainage. Am J Surg 2016; 212(4):794–8.
32. Darwazeh G, Cunningham SC, Kowdley GC. A systematic review of perforated appendicitis and phlegmon: interval appendectomy or wait-and-see? Am Surgeon 2016;82(1):11–5.
33. Senekjian L, Nirula R, Bellows B, et al. Interval appendectomy: finding the breaking point for cost-effectiveness. J Am Coll Surg 2016;223(4):632–43.
34. Carpenter SG, Chapital AB, Merritt MV, et al. Increased risk of neoplasm in appendicitis treated with interval appendectomy: single-institution experience and literature review. Am Surgeon 2012;78(3):339–43.
35. Son J, Park YJ, Lee SR, et al. Increased Risk of Neoplasms in Adult Patients Undergoing Interval Appendectomy. Ann Coloproctol 2020;36(5):311.
36. Hayes D, Reiter S, Hagen E, et al. Is interval appendectomy really needed? A closer look at neoplasm rates in adult patients undergoing interval appendectomy after complicated appendicitis. Surg Endosc 2020;35(7):3855–60.
37. Fouad D, Kauffman JD, Chandler NM. Pathology findings following interval appendectomy: Should it stay or go? J Pediatr Surg 2020;55(4):737–41.
38. Mällinen J, Rautio T, Grönroos J, et al. Risk of appendiceal neoplasm in periappendicular abscess in patients treated with interval appendectomy vs follow-up with magnetic resonance imaging: 1-year outcomes of the peri–appendicitis acuta randomized clinical trial. JAMA Surg 2019;154(3):200–7.

39. Sylthe E, Stornes T, Rekstad LC, et al. Is there a role for routine colonoscopy in the follow-up after acute appendicitis? Scand J Gastroenterol 2018;53(8):1008–12.
40. Lai HW, Loong CC, Tai LC, et al. Incidence and odds ratio of appendicitis as first manifestation of colon cancer: a retrospective analysis of 1873 patients. J Gastroenterol Hepatol 2006;21(11):1693–6.
41. Seretis C, Gill J, Lim P, et al. Surveillance colonoscopy after appendicectomy in patients over the age of 40: targeted audit of outcomes and variability in practice. Chirurgia (Bucur) 2020;115(5):595–9.
42. Jaschinski T, Mosch C, Eikermann M, et al. Laparoscopic versus open appendectomy in patients with suspected appendicitis: a systematic review of meta-analyses of randomised controlled trials. BMC Gastroenterol 2015;15(1):1–10.
43. Markar SR, Penna M, Harris A. Laparoscopic approach to appendectomy reduces the incidence of short-and long-term post-operative bowel obstruction: systematic review and pooled analysis. J Gastrointest Surg 2014;18(9):1683–92.
44. Quah GS, Eslick GD, Cox MR. Laparoscopic appendicectomy is superior to open surgery for complicated appendicitis. Surg Endosc 2019;33(7):2072–82.

Controversies in Breast Cancer Surgery

Lily Gutnik, MD, MPH[a], Oluwadamilola M. Fayanju, MD, MA, MPHS[b],*

KEYWORDS

- Axilla • Breast cancer • Chemotherapy • Contralateral prophylactic mastectomy
- Endocrine therapy • Neoadjuvant

KEY POINTS

- Contralateral prophylactic mastectomy (CPM) in women with unilateral breast cancer confers no survival advantage, can be associated with more complications, and represents a preference-sensitive decision.
- Neoadjuvant chemotherapy (NACT) should be used in locally advanced, inflammatory, and higher-stage HER2+ and triple-negative breast cancers, when breast conservation is strongly desired, and to facilitate axillary downstage.
- Neoadjuvant endocrine therapy (NET) in select postmenopausal women with hormone receptor-positive cancer is comparably effective to NACT.
- Patients who are clinically node-positive and become clinically node-negative after NACT are eligible for sentinel lymph node biopsy, which should be done with dual tracer and ideally yields the retrieval of at least 3 nodes and the previously biopsied node. If these nodes are negative, then further axillary surgery can potentially be omitted.

INTRODUCTION

Breast surgical oncology is a rapidly evolving field shaped by decades of practice-changing research and public health initiatives. Widespread dissemination of screening in the United States enabled increased detection of early-stage disease and transformed breast cancer into a largely curable entity, although significant disparities in screening, stage at diagnosis, and survival persist.[1–3] For late-stage and biologically aggressive subtypes including HER2-enriched (HER2+) and triple-negative breast cancer (TNBC), increased use of neoadjuvant systemic therapy (NST) has enabled de-escalation of surgical treatment in the breast and axilla.[4,5] Nevertheless, women in the United States continue to undergo contralateral prophylactic mastectomy (CPM) for unilateral disease at high rates compared with several other countries, with many average-risk women undergoing CPM even when breast-conserving therapy (BCT) is feasible.[6]

[a] Duke University School of Medicine, DUMC 3513, Durham, NC 27707, USA; [b] Penn Medicine, 3400 Spruce Street, Silverstein 4, Philadelphia, PA 19104, USA
* Corresponding author.
E-mail addresses: Oluwadamilola.Fayanju@pennmedicine.upenn.edu
Twitter: @LGutnik (L.G.); @DrLolaFayanju(O."L".F.)

Surg Clin N Am 101 (2021) 1033–1044
https://doi.org/10.1016/j.suc.2021.06.002
0039-6109/21/© 2021 Elsevier Inc. All rights reserved.

Ironically, higher rates of CPM are observed among recipients of neoadjuvant chemotherapy (NACT) than among recipients of adjuvant or no chemotherapy.[7] Thus, the benefit of NACT as a means of facilitating BCT in place of mastectomy is realized less often than it could be, prompting exploration of less toxic neoadjuvant systemic alternatives such as neoadjuvant endocrine therapy (NET), which is less commonly used in the United States. Notably, however, there is a strong trend toward using NACT to de-escalate locoregional treatment of the axilla given the morbidity associated with axillary lymph node dissection (ALND) with or without the addition of axillary radiation (ART).

Here, we discuss the 3 important yet controversial topics described earlier, specifically (1) high rates of CPM despite unclear benefit, (2) shifting indications for NST (ie, NACT and/or NACT), and (3) evolving approaches to surgical management of the axilla.

DISCUSSION
Contralateral Prophylactic Mastectomy

Breast cancer risk assessment is critical to surgical decision making, particularly with regard to the appropriateness of CPM. Breast cancer risk factors can be divided into modifiable (ie, alcohol use) and nonmodifiable (ie, age) factors. Several risk calculators are available to help counsel patients on their estimated lifetime breast cancer risk.[8] These tools help guide discussions on surgery choice in patients who may be considering prophylactic, also referred to as *risk-reducing*, mastectomy.

Improved radiographic technology and increased use of adjuvant endocrine therapy contributed to a decrease in contralateral breast cancer incidence among patients with unilateral breast cancer since 1985, with the annual risk of contralateral breast cancer estimated to be only 0.2% to 0.5%.[9,10] CPM rates have been increasing over the last 20 years despite unclear and even contradictory evidence of survival benefit.[11–16] The most commonly cited reason for CPM is patient preference, often driven by fear and anxiety about future breast cancer diagnosis and cosmetic concerns, such as asymmetry after unilateral mastectomy.[10,17] Women who are young, white, more educated, and have a family history of breast cancer are more likely to choose CPM.[18] Although some studies have shown concomitant postoperative decrease in cancer-related anxiety after CPM, it is associated with increased risk of surgical complications and sometimes negative psychological outcomes including decision regret, compromised body image, and unsatisfactory sexual function.[10,11,15] The option for CPM is of greatest import for women deemed to have a high (>20%) lifetime risk of metachronous breast cancer. For these women, nonsurgical options for breast cancer risk reduction include endocrine therapy chemoprevention and specialized radiographic surveillance protocols.

Evidence-based counseling, formal risk assessment, and, if needed, engagement of psychosocial support services should all be a part of shared decision making (SDM) for CPM. Once the decision to pursue CPM has been made, the next steps in SDM involve type of mastectomy (nipple-sparing, skin-sparing, or simple), type of reconstruction (autologous, implant-based, or both), and indications for sentinel lymph node biopsy (SLNB). Nipple-sparing mastectomy is oncologically safe, with no difference in survival compared with traditional mastectomy. Furthermore, it has a similar complication profile but improved esthetic outcomes compared with other forms of mastectomy.[19] However, although promising, long-term data regarding future breast cancer risk and survival are relatively sparse.[20]

Increased access to reconstructive surgery has been linked to increased use of CPM.[21] Two important decisions must be made once a patient chooses reconstruction: the timing of reconstruction relative to mastectomy (immediate vs delayed) and type of reconstruction (autologous vs implant based). Most CPM recipients undergo immediate, implant-based reconstruction.[22] Immediate reconstruction can be done in one stage (direct to implant or upfront autologous reconstruction) or 2 stages (tissue expander followed by later exchange for implant or autologous reconstruction). Immediate reconstruction is associated not only with improved psychosocial well-being, lower costs, and improved cosmesis but also with increased implant and flap failure rates compared with delayed reconstruction.[23–26] Data are conflicting with regard to overall surgical and medical complication rates after delayed versus immediate reconstruction.[23,24]

Implant-based reconstruction is a less-invasive procedure with quicker recovery compared with autologous reconstruction while still resulting in excellent cosmetic outcomes. However, risks include capsular contracture, implant failure, and a small risk of breast implant-associated anaplastic large cell lymphoma, all of which may require additional future surgeries.[27,28] In contrast, autologous reconstruction uses a patient's own tissue, usually abdominal, to create a more natural appearance with good longevity and higher satisfaction on patient reported outcomes.[28,29] It is, however, a more invasive procedure with longer recovery, potentially catastrophic complications of flap loss, and additional donor site morbidity.[28]

Among mutation carriers, performing SLNB is rationalized by the concern for the difficulty of performing sentinel node mapping after mastectomy in the event of unexpected occult invasive cancer (1%–3%). Thus, although the chance of a positive lymph node in such a scenario is estimated to be only 0.5%,[11] some advocate for SLNB in all mutation carriers undergoing CPM, whereas others do not believe that the risk of occult cancer justifies the risks, albeit low, of SLNB. MRI has been used to screen for breast cancer before surgery, thus lessening the risk of occult cancer that would require SLNB, but the high cost-benefit ratio of this approach has called this strategy into question.[11]

In conclusion, CPM has become increasingly common without clear evidence of survival benefit. Among women with clinically actionable genetic mutations, CPM is associated with decreased risk of a future breast cancer, but there are nonoperative strategies that may confer similar levels of risk reduction. Both evidence-based risk assessment and an accurate capture of patient preferences are important components of the SDM process for CPM.

Neoadjuvant Systemic Therapy

NACT was first used in the 1970s in the treatment of locally advanced breast cancers.[30] In the 1980s and 1990s, 2 large randomized controlled trials (National Surgical Adjuvant Breast and Bowel Project [NSABP] B-18 and B-27) demonstrated no survival difference between neoadjuvant and adjuvant chemotherapy.[31] Subsequent randomized trials confirmed substantial tumor response and increased rates of BCT after NACT but, likewise, no significant difference in mortality between neoadjuvant and adjuvant chemotherapy treatment groups.[32] Notably, pathologic complete response (pCR) rates among NACT recipients varies by tumor subtype, with high pCR rates among hormone receptor-negative (HR-), high grade, and/or HER2+ tumors and low pCR rates among low-intermediate grade and hormone receptor-positive (HR+) tumors.[33] Furthermore, not only does pCR vary with tumor subtype but also anatomic extent of pCR (ie, whether it occurs in the breast, axilla, or both) predicts survival for less chemosensitive (eg, HR+/HER2-) and more aggressive (eg, TNBC) subtypes.[34]

Over the past 30 years, NACT use has increased. Indications for NACT include the intention of downstaging large primary and/or node-positive tumors to enable less morbid operations and opportunities to preserve the breast. NACT also enables in vivo demonstration of tumor chemosensitivity or chemoresistance, information that can subsequently guide treatment. However, in the event of chemoresistance, there is the theoretically increased risk of metastasis or local tumor enlargement from delay in surgery, with concomitantly worse prognosis or unavoidable mastectomy.[35,36] In fact, a meta-analysis of randomized trials evaluating neoadjuvant versus adjuvant chemotherapy found an increased risk of local recurrence in the NACT group, but there was no association with increased risk of distant recurrence or survival.[32] Furthermore, tumor progression during NACT, although relatively uncommon, is associated with decreased overall survival.[37]

Data regarding tumor response to NACT can help guide adjuvant therapy decision making. For example, the KATHERINE trial demonstrated that in women with early-stage HER2+ breast cancer treated with NACT in combination with anti-HER2 targeted therapy but who still had residual disease on final post-NACT surgical pathology, treatment with adjuvant ado-trastuzumab emtansine (T-DM1, also known as Kadcyla [Genentech]) decreased risk of recurrence or death by 50%.[38]

Unfortunately, NACT has been proved to be less effective at breast and axillary downstage for HR+ tumors, which constitute nearly 75% of all invasive breast cancer.[30] Adjuvant endocrine therapy for HR+ breast cancer is known to improve survival, but less is known about the impact of NET as a single agent or in combination with chemotherapy. A recent analysis of US practice patterns showed a 20% utilization rate of NET.[40] At present, it is most commonly used among elderly patients or those deemed unable to tolerate chemotherapy.[39] Notably, there is no significant difference in BCT rate between NET and NACT recipients, but NET is significantly less toxic.[39]

The optimal NET regimen with regard to composition and timing has been explored in several trials. The P024 trial compared 4 months of neoadjuvant tamoxifen with the aromatase inhibitor (AI) letrozole in postmenopausal women with HR+ breast cancers who were ineligible for BCT. The letrozole group had higher rates of BCT than the tamoxifen group.[41] The IMPACT trial compared neoadjuvant tamoxifen, anastrozole, and a combination of tamoxifen and anastrozole administered for 3 months in postmenopausal women with estrogen receptor-positive (ER+) invasive breast cancer. BCT rates were increased in the anastrozole groups relative to the tamoxifen-only group, although all groups exhibited some response.[42] The American College of Surgeons Oncology Group (ACOSOG) Z1031 found that all AIs (letrozole, anastrozole, and exemestane) used in the neoadjuvant setting among postmenopausal women with ER+ breast cancer facilitated increased BCT rates.[43] The PTEX46 trial found no difference in clinical response rate between neoadjuvant exemestane administered for 4 versus 6 months.[44] Several other studies evaluating optimal length of NET support 4 to 6 months, although longer times may be acceptable if patients show continued response.[45]

Most NET trials have been conducted among postmenopausal women, thus less is known about the safety and efficacy of NET in premenopausal women. The STAGE trial, focusing on premenopausal women, demonstrated that 6 months of ovarian suppression plus an AI in the neoadjuvant setting had more clinical response than neoadjuvant tamoxifen.[46] The ALTERNATE trial found no significant difference in the clinical response rate between premenopausal women randomized to NET with either fulvestrant or fulvestrant plus anastrozole with stage II/III ER+, HER2- breast cancer.[47] In addition, little is known about the effect of NET on HR+ disease that is also HER2+, because most NET trials have been limited to individuals with ER+/HER2- disease. There were some women with this subtype included in both the aforementioned IMPACT and ASCOG Z1031 trials, and in both, AIs yielded slightly better response rates than tamoxifen among patients with HR+, HER2+ disease.[42,43]

During neoadjuvant therapy, patients should be followed with regular clinical breast examinations to monitor response. Imaging may be obtained at the treating physicians' discretion and should be the same modality as baseline pretreatment imaging.[48] The early months of the coronavirus disease 2019 pandemic saw increased neoadjuvant therapy use, largely in response to the Society of Surgical Oncology and the American Society of Breast Surgeons recommending 3 to 6 months of NET in women with early-stage HR+/HER2-breast cancer and NACT in TNBC or HER2+ breast cancer instead of upfront surgery.[49,50] The rapid but heterogeneous adoption of these recommendations has provided an unprecedented opportunity to observe and analyze adherence, outcomes, and side effects for previously underutilized neoadjuvant care pathways. Between pandemic-related natural history studies and upcoming trials aimed at risk stratifying premenopausal women with HR+ disease, the next decade holds promise for expanding our understanding of how best to use NACT and NET among diverse women with breast cancer.

Management of the Axilla

Since the era of the Halstead radical mastectomy, surgery of the breast has been de-escalated to simple mastectomy and, for eligible patients, BCT. Similarly, there has been increased movement toward de-escalating locoregional treatment of the axilla.

Axillary surgery is performed to optimize control of regional disease and to stage the axilla, thereby providing information to guide adjuvant therapy and inform prognosis. In the 1990s and 2000s, significant progress was made in decreasing unnecessary ALNDs and their associated morbidity. The NSABP B-32 trial randomized women with clinically node-negative invasive breast cancer to SLNB and ALND or SLNB alone. The SLNB false-negative rate (FNR) was 9.8%. At 8-year follow-up, there was no significant difference in survival (91.8% ALND vs 90.3% SLNB) or regional recurrence (0.4% ALND vs 0.7% SLNB). However, ALND had nearly twice the rate of lymphedema (14%) as SLNB (8%).[51] This trial proved that SLNB is as safe and effective as ALND in staging the axilla in patients with clinically node-negative disease.

ACOSOG Z0011 built upon the findings of NSABP B-32 and examined whether women with 1 or 2 positive sentinel lymph nodes (SLNs) needed to undergo completion ALND. Women undergoing BCT with cT1-T2, cN0 invasive tumors but found to have 1 or 2 positive SLNs on final surgical pathologic review were randomized to ALND or no further surgery.[52] At 10-year follow-up, neither the cumulative incidence of nodal recurrences (0.5% ALND vs 1.5% SLNB)[53] nor overall survival (83.6% ALND vs 86.3% SLNB) was significantly different.[54] Notably, most patients in both groups received some form of systemic therapy and whole-breast radiation. Furthermore, 27% of patients in the ALND group had additional positive nodes in the final tissue sample. Given the randomized study design and presumed balance between the groups, this finding suggests that there were similar levels of unresected nodal disease among patients who underwent SLNB alone, but this residual tumor did not adversely impact recurrence or survival.[52] Consistent with these findings, in ACOSOG Z0010, which included patients with cT1-2, cN0 invasive tumor, occult micrometastases were found in 10.5% of SLNB specimens, but this level of involvement had no impact on survival.[55] Similarly, the International Breast Cancer Study Group (IBCSG) 23-01 trial randomized patients with one or more micrometastatic ($\leq$2 mm) SLNs to ALND or no ALND. Ten-year survival was not significantly different between the 2 arms (74.9% in ALND vs 76.8% in no ALND). As seen in prior studies, the lymphedema rate was higher (13%) among ALND recipients versus nonrecipients (6%).[56]

Z0011 examined whether additional axillary surgery is necessary when patients are found to have positive SLNs, whereas the AMAROS trial sought to determine whether positive SLNs can be as effectively treated with radiation alone as opposed to ALND. Women with cT1-2, cN0 tumors undergoing BCT or mastectomy who had a positive SLN were randomized to ALND or ART. At 5 years posttreatment, there was no significant difference in axillary recurrence (0.43% ALND vs 1.19% ART) or overall survival (93.3% ALND vs 92.5% ART). However, clinical signs of lymphedema were more common after ALND (23%) than after radiation (11%).[57] Thus, these trials support the current practice of performing SLNB in women with cN0 disease and of not routinely recommending further axillary surgery if they have less than 3 positive SLNs.

Axillary management in the context of neoadjuvant therapy is controversial. It remains unclear whether to treat patients based on clinical stage at presentation (cTN) or on their clinical (ycTN) and/or pathologic (ypTN) stages following neoadjuvant treatment. There are 3 main groups of patients who warrant nuanced consideration with regard to surgical management of the axilla after NST: (1) those who are clinically node-negative (cN0) before and remain node-negative after NST, (2) those who are clinically node-positive with low burden of disease (cN1) who remain so after NST (ie, ycN1), and (3) those who present with cN1 disease but become node-negative (ie, ycN0) after NST. Significant axillary downstage is uncommon after NET, thus incorporating axillary response after NST into surgical decision making is most relevant for those undergoing NACT. For patients who are cN0 before and after NACT, SLNB is appropriate. If SLNB is negative, then no further surgery is needed. If it is positive, ALND remains standard of care. Notably, these patients are *not* analogous to patients who are cN0 with positive SLNs in Z0011 and AMAROS because ypN1 disease in a patient who is cN0 suggests either previously undiagnosed, chemoresistant disease or new disease that developed while on treatment.[58] For patients who have nodal disease before NACT and remain node-positive after, ALND is standard of care.[59]

The greatest controversy surrounds those who are cN1 at presentation but downstage by imaging and examination to ycN0. Several trials were developed to determine whether SLN mapping was possible and reliable after NACT for cN1 disease. The SENTINA trial in Europe examined the accuracy of SLNB in patients who were cN1 after NACT and had 4 study arms, 2 for patients who were cN0 (arms A and B) and 2 for patients who were cN1 (arms C and D). After NACT, patients who were cN1 were clinically restaged as ycN0 (arm C) or ycN1 (arm D), with the former undergoing SLNB and ALND whereas the patients who were ycN1 went straight to ALND. In arm C, the SLN detection rate was 80% and overall FNR was 14.2%, with rates decreasing to 8.6% with use of dual tracer (blue dye and radiocolloid) mapping and to 7.3% when at least 3 nodes were retrieved.[60] ACOSOG (Alliance) Z1071 trial exhibited a 90% detection rate and 12.6% FNR. The latter decreased to 10.8% with dual tracer mapping and 9.1% when 3 or more nodes were identified.[61] Finally, in the SN-FNAC (Sentinel Node Biopsy Following Neoadjuvant Chemotherapy in Biopsy Proven Node Positive Breast Cancer) trial, the node detection rate was 87.6%, and the FNR was 8.4%.[62]

To assess whether the FNRs from Z1071, SENTINA, and SN-FNAC could be improved, MD Anderson created a registry for targeted axillary dissection (TAD), which is the post-NACT identification and removal of both any SLNs identified via dual tracer mapping and any lymph nodes clipped and biopsied before NACT. To facilitate TAD, the clipped node was localized with an I-125 impregnated seed immediately before surgery. It was observed that the clipped node was not the sentinel node in 23% of patients. In patients undergoing SLNB alone, the FNR was 10.1%, but adding the clipped node decreased the FNR to 1.4%.[63] If the SLNBs and/or previously clipped node are positive, ALND is recommended.[59] TAD is increasingly being used in practice, but long-term data on post-TAD outcomes are sparse.

There are 2 large ongoing clinical trials exploring the role of radiation in patients who are cN1 who had NACT and have a positive SLNB. The Alliance A11202 is randomizing women with positive SLNB after NACT to ALND or ART and measuring recurrence-free and overall survival. At the same time, NRG Oncology NSABP B-51 (also known as Radiation Therapy Oncology Group [RTOG] 1304) is a companion trial in which patients who are cN1 found to be ypN0 on post-NACT SLNB are randomized to undergo or forego nodal radiation with the primary outcome being invasive breast cancer recurrence-free interval.[64]

There has also been a move toward de-escalating axillary treatment of elderly patients with early-stage, nonaggressive breast cancer, potentially omitting SLNB in some. IBCSG 10-93 randomized women older than 60 years with cN0, HR+ cancer to breast surgery and axillary clearance (SLNB and ALND) or breast surgery alone. At 6-year follow-up, there were no significant differences in overall survival (75% axillary surgery vs 73% no axillary surgery) or axillary recurrences (2 axillary recurrences in the axillary surgery group and 3 in the no axillary surgery group).[65] Another randomized trial of elderly patients older than 70 years undergoing breast surgery with or without ALND found a 15-year recurrence rate of only 5.8% in the no axillary surgery group and no significant difference in mortality (14% in no ALND vs 13.6% in ALND), although more patients in the ALND group had received radiation.[66] It is also important to note that women in all these trials were taking adjuvant endocrine therapy. Nevertheless, despite these findings, and even Choosing Wisely recommendations that SLNB can be safely omitted in elderly women with early-stage cN0 breast cancer, a recent analysis demonstrated that 91% of patients with early-stage breast cancer older than 65 years have undergone some sort of axillary surgery.[67]

In summary, there is evidence to suggest that ALND may be omitted in select node-positive patients after NACT and safely omitted among elderly women with low-risk in-breast disease.

SUMMARY

In conclusion, use of CPM, indications for NST, and surgical management of the axilla represent areas of current debate and active research. Although much of breast surgical oncology is moving toward de-escalating surgical care both in the breast and the axilla, particularly with the use of NST, CPM represents an area of potential overuse despite unclear benefit for many recipients. Future research should focus on delineating the populations in whom CPM and de-escalation of locoregional treatment are most appropriate and on exploring NET as a less toxic but potentially comparable alternative to NACT in some women with breast cancer.

CLINICS CARE POINTS

- CPM confers no survival advantage and has increased risk of complications but may be appropriate in some high-risk individuals. Appropriate counseling and SDM is encouraged.
- NACT can be used to improve candidacy for BCT, downstage the axilla, and prevent distant metastases in locally advanced, inflammatory, HER2+, and TNBCs.
- NET is an effective, less toxic but currently underutilized alternative to NACT for postmenopausal women with ER+ breast cancers who wish to improve candidacy for BCT.

- Clinically node-positive patients who become clinically node-negative after NACT are eligible for SLNB. Use of dual tracer mapping, retrieval of at least 3 lymph nodes, and identification of the previously biopsied node significantly decrease the FNRs of post-NACT axillary staging. If SLNB, or, ideally, TAD, is negative, ALND can be omitted. If SLNB is positive, proceed to ALND.

DISCLOSURE

The authors have no relevant conflicts of interest to disclose.

REFERENCES

1. Lauby-Secretan B, Scoccianti C, Loomis D, et al. Breast-cancer screening–viewpoint of the IARC Working Group. N Engl J Med 2015;372(24):2353–8.
2. Chen L, Li CI. Racial disparities in breast cancer diagnosis and treatment by hormone receptor and HER2 status. Cancer Epidemiol Biomarkers Prev 2015; 24(11):1666–72.
3. Ahmed AT, Welch BT, Brinjikji W, et al. Racial disparities in screening mammography in the united states: a systematic review and meta-analysis. J Am Coll Radiol 2017;14(2):157–165 e159.
4. Hayes DF. HER2 and breast cancer—a phenomenal success story. N Engl J Med 2019;381(13):1284–6.
5. Mougalian SS, Soulos PR, Killelea BK, et al. Use of neoadjuvant chemotherapy for patients with stage I to III breast cancer in the United States. Cancer 2015; 121(15):2544–52.
6. Yao K, Sisco M, Bedrosian I. Contralateral prophylactic mastectomy: current perspectives. Int J Womens Health 2016;8:213–23.
7. Christian N, Zabor EC, Cassidy M, et al. Contralateral prophylactic mastectomy use after neoadjuvant chemotherapy. Ann Surg Oncol 2020;27(3):743–9.
8. Amir E, Freedman OC, Seruga B, et al. Assessing women at high risk of breast cancer: a review of risk assessment models. J Natl Cancer Inst 2010;102(10): 680–91.
9. Nichols HB, Berrington de Gonzalez A, Lacey JV Jr, et al. Declining incidence of contralateral breast cancer in the United States from 1975 to 2006. J Clin Oncol 2011;29(12):1564–9.
10. Ager B, Butow P, Jansen J, et al. Contralateral prophylactic mastectomy (CPM): a systematic review of patient reported factors and psychological predictors influencing choice and satisfaction. Breast 2016;28:107–20.
11. Hunt KK, Euhus DM, Boughey JC, et al. Society of surgical oncology breast disease working group statement on prophylactic (Risk-Reducing) mastectomy. Ann Surg Oncol 2017;24(2):375–97.
12. Kruper L, Kauffmann RM, Smith DD, et al. Survival analysis of contralateral prophylactic mastectomy: a question of selection bias. Ann Surg Oncol 2014; 21(11):3448–56.
13. Yao K, Stewart AK, Winchester DJ, et al. Trends in contralateral prophylactic mastectomy for unilateral cancer: a report from the National Cancer Data Base, 1998-2007. Ann Surg Oncol 2010;17(10):2554–62.
14. Wong SM, Freedman RA, Sagara Y, et al. Growing use of contralateral prophylactic mastectomy despite no improvement in long-term survival for invasive breast cancer. Ann Surg 2017;265(3):581–9.

15. Carbine NE, Lostumbo L, Wallace J, et al. Risk-reducing mastectomy for the prevention of primary breast cancer. Cochrane Database Syst Rev 2018;4: CD002748.
16. Nash R, Goodman M, Lin CC, et al. State variation in the receipt of a contralateral prophylactic mastectomy among women who received a diagnosis of invasive unilateral early-stage breast cancer in the United States, 2004-2012. JAMA Surg 2017;152(7):648–57.
17. Fairbairn K, Cervantes A, Rayhrer C, et al. Trends in contralateral prophylactic mastectomy. Aesthet Plast Surg 2020;44(2):323–9.
18. Tracy MS, Rosenberg SM, Dominici L, et al. Contralateral prophylactic mastectomy in women with breast cancer: trends, predictors, and areas for future research. Breast Cancer Res Treat 2013;140(3):447–52.
19. Mota BS, Riera R, Ricci MD, et al. Nipple- and areola-sparing mastectomy for the treatment of breast cancer. Cochrane database Syst Rev 2016;11:CD008932.
20. Elmore LC, Dietz JR, Myckatyn TM, et al. The landmark series: mastectomy trials (skin-sparing and nipple-sparing and reconstruction landmark trials). Ann Surg Oncol 2021;28(1):273–80.
21. Hawley S, Jagsi R, Morrow M, et al. Correlates of contralateral prophylactic mastectomy in a population-based sample. J Clin Oncol 2011;29(15_suppl):6010.
22. Plastic Surgery Statistics Report. American Society of Plastic Surgeons 2018. https://www.plasticsurgery.org/documents/News/Statistics/2018/plastic-surgery-statistics-full-report-2018.pdf. Accessed 28 February, 2021.
23. Sanati-Mehrizy P, Massenburg BB, Rozehnal JM, et al. A comparison of postoperative outcomes in immediate versus delayed reconstruction after mastectomy. Eplasty 2015;15:e44.
24. Yoon AP, Qi J, Brown DL, et al. Outcomes of immediate versus delayed breast reconstruction: results of a multicenter prospective study. Breast 2018;37:72–9.
25. Al-Ghazal S, Sully L, Fallowfield L, et al. The psychological impact of immediate rather than delayed breast reconstruction. Eur J Surg Oncol 2000;26(1):17–9.
26. Elkowitz A, Colen S, Slavin S, et al. Various methods of breast reconstruction after mastectomy: an economic comparison. Plast Reconstr Surg 1993;92(1):77–83.
27. Doren EL, Miranda RN, Selber JC, et al. US epidemiology of breast implant–associated anaplastic large cell lymphoma. Plast Reconstr Surg 2017;139(5): 1042–50.
28. Serletti JM, Fosnot J, Nelson JA, et al. Breast reconstruction after breast cancer. Plast Reconstr Surg 2011;127(6):124e–35e.
29. Toyserkani NM, Jørgensen MG, Tabatabaeifar S, et al. Autologous versus implant-based breast reconstruction: a systematic review and meta-analysis of Breast-Q patient-reported outcomes. J Plast Reconstr Aesthet Surg 2020;73(2): 278–85.
30. Rubens RD, Sexton S, Tong D, et al. Combined chemotherapy and radiotherapy for locally advanced breast cancer. Eur J Cancer 1980;16(3):351–6.
31. Rastogi P, Anderson SJ, Bear HD, et al. Preoperative chemotherapy: updates of national surgical adjuvant breast and bowel project protocols B-18 and B-27. J Clin Oncol 2008;26(5):778–85.
32. Long-term outcomes for neoadjuvant versus adjuvant chemotherapy in early breast cancer: meta-analysis of individual patient data from ten randomised trials. Lancet Oncol 2018;19(1):27–39.
33. Cortazar P, Zhang L, Untch M, et al. Pathological complete response and long-term clinical benefit in breast cancer: the CTNeoBC pooled analysis. Lancet 2014;384(9938):164–72.

34. Fayanju OM, Ren Y, Thomas SM, et al. The clinical significance of breast-only and node-only pathologic complete response (pCR) after neoadjuvant chemotherapy (NACT): a review of 20,000 breast cancer patients in the national cancer data base (NCDB). Ann Surg 2018;268(4):591–601.

35. van der Hage JH, van de Velde CC, Mieog SJ. Preoperative chemotherapy for women with operable breast cancer. Cochrane Database Syst Rev 2007;(2):CD005002.

36. Prakash I, Thomas SM, Greenup RA, et al. Time to surgery among women treated with neoadjuvant systemic therapy and upfront surgery for breast cancer. Breast Cancer Res Treat 2020;186(2):535–50.

37. Caudle AS, Gonzalez-Angulo AM, Hunt KK, et al. Predictors of tumor progression during neoadjuvant chemotherapy in breast cancer. J Clin Oncol 2010;28(11): 1821–8.

38. von Minckwitz G, Huang CS, Mano MS, et al. Trastuzumab emtansine for residual invasive HER2-positive breast cancer. N Engl J Med 2019;380(7):617–28.

39. Spring LM, Gupta A, Reynolds KL, et al. Neoadjuvant endocrine therapy for estrogen receptor-positive breast cancer: a systematic review and meta-analysis. JAMA Oncol 2016;2(11):1477–86.

40. Weiss A, Wong S, Golshan M, et al. Patterns of axillary management in stages 2 and 3 hormone receptor-positive breast cancer by initial treatment approach. Ann Surg Oncol 2019;26(13):4326–36.

41. Ellis MJ, Coop A, Singh B, et al. Letrozole is more effective neoadjuvant endocrine therapy than tamoxifen for ErbB-1- and/or ErbB-2-positive, estrogen receptor-positive primary breast cancer: evidence from a phase III randomized trial. J Clin Oncol 2001;19(18):3808–16.

42. Smith IE, Dowsett M, Ebbs SR, et al. Neoadjuvant treatment of postmenopausal breast cancer with anastrozole, tamoxifen, or both in combination: the Immediate Preoperative Anastrozole, Tamoxifen, or Combined with Tamoxifen (IMPACT) multicenter double-blind randomized trial. J Clin Oncol 2005;23(22):5108–16.

43. Ellis MJ, Suman VJ, Hoog J, et al. Randomized phase II neoadjuvant comparison between letrozole, anastrozole, and exemestane for postmenopausal women with estrogen receptor-rich stage 2 to 3 breast cancer: clinical and biomarker outcomes and predictive value of the baseline PAM50-based intrinsic subtype–ACOSOG Z1031. J Clin Oncol 2011;29(17):2342–9.

44. Hojo T, Kinoshita T, Imoto S, et al. Use of the neo-adjuvant exemestane in postmenopausal estrogen receptor-positive breast cancer: a randomized phase II trial (PTEX46) to investigate the optimal duration of preoperative endocrine therapy. Breast 2013;22(3):263–7.

45. Grossman J, Ma C, Aft R. Neoadjuvant endocrine therapy: who benefits most? Surg Oncol Clin N Am 2018;27(1):121–40.

46. Masuda N, Sagara Y, Kinoshita T, et al. Neoadjuvant anastrozole versus tamoxifen in patients receiving goserelin for premenopausal breast cancer (STAGE): a double-blind, randomised phase 3 trial. Lancet Oncol 2012;13(4):345–52.

47. Ma CX, Suman VJ, Leitch AM, et al. ALTERNATE: neoadjuvant endocrine treatment (NET) approaches for clinical stage II or III estrogen receptor-positive HER2-negative breast cancer (ER+ HER2- BC) in postmenopausal (PM) women: alliance A011106. J Clin Oncol 2020;38(15_suppl):504.

48. Korde LA, Somerfield MR, Carey LA, et al. Neoadjuvant chemotherapy, endocrine therapy, and targeted therapy for breast cancer: ASCO guideline. J Clin Oncol 2021;39(13):1485–505.

49. Resource for management options of breast cancer during COVID-19. Available at: https://www.surgonc.org/wp-content/uploads/2020/03/Breast-Resource-during-COVID-19-3.30.20.pdf. Accessed December 20, 2021.

50. Dietz JR, Moran MS, Isakoff SJ, et al. Recommendations for prioritization, treatment, and triage of breast cancer patients during the COVID-19 pandemic. the COVID-19 pandemic breast cancer consortium. Breast Cancer Res Treat 2020; 181(3):487–97.

51. Krag DN, Anderson SJ, Julian TB, et al. Sentinel-lymph-node resection compared with conventional axillary-lymph-node dissection in clinically node-negative patients with breast cancer: overall survival findings from the NSABP B-32 randomised phase 3 trial. Lancet Oncol 2010;11(10):927–33.

52. Giuliano AE, Hunt KK, Ballman KV, et al. Axillary dissection vs no axillary dissection in women with invasive breast cancer and sentinel node metastasis: a randomized clinical trial. JAMA 2011;305(6):569–75.

53. Giuliano AE, Ballman K, McCall L, et al. Locoregional recurrence after sentinel lymph node dissection with or without axillary dissection in patients with sentinel lymph node metastases: long-term follow-up from the American College of Surgeons Oncology Group (Alliance) ACOSOG Z0011 randomized trial. Ann Surg 2016;264(3):413–20.

54. Giuliano AE, Ballman KV, McCall L, et al. Effect of axillary dissection vs no axillary dissection on 10-year overall survival among women with invasive breast cancer and sentinel node metastasis: the ACOSOG Z0011 (Alliance) randomized clinical trial. JAMA 2017;318(10):918–26.

55. Giuliano AE, Hawes D, Ballman KV, et al. Association of occult metastases in sentinel lymph nodes and bone marrow with survival among women with early-stage invasive breast cancer. JAMA 2011;306(4):385–93.

56. Galimberti V, Cole BF, Viale G, et al. Axillary dissection versus no axillary dissection in patients with breast cancer and sentinel-node micrometastases (IBCSG 23-01): 10-year follow-up of a randomised, controlled phase 3 trial. Lancet Oncol 2018;19(10):1385–93.

57. Donker M, van Tienhoven G, Straver ME, et al. Radiotherapy or surgery of the axilla after a positive sentinel node in breast cancer (EORTC 10981-22023 AMAROS): a randomised, multicentre, open-label, phase 3 non-inferiority trial. Lancet Oncol 2014;15(12):1303–10.

58. Esposito E, Di Micco R, Gentilini OD. Sentinel node biopsy in early breast cancer. A review on recent and ongoing randomized trials. Breast 2017;36:14–9.

59. Telli ML, Gradishar WJ, Ward JH. NCCN guidelines updates: breast cancer. J Natl Compr Cancer Netw 2019;17(5):552–5.

60. Kuehn T, Bauerfeind I, Fehm T, et al. Sentinel-lymph-node biopsy in patients with breast cancer before and after neoadjuvant chemotherapy (SENTINA): a prospective, multicentre cohort study. Lancet Oncol 2013;14(7):609–18.

61. Boughey JC, Suman VJ, Mittendorf EA, et al. Sentinel lymph node surgery after neoadjuvant chemotherapy in patients with node-positive breast cancer: the ACOSOG Z1071 (Alliance) clinical trial. JAMA 2013;310(14):1455–61.

62. Boileau JF, Poirier B, Basik M, et al. Sentinel node biopsy after neoadjuvant chemotherapy in biopsy-proven node-positive breast cancer: the SN FNAC study. J Clin Oncol 2015;33(3):258–64.

63. Caudle AS, Yang WT, Krishnamurthy S, et al. Improved axillary evaluation following neoadjuvant therapy for patients with node-positive breast cancer using selective evaluation of clipped nodes: implementation of targeted axillary dissection. J Clin Oncol 2016;34(10):1072–8.

64. Mamounas EP, Bandos H, White JR, et al. NRG Oncology/NSABP B-51/RTOG 1304: phase III trial to determine if chest wall and regional nodal radiotherapy (CWRNRT) post mastectomy (Mx) or the addition of RNRT to whole breast RT post breast-conserving surgery (BCS) reduces invasive breast cancer recurrence-free interval (IBCR-FI) in patients (pts) with pathologically positive axillary (PPAx) nodes who are ypN0 after neoadjuvant chemotherapy (NC). J Clin Oncol 2019;37(15_suppl):TPS600.

65. Rudenstam CM, Zahrieh D, Forbes JF, et al. Randomized trial comparing axillary clearance versus no axillary clearance in older patients with breast cancer: first results of International Breast Cancer Study Group Trial 10-93. J Clin Oncol 2006;24(3):337–44.

66. Martelli G, Miceli R, Daidone MG, et al. Axillary dissection versus no axillary dissection in elderly patients with breast cancer and no palpable axillary nodes: results after 15 years of follow-up. Ann Surg Oncol 2011;18(1):125–33.

67. Dominici LS, Sineshaw HM, Jemal A, et al. Patterns of axillary evaluation in older patients with breast cancer and associations with adjuvant therapy receipt. Breast Cancer Res Treat 2018;167(2):555–66.

Small Bowel Obstruction in the Virgin Abdomen

Sarah Baker, MD[a], Kimberly Miller-Hammond, MD[b], Erin King-Mullins, MD[a],*

KEYWORDS

- Small bowel obstruction • General surgery • Virgin abdomen • Interval laparoscopy

INTRODUCTION

Small bowel obstruction (SBO) is one the most common clinical diagnoses general surgeons will encounter during their career. Despite there being no other obvious clinical or radiographic cause for the obstruction, most surgeons feel very comfortable nonoperatively managing this common condition in the typical patient who has had previous abdominal or pelvic surgery, knowing that the etiology is most frequently due to postsurgical adhesions. SBO in the virgin abdomen (one without prior abdominopelvic surgery), however, has long been a controversial and perplexing topic among general surgeons, and there is no standard of care in regard to the evaluation and management of these patients. We present a review of the current literature and controversies surrounding this less frequently encountered patient population, and then will finish with a series of case presentations.

INCIDENCE

There are approximately 300,000 inpatient admissions for SBO annually in the United States, with the large majority of these being related to adhesions from prior surgery (approximately 70%).[1] Around 4.6% of patients with a history of abdominopelvic surgery develop an SBO, and the risk can vary widely depending on the type and technique of the surgical procedure, with the highest rates seen after open colectomy and pelvic surgery. Barmparas and colleagues[2] found the highest incidence of adhesive SBO to be in patients who have undergone ileal pouch–anal anastomosis at 19.3%. A study by Collom and colleagues[3] looked at the administration of diatrizoate (Gastrografin) in decreasing the need for operative management and compared this in patients who did and did not have a history of prior abdominal surgery. A total of 601 patients were included in their study, 500 with prior abdominal surgery and 101 without. This study demonstrated that 16.8% of the patients in this study had no prior history of abdominal surgery, 8.9% had a prior SBO admission, and 38.6% overall

[a] Georgia Colon and Rectal Surgical Associates, Northside Hospital, 5445 Meridian Mark Road, Suite 180, Atlanta, GA 30342, USA; [b] Atlanta Surgery Associates, 1430 Peachtree Street Suite 1430, Atlanta, GA 30308, USA
* Corresponding author.
E-mail address: erin.king@northside.com

Surg Clin N Am 101 (2021) 1045–1052
https://doi.org/10.1016/j.suc.2021.06.003
0039-6109/21/© 2021 Elsevier Inc. All rights reserved.

surgical.theclinics.com

required operative exploration.[3] This study found that both patients with and without prior abdominal surgery who received diatrizoate had a significantly lower rate of operative intervention.

CAUSES

Although the majority of evidence is low quality, recent studies have shown that a very significant percentage of SBO in patients with no prior abdominopelvic surgery have a benign etiology. Approximately 60% of cases have been found to be due to congenital de novo or inflammatory adhesions, with the next most common cause being hernia. Less common causes of SBO in the virgin abdomen include metastatic disease, Crohn's disease, foreign body obstructions, gallstone ileus, Meckel's diverticulum, internal hernia, volvulus, endometriosis, and sclerosing encapsulating peritonitis.[2,4] Several small retrospective studies have shown the risk of having an undiagnosed malignancy as the cause of SBO in patients without prior abdominopelvic surgery to be approximately 10% to 13%.[1,4–6]

APPROACH AND THRESHOLD FOR URGENT SURGERY

A methodical, common sense approach with good clinical judgment based on experience will likely guide the clinician to successful, appropriate care, while keeping in mind certain considerations. Most important, the indications for urgent surgery are similar to any patient who presents with an acute abdomen and findings of SBO warranting immediate exploration: concern for bowel ischemia or strangulation, incarcerated hernia, closed loop obstruction, pneumatosis intestinalis, pneumoperitoneum, and/or clinical findings consistent with peritonitis. Decisions on surgical technique should incorporate the patient's clinical status, physical examination, radiographic findings, and the expertise of the surgeon.

Worth noting is that at least 2 studies have shown diatrizoate challenge to be safe in patients without prior surgical history. The previously referenced study by Collom and colleagues[3] showed that the use of diatrizoate decreased the need for surgical intervention in patients admitted with SBO without prior surgical history from 50% to 17%. In general, the trend for management of patients with or without prior abdominal surgery tends to rely on good clinical judgment, patient history, and radiographic findings. Definitive indications for immediate operative intervention are unchanged, and high clinical suspicion should always be maintained in patients with any history of malignancy or findings suspicious for malignancy on computed tomography scans.

A study out of the Mayo Clinic by Stragina and colleagues specifically looked at patients admitted with SBO in a virgin abdomen while excluding patients with indications for urgent surgery.[1] A total of 60 patients were included, and 8 (13%) were ultimately diagnosed with a malignancy. Fifty patients (83%) underwent operative exploration and 10 patients (17%) were managed nonoperatively. Twenty patients (40%) in the operative group had a negative exploration, with no recent weight loss and leukocytosis being associated with negative findings at surgery ($P = .04$). Upon retrospective review, 3 of the 8 patients ultimately diagnosed with malignancy had signs visible on initial imaging, leading to their conclusion, which emphasizes that patients with malignant SBO had either imaging or clinical clues, which should have led to their malignancy diagnosis. Therefore, a high index of suspicion should be maintained when reviewing patient history and computed tomography imaging findings.

NEED FOR INTERVAL LAPAROSCOPY

There is no universally agreed upon algorithm or indication for interval laparoscopy or surgical intervention, however, some populations have been considered to be at higher risk compared with others on recent studies. There are no randomized controlled trials available to indicate the safety of forgoing operative intervention, or the timing in which operative intervention should occur. A systematic review and meta-analysis by Choi and colleagues[5] published in 2020 found the prevalence of malignancy ranged from 7.7% to 13.4% (95% confidence interval, 7.6–20.3) on sensitivity analysis.[4] This percentage indicates the risk of having an undiagnosed malignancy in patients who do not ultimately undergo further diagnostic work-up or surgical intervention. In this study, of the 442 patients ultimately included in the analysis, 225 (59%) were managed nonoperatively. A particular point of interest in the study is that patients found to have a malignant etiology were more likely to have reported a previous admission for bowel obstruction (40% compared with 10% nonmalignant).

The aforementioned retrospective review by Stragina and colleagues identified 60 patients over a 10-year period who were classified as having an acute SBO and no previous history of abdominopelvic surgery.[1] Ten patients were managed nonoperatively, almost one-half (29) underwent therapeutic exploration, and one-third (20) underwent negative exploration. One patient underwent a nontherapeutic exploration as carcinomatosis was identified. All who underwent exploration did so during the same admission. The most common etiologies for the SBO in the therapeutic group were adhesive disease, stricture, and malignancy (**Fig. 1**). Of the patients who had a negative exploration, 3 developed a recurrent SBO. For these patients, a small bowel

		n = 60
Non-operative		**10**
	colon cancer	1
	endometriosis	1
	NSAID related stricture	1
Therapeutic exploration		**29**
	adhesions	
	stricture	
	malignancy	
Non-therapeutic exploration (carcinomatosis)		**1**
Negative Exploration		**20**
	recurrent SBO	**3**

Fig. 1. Patients presenting with an SBO. (*From* Choi J, Fisher AT, Mulaney B, Anand A, Carlos G, Stave CD, Spain DA, Weiser TG. Safety of Foregoing Operation for Small Bowel Obstruction in the Virgin Abdomen: Systematic Review and Meta-Analysis. J Am Coll Surg. 2020 Sep;231(3):368-375.e1. https://doi.org/10.1016/j.jamcollsurg.2020.06.010. Epub 2020 Jun 20. PMID: 32574687.)

neuroendocrine tumor was ultimately identified in one, another required laparotomy 2 years later for adhesive disease, and the last recurred at 3 years and was also managed nonoperatively. Finally, of the 10 who did not undergo surgery at initial presentation, a transverse colon cancer was identified in one patient on outpatient colonoscopy 3 months later, another required a small bowel resection owing to endometriosis, and another required resection of a stricture associated with prolonged NSAID use. Overall 8 of the 60 included patients (13.3%) were diagnosed with a malignant SBO, which is consistent with other studies that have been conducted.[1]

To answer the question regarding the role of interval laparoscopy, more long-term cohort studies would be needed to truly understand the natural history of this disease. In general, there must be adequate communication between surgeon and radiologist to paint a clearer clinical picture, and elucidate any findings that would implicate the culprit of the obstruction. Although it is clear immediate surgery is not always necessary in the absence of acute surgical indications (peritonitis, ischemia, closed loop obstruction, hemodynamic instability), the case can be made that surgical intervention should be a part of the diagnostic armamentarium. The authors have provided their algorithm for evaluation and management in **Fig. 2**.

Case Presentations

Case 1

A 66 year-old woman with history of bipolar schizophrenia presents with 3 days of constipation and obstipation per caregiver. Computed tomography scans (**Figs. 3** and **4**) demonstrate SBO with transition point in mid small bowel anterior upper pelvis and was reported as low-grade distal jejunal SBO. The patient has audible gas upon evaluation. A diatrizoate small bowel series is negative for obstruction. Bowel function resumes after diatrizoate challenge. Reportedly the patient had a previous admission for obstruction 4 to 5 years prior, which was also managed nonoperatively. She has a

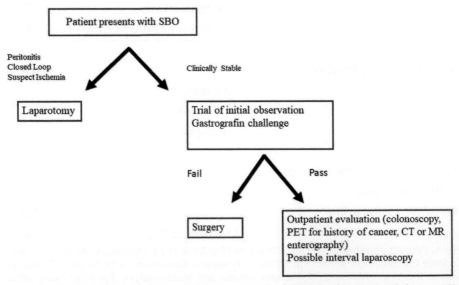

Fig. 2. Algorithm for evaluation and management of SBO in the virgin abdomen. CT, computed tomography.

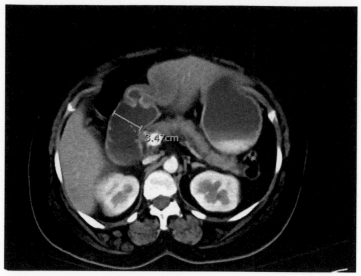

Fig. 3. Axial imaging demonstrating dilation up to 3.47 cm.

remote history of breast cancer and no evidence of recurrence or metastatic disease on her current surveillance regimen.

Case 2

A 55-year-old woman presents with 4 days of constipation, minimal flatus, nausea, vomiting, and epigastric pain. She has no previous history of abdominopelvic surgery.

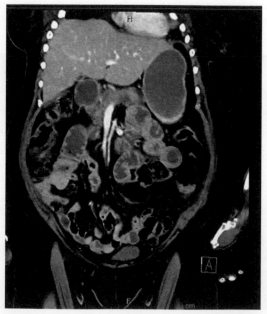

Fig. 4. Coronal imaging demonstrating transition point in right pelvis.

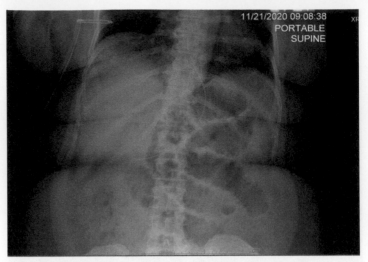

Fig. 5. Abdominal radiograph consistent with an SBO.

A computed tomography scan demonstrates high-grade mid-SBO with transition point in the lower pelvis. Patient desired to avoid surgery therefore a nasogastric tube was placed. Abdominal plain films (**Fig. 5**) showed no improvement over 2 days. At abdominal exploration inflammatory bands were identified in the pelvis without bowel compromise.

Case 3
A 62-year-old man presents with several hours of persistent abdominal pain. The patient reports similar episodic pains for 6 months. A computed tomography scan (**Fig. 6**) reveals a swirled appearance of the small bowel mesentery, concerning for a mid-gut

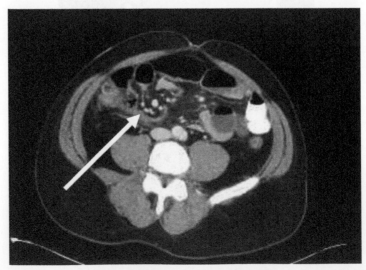

Fig. 6. Computed tomography scan demonstrating whirling of the mesentery (*white arrow*).

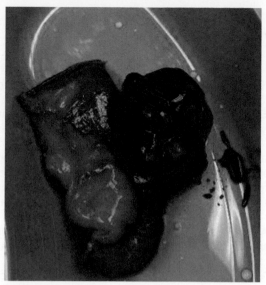

Fig. 7. Exophytic mass of the small bowel, a gastrointestinal stromal tumor. (Photo courtesy of Michael Hoffman, MD, FACS.)

volvulus. A diagnostic laparoscopy was performed demonstrating an exophytic mass of the small bowel (**Fig. 7**) necessitating a small bowel resection. Pathology consistent with a gastrointestinal stromal tumor.

SUMMARY

Of the 300,000 patients who present annually with an SBO, the overwhelming majority of them will have a history of previous abdominopelvic surgery. In considering the management and treatment of these patients, the first priority is determining if there is a need for urgent surgery. Here, standard rules apply—an acute surgical abdomen requires acute surgical intervention. Beyond the determination of treatment at initial presentation, keen clinical judgment is necessary to continue the diagnostic process concurrent with management to determine definitive therapeutic options.

CLINICS CARE POINTS

- SBO in the virgin abdomen remains a controversial topic and currently there is no standard of care regarding evaluation and management.

- Recent studies have shown that a large number of these patients have benign etiologies and may be managed nonoperatively, contrary to previous surgical dogma.

- The indications for urgent surgical exploration remain unchanged from those in patients with a history of prior abdominopelvic surgery.

- The rate of malignancy is 10% to 13% in patients presenting with SBO and no previous history of abdominopelvic surgery. Imaging should be thoroughly examined for any subtle findings concerning for malignancy. Short-term follow-up should be implemented in patients managed nonoperatively, including consideration for adjunct diagnostic studies such as colonoscopy and even diagnostic laparoscopy.

DISCLOSURE

The authors have no relevant financial or other disclosures.

REFERENCES

1. Stragina V, Kim B, Zielinski M. Small bowel obstruction in the virgin abdomen. Am J Surg 2019;218:521–6.
2. Barmparas G, Branco BC, Schnüriger B, et al. The incidence and risk factors of post-laparotomy adhesive small bowel obstruction. J Gastrointest Surg 2010;14: 1619–28.
3. Collom ML, Duane TM, Campbell-Furtick M, et al. Deconstructing dogma: nonoperative management of small bowel obstruction in the virgin abdomen. J Trauma Acute Care Surg 2018;85:33e36.
4. Bower KL, Lollar DI, Williams SL, et al. Small bowel obstruction. Surg Clin North Am 2018;98(5):945–71.
5. Choi J, Fisher AT, Mulaney B, et al. Safety of foregoing operation for small bowel obstruction in the virgin abdomen: systematic review and meta-analysis. J Am Coll Surg 2020;231(3):368–75.e1.
6. Beardsley C, Furtado R, Mosse C, et al. Small bowel obstruction in the virgin abdomen: the need for a mandatory laparotomy explored. Am J Surg 2014; 208(2):243–8.

The Bad Gallbladder

Miloš Buhavac, MD*, Ali Elsaadi, MD, Sharmila Dissanaike, MD

KEYWORDS

- Laparoscopic cholecystectomy • Open cholecystectomy
- Intraoperative cholangiogram • Acute cholecystitis • Bad/difficult gallbladder
- Percutaneous cholecystostomy tube • Subtotal cholecystectomy
- Common bile duct stones

KEY POINTS

- The Bad Gallbladder is a difficult problem not only to define but also to manage.
- Surgeons should be familiar with bailout procedures and adjuncts to surgery to avoid damage to vital structures when the Bad Gallbladder is encountered.
- Surgeons should know how to perform both an open cholecystectomy and how to manage common bile duct stones depending on their technical comfort and available resources.

WHAT IS A "BAD" GALLBLADDER?

According to the 2018 Tokyo guidelines, cholecystitis can be stratified into grades I, II, and III based on the severity of the illness as well as patient comorbidities.[1] Using the American Society of Anesthesiologists physical status classification and Charlson co-morbidity index, patients can be categorized into how sick they are, which will help the surgeon to decide on which management option is safest for the patient. Ashfaq and colleagues[2] defined the "bad gallbladder" as one that is necrotic or gangrenous, contains Mirizzi syndrome, has extensive adhesions, required conversion to an open operation, an operation that lasted more than 120 minutes, had prior tube cholecystostomy or has known gallbladder perforation.[2] Other definitions include the Parkland Grading Scale for Cholecystitis and the American Association for the Surgery of Trauma grading scale for acute cholecystitis.[3,4] A recent multicenter validation study found that the Parkland Grading Scale outperformed the American Association for the Surgery of Trauma grading scale in correctly predicting the need for a surgical "bailout" (subtotal or fenestrated cholecystectomy, or cholecystostomy), conversion to open, surgical complications (bile leak, surgical site infection, bile duct injury), all complications, and operative time.[5] Definitions like these are a step in the right

The authors have nothing to disclose.
Texas Tech University Health Sciences Center, Department of Surgery, 3601 4th Street, Lubbock, TX 79430, USA
* Corresponding author.
E-mail address: milos.buhavac@ttuhsc.edu

direction to inform us on how technically challenging the surgery may be and will allow us to have more informed conversations with our patients about the potential outcomes of their operation.

IF WE PLAN TO PERFORM LAPAROSCOPIC CHOLECYSTECTOMY FOR ACUTE CHOLECYSTITIS, SHOULD WE DO IT SOONER RATHER THAN LATER?

Many studies have looked at early versus late laparoscopic cholecystectomy, with data to be found supporting both approaches. Vaccari and colleagues[6] looked at patients who underwent cholecystectomy 72 hours after symptom onset and showed a higher mortality rate, longer hospital stay, and higher rate of conversion to open in this subset of patients, compared with patients who waited 6 weeks after symptoms onset for an interval cholecystectomy. This group had no mortality (vs 5% mortality in the urgent cholecystectomy group), and a conversion rate of only 4% compared with the 18% seen in the early group.[6] There is, however, a much larger body of literature, including randomized prospective studies and meta-analyses that show significantly lower morbidity, length of stay and hospital costs for immediate/early laparoscopic cholecystectomy versus delayed.[7] Gurusamy and colleagues[8] have performed meta-analyses and Cochrane reviews that confirm the safety of early laparoscopic cholecystectomy, showing no difference in bile duct injuries or conversion to open cholecystectomy.

One of the challenges in evaluating all this data is that there is no standard definition for early versus late, with studies variously defining early intervention as during the initial hospital admission, versus within 72 hours from symptom onset, to 24 hours from admission.

Taking into account all the available literature, it is our practice and opinion that there is little benefit in waiting up to 6 weeks for inflammation to subside and that it is preferable to operate as soon as it is safe to do so. Using basic principles derived from trauma and sepsis management, 2 conditions familiar to acute care surgeons, performing surgery to obtain definitive source control as soon as physiologic derangements have been addressed with adequate resuscitation seems to be the logical approach. In the authors' experience, although difficult to quantify in the literature, adhesions in the very early stages of infection tend to be edematous rather than fibrous, and clear instead of thick, allowing easier and safer dissection. Theoretically, the sooner the operation is performed, the shorter the hospital stay may have to be, which represents significant cost savings in today's cost-conscious world of health care. The next step forward would be to perform a randomized control trial to compare laparoscopic cholecystectomy within 24 hours and 72 hours to redefine early cholecystectomy, and the potential benefits of performing the surgery as soon as possible.

There used to be a theory that, beyond 72 hours from symptom onset in acute cholecystitis, patients should not undergo cholecystectomy. This theory was partly based on observations that, during the first 2 to 4 days of symptoms, there would be edematous cholecystitis, followed by necrotizing and then suppurative cholecystitis, which could make laparoscopic cholecystectomy more dangerous.[9] However, retrospective case control studies have shown that even beyond 72 hours laparoscopic cholecystectomy seems to be safe.[10–12] In a single-center, randomized trial from Switzerland that specifically looked at operating after 72 hours of symptoms versus operating after initial antibiotics and 6 weeks to allow for inflammation to resolve, the patients who were operated on after 72 hours still had less overall morbidity, a shorter hospital stay and duration of antibiotics, and decreased costs when compared with the delayed cholecystectomy group.[13] Although these data may be encouraging, the body mass index of these patients, and their overall health is starkly different from the patient population that many surgeons in America have to deal with. It is our practice to take all patients who are medically fit enough for surgery to the operating room, regardless of symptom duration.

WHEN SHOULD WE PROCEED WITH A LAPAROSCOPIC CHOLECYSTECTOMY VERSUS PLACING A PERCUTANEOUS CHOLECYSTOSTOMY TUBE?

The first decision branch point we encounter as surgeons is often whether or not to operate; should we "heal with steel," or would a nonoperative approach be safer for the patient? When source control is required and the patient cannot tolerate the added risk of surgical intervention, a percutaneous cholecystostomy tube is often used. After the publication and adoption of the Tokyo guidelines, it became common for critically ill patients to undergo percutaneous cholecystostomy tube placement instead of laparoscopic cholecystectomy.

Turiño and colleagues[14] implemented nonoperative measures for 201 patients with acute calculous cholecystitis. Of these patients, 97 underwent a cholecystostomy tube placement. These patients typically had more comorbidities, were older, and had worse inflammatory markers on admission. Of the 97, the rate of readmission was 38%, and the rate of recurrent cholecystitis was 25%.[14] A retrospective analysis from 2019 looking at more than 180,000 cases of cholecystitis showed somewhat similar outcomes. In 3167 patients undergoing cholecystostomy tube placement for acute cholecystitis, the readmission rate was just over 20%. Patients who underwent cholecystectomy had a readmission rate of 6.7% with a lower in-hospital mortality and cost. Factors contributing to the decision to place a cholecystostomy tube included cirrhosis, congestive heart failure, chronic atrial fibrillation, and sepsis.[15] Similar outcomes were seen by Dimou and colleagues,[16] who showed higher readmission rates at 30 days, 90 days, and 2 years after cholecystostomy tube placement. Considering these data, a cholecystostomy tube is not necessarily causative, and it may instead be a marker for a sicker patient population.

Another nonoperative route is antibiotic therapy alone, which is usually reserved for patients with milder disease. The pitfalls of this approach include the risk of recurrent symptoms that may lead to readmission and a more difficult operation later on. In a systematic review and pooled analysis of 1841 patients treated nonoperatively for acute calculous cholecystitis, 87% of patients responded favorably initially; however, 22% developed a subsequent gallstone-related problem.[17] Two Norwegian randomized controlled trials involving 201 patients showed that 45% required interval surgery, which was also associated with higher overall costs.[18]

DOES THE PRESENCE OF ANTITHROMBOTIC THERAPY INFLUENCE OUTCOMES AND SHOULD IT AFFECT THE SURGEON'S TREATMENT STRATEGY?

The presence of antithrombotic therapy may influence the surgeon to consider a nonoperative strategy owing to the concern for surgical bleeding. Multiple studies have looked at the impact of antithrombotic therapy in patients with acute cholecystitis. In a 2017 study by Yun and colleagues,[19] 67 patients on antithrombotic therapy were separated into an emergency versus elective group; the elective group stopped antithrombotic therapy 7 days before surgery, whereas the emergent group either did not stop or stopped within 3 days of surgery. Patient outcomes were similar in terms of morbidity, hospital stay, and mortality. The major difference was that 6 patients in the emergent group developed acute blood loss anemia and 3 required a postoperative blood transfusion.[19] Another single-institution experience actually showed similar results with 21 patients on anticoagulation or antiplatelet therapy. In this study, no significant difference in complications, blood loss, or conversion to open were noted in patients operated on while on therapeutic anticoagulation.[20]

Although underpowered studies cannot provide strong recommendations, they do provide the framework for larger studies to be conducted. A 2020 systematic review by Sagami and colleagues[21] looked at the use of various endoscopic drainage procedures versus laparoscopic cholecystectomy in patients on antithrombotic therapy. Of 2578 patients undergoing laparoscopic cholecystectomy, 354 were receiving antithrombotic therapy. The results showed no significant differences between patients with continued and discontinued antiplatelet therapy (aspirin and/or thienopyridine) in intraoperative blood loss, operative time, conversion rate to open surgery, 30-day morbidity, or bleeding complications requiring blood transfusion.[21]

It is these authors' practice to continue antiplatelet therapy without interruption in patients undergoing laparoscopic cholecystectomy. Many patients are on these drugs to prevent thrombosis of drug-eluting cardiac stents, a potentially lethal complication that can be harder to correct than postoperative bleeding. For patients who are on therapeutic anticoagulation for atrial fibrillation, cardiac valve replacement, or coagulation disorders, we routinely transition these agents to either low-molecular-weight heparin or intravenous heparin and perform the operation during a short, planned window off anticoagulation. The duration of this window and the timing of resumption of anticoagulation after surgery are predicated on balancing the risk of stroke and thrombosis (which varies greatly based on underlying disease, but can usually be approximated based on established calculations such as CHADS score for atrial fibrillation) against the risk of bleeding, in each individual case.

SHOULD A POTENTIAL "BAD" GALLBLADDER OPERATION BE STARTED LAPAROSCOPICALLY?

Once the decision for surgery has been made, an operative plan needs to be discussed and implemented. Should one initially start with laparoscopic surgery for the "bad gallbladder"? If a laparoscopic approach is taken, when should bail-out maneuvers be attempted? Is converting to open operation still the standard next step?

A 2016 study published by Ashfaq and colleagues[2] sheds some light on our first question. They studied 2212 patients who underwent laparoscopic cholecystectomy, of which 351 were considered "difficult gallbladders." A difficult gallbladder was considered one that was necrotic or gangrenous, involved Mirizzi syndrome, had extensive adhesions, was converted to open, lasted more than 120 minutes, had a prior tube cholecystostomy, or had known gallbladder perforation. Seventy of these 351 operations were converted to open.[2] The indications for conversion included severe inflammation and adhesions around the gallbladder rendering dissection of triangle of Calot difficult (n = 37 [11.1%]), altered anatomy (n = 14 [4.2%]), and intraoperative bleeding that was difficult to control laparoscopically (n = 6 [1.8%]). The remaining 13 patients (18.5%) included a combination of cholecystoenteric fistula, concern for malignancy, common bile duct exploration for stones, and inadvertent enterotomy requiring small bowel repair. Comparing the total laparoscopic cholecystectomy group and the conversion groups, operative time and length of hospital stay were significantly different; 147 ± 47 minutes versus 185 ± 71 minutes ($P<.005$) and 3 ± 2 days versus 5 ± 3 days ($P = .011$), respectively. There was no significant difference in postoperative hemorrhage, subhepatic collection, cystic duct leak, wound infection, reoperation, and 30-day mortality.[2] From these findings, we can glean that most cholecystectomies should be started laparoscopically, because it is safe to do so. It is the authors' practice to start laparoscopically in all cases.

BAILOUT PROCEDURES: WHAT, WHERE AND WHEN?

Despite the best efforts of experienced surgeons, it is sometimes impossible to safely obtain the critical view of safety in a bad gallbladder with dense inflammation and even scarring in the hepatocystic triangle. Continued attempts to dissect in this hazardous region can lead to devastating injury, including transection of 1 or both hepatic ducts, the common bile duct, and/or a major vascular injury (usually the right hepatic artery). Therefore, it is imperative that any surgeon faced with a bad gallbladder have a toolkit of procedures to safely terminate the operation while obtaining maximum symptom and source control, rather than continue to plunge blindly into treacherous terrain.

If the critical view of safety cannot be achieved owing to inflammation, and when further dissection in the hepatocystic triangle is dangerous, these authors default to laparoscopic subtotal cholecystectomy as our bail-out procedure of choice. The rationale for this approach is that it resolves symptoms by removing the majority of the gallbladder, leading to low (although not zero) rates of recurrent symptoms. It is safe, and can be easily completed laparoscopically, thus avoiding the longer hospital stay and morbidity of an open operation.[22]

There is now significant data supporting this approach. In a series of 168 patients (of whom 153 were laparoscopic) who underwent subtotal cholecystectomy for bad gallbladders, the mean operative time was 150 minutes (range, 70–315 minutes) and the average blood loss was 170 mL (range, 50–1500 mL). The median length of stay for these patients was 4 days (range, 1–68 days), and there were no common bile duct injuries.[23] There were 12 postoperative collections (7.1%), 4 wound infections (2.4%), 1 bile leak (0.6%), and 7 retained stones (4.2%), but the 30-day mortality was similar to those who underwent a total laparoscopic cholecystectomy.[23] A systematic review and meta-analysis by Elshaer and colleagues[24] showed that subtotal cholecystectomy achieves comparable morbidity rates compared with total cholecystectomy. These data support the idea that we should move away from the idea that the only acceptable outcome for a cholecystectomy is the complete removal of a gallbladder, especially when it is not safe to do so. This shift toward subtotal cholecystectomy has been appropriately referred to as the safety first, total cholecystectomy second approach.[25]

FENESTRATED VERSUS RECONSTITUTING SUBTOTAL CHOLECYSTECTOMY

When performing a subtotal cholecystectomy, the next decision point is which type of subtotal cholecystectomy is best: fenestrated or reconstituting? In a fenestrating subtotal cholecystectomy, the gallbladder is excised except for a small rim of infundibulum around the cystic orifice and the posterior wall adherent to the liver. This remainder of gallbladder acts as a shield over the hepatocystic triangle, preventing iatrogenic injury. Stones and other debris are extracted (**Fig. 1**). In the reconstituting subtype, the gallbladder is excised down to just above the infundibulum and stapled off. This strategy creates a small residual infundibulum (**Fig. 2**). While preventing the bile leak that is almost inevitable with the fenestrating variety, it has been hypothesized that the creation of a residual gallbladder remnant may lead to recurrence of cholecystitis. A 2016 article published by Van Dijk and associates[26] showed there to be no difference in reintervention rates between the 2 types: 32% in the fenestrating subtotal cholecystectomy group and 26% in the reconstituting subtotal cholecystectomy group ($P = .211$). However after 6 years follow-up (interquartile range, 5–10 years), the recurrence rate of biliary events was lower after fenestrating than reconstituting subtotal cholecystectomy (9% vs 18%, respectively; $P<.022$). Completion cholecystectomy was performed significantly more in patients after fenestrating subtotal cholecystectomy (9% vs 4%; $P<.022$).[26] A 2017 study by Santos and colleagues[27]

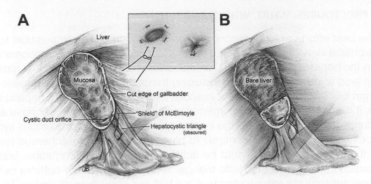

Fig. 1. Subtotal fenestrated cholecystectomy, reproduced with permission from Elsevier.[46]

suggests that the fenestrating subtype is preferred owing to the lower risk of biliary stone formation and the chance for an even more difficult completion cholecystectomy with a reconstituting type. In general, it seems to be a matter of technical ability and preference whether one opts to do a fenestrating versus reconstituting subtotal cholecystectomy. Complication profiles varies with reconstituting cholecystectomy leading to recurrent stones and symptoms, and fenestration leads to increase risk of bile leak. Matsui and colleagues[28] showed that, by modifying the fenestration technique with a free omental patch, they could decrease the bile leak rate to 1% versus 44% in the no omental plug group. It is our practice to perform a laparoscopic fenestrated subtotal cholecystectomy and then suture a piece of pedicled omentum into the gallbladder infundibulum to help obliterate the cystic duct opening and decrease our risk of bile leak. We routinely leave drains to manage any bile leak that may result, and in cases of persistent or high volume bile leak we use biliary stenting via endoscopic retrograde cholangiopancreatography to decrease this duration. In general, drains can be removed in clinic approximately 2 to 6 weeks after the procedure, with a few patients requiring longer periods to control drainage and develop a tract to prevent recurrent biloma. To encourage the formation of a defined fibrous tract around the drain, we tend to use latex or rubber drains rather than the more common silicon drains.[22]

WHAT IS THE ROLE OF OPEN CHOLECYSTECTOMY?

Another important question that must be asked is whether there is even a role for open cholecystectomy as a fallback option in the modern laparoscopic era, when resident

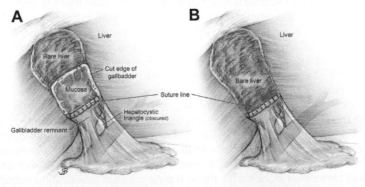

Fig. 2. Subtotal reconstituting cholecystectomy, reproduced with permission from Elsevier.[46]

experience with open cholecystectomies is ever decreasing? A 2013 retrospective analysis by McCoy and coworkers[29] showed that resident experience with open cases overall has decreased significantly in the past 12 years, with the average resident performing only 10 open cholecystectomies. This trend is well-documented with regard to open operations, because minimally invasive approaches become the norm.

The crucial question: has this decrease in operative experience affected the ability of young surgeons to perform open cholecystectomy safely and effectively? Using a cadaveric animal model, residents' open versus laparoscopic skills were tested by board-certified surgeons. Twenty-two percent of the trainees had no previous laparoscopic and 62% had no previous open cholecystectomy experience. Significant differences were found in the overall score (median difference of 1; 95% confidence interval, 1–1; $P<.001$), gallbladder perforation rate (73% vs 29%, $P<.001$), safe dissection of Calot's triangle (98% vs 90%; $P = .001$), and duration of surgery (42 ± 13 minutes vs 26 ± 10 minutes; mean differences, 17.22; 95% confidence interval, 15.37–19.07; $P<.001$), all favoring open surgery.[30] Therefore, it seems that even without much clinical experience, residents were able to perform open cholecystectomy safely. It could therefore be argued that, when absolutely necessary, open cholecystectomy can be performed safely, even by the surgeons of tomorrow. Nonetheless, given that these were cadaveric animal bench models that were unlikely to have severe inflamed acute cholecystitis, these findings are perhaps more generalizable to an incidental cholecystectomy for gallstone disease during an open abdominal operation, versus as a rescue procedure in a difficult bad gallbladder.

It is our practice to opt for open cholecystectomy in cases where there are dense adhesions to the colon, duodenum, or other fragile structures that may be injured by prolonged laparoscopic dissection and where the additional benefit of tactile feedback may be invaluable in avoiding iatrogenic injury. We also convert to open for any case where there is a suspicion of cancer or for bleeding that cannot be quickly and completely controlled laparoscopically. Open cholecystectomy remains an important skillset for the general surgeon; however, we prefer to use it for the indications mentioned elsewhere in this article, rather than as the default for severe inflammation.

WHEN SHOULD WE USE AN INTRAOPERATIVE CHOLANGIOGRAM?

The next question to address is the role of intraoperative cholangiogram (IOC). Although it could be argued that IOC is not necessary for routine cases, there may be some benefits in identifying unsuspected stones in the CBD. A study by Andrews and colleagues[31] found that in 1085 routine cholecystectomies, 2.3% had retained stones, with a median stone size of 5 mm. In a smaller retrospective study looking at 61 patients who underwent laparoscopic cholecystectomy without IOC, the median time to presentation for a retained stone was 4 years after surgery.[32] Therefore, it could be argued that routine IOC may prevent missed CBD stones, albeit in a very small (<5%) proportion of cases. This benefit has to be weighed against the additional effort, time, cost, and radiation required to perform a routine IOC.

Apart from identifying stones, IOC is used to avoid or detect inadvertent common bile duct injury. A study published by Flum and colleagues[33] looking at the rate of common bile duct injury in laparoscopic cholecystectomy with IOC versus without IOC showed that IOC significantly decreased the incidence of common bile duct injury from 0.33% to 0.20%. Interestingly, as a surgeon uses IOC more, their rate of common bile duct injury goes down. Comparing surgeons who performed IOC more than 75% of the time versus those who did not, the rate of common bile duct injury was 1.6% compared with 6.3%, respectively.[33] A 2016 study by Zang and colleagues[34] showed that selective magnetic resonance cholangiopancreatography can be used similar to IOC when it comes to common bile duct stones and bile duct injuries. In their study, patients randomized to having preoperative magnetic resonance cholangiopancreatography had a 0.13% of bile duct injuries compared with 0.20% in the IOC group. No patients with preoperative magnetic resonance cholangiopancreatography returned in 1 year with symptomatic common bile duct stones.[34] One study found that, even after preoperative magnetic resonance cholangiopancreatography followed by endoscopic retrograde cholangiopancreatography to remove stones before laparoscopic cholecystectomy, IOC still helped to identify retained common bile duct stones. The study reported that of 56 of the 405 patients who underwent preoperative magnetic resonance cholangiopancreatography and endoscopic retrograde cholangiopancreatography with sphincterotomies for common bile duct stones, 7 patients still had stones seen on IOC.[35] All this being said, should one not use IOC, the rates of bile duct injury and retained stones are still acceptably low with 1 study of more than 1000 patients by Lill and colleagues[36] showing bile duct injury rates of 0.5% and retained stones of 0.9%.

At our institution, we perform selective IOC in cases where we have suspicion of a common bile duct stone such as a persistently elevated total bilirubin, liver function enzymes 3 times the upper limit of normal, presence of pancreatitis on computed tomography scans, lipase levels 3 times the upper limit of normal, and a dilated duct on ultrasound imaging.

One interesting emerging technology that presents an alternative option is laparoscopic ultrasound. Support for this technique includes its speed of use (9.8 minutes vs 17 minutes) compared with IOC, cost effectiveness, and the ease of its use.[37] It is also thought to be more specific than IOC and can even detect abnormalities such as hemobilia, diverticulum, or polyps that would likely be missed or incorrectly characterized by IOC.[37]

Another emerging technology is the use of indocyanine green (ICG), either laparoscopically or robotically, to define biliary anatomy. In a study by Maker and Kunda,[38] 2.5 mg of ICG was given at intubation and the Da Vinci robot's "firefly" was used to toggle between near-infrared fluorescent cholangiography and bright light illumination to determine the extrahepatic biliary anatomy. In 35 robotic cholecystectomies, patients tolerated ICG well without adverse effects, no biliary injuries occurred, and cases were completed completely robotically.[38] In another larger study of 184 robotic cholecystectomies using ICG 45 minutes before the procedure, no biliary injuries were seen nor were conversions to open or laparoscopic surgery.[39] The cystic duct, the common bile duct, and the common hepatic duct were successfully visualized with ICG in 97.8%, 96.1%, and 94% of cases, respectively.[39] The ability to quickly toggle to and from near-infrared fluorescence as well as the minimal requirement for extra preoperative and intraoperative preparation makes ICG an attractive option in robotic cholecystectomies with a difficult anatomy.

MANAGEMENT OF COMMON BILE DUCT STONES DISCOVERED INTRAOPERATIVELY

Regardless of whether one performs selective or routine IOCs, every surgeon will at some point be confronted with a common bile duct stone that is, discovered intraoperatively, because 10% to 15% of patient undergoing cholecystectomy for uncomplicated, symptomatic cholelithiasis will have choledocholithiasis. The management algorithm will depend on the surgeon's training and available amenities. Taking a systematic approach, we usually define the anatomy with a cholangiogram, then start with flushing the duct with saline. The administration of 1 mg of intravenous glucagon can also help to relax the sphincter and allow the stones to be flushed into the duodenum.

If this procedure is unsuccessful, the surgeon can either proceed with laparoscopic common bile duct exploration, delayed endoscopic retrograde cholangiopancreatography, or on-table endoscopic retrograde cholangiopancreatography. If the surgeon decides to proceed with laparoscopic common bile duct exploration, a decision must be made on the transcystic approach versus a choledochotomy. Number, size, cystic duct anatomy, and the location of the stones are the most important factors when it comes to determining operative approach.[40] As a general rule, small distal stones are approached transcystically, whereas large proximal stones are approached via a choledochotomy. Multiple stones, as long as they are distal and less than 6 mm in size, can be approached transcystically. Stones larger than this size, no matter the location, require a choledochotomy. A cystic duct size of greater than 4 mm will also allow a transcystic approach.

Another important consideration is the diameter of the common bile duct. The recommendation is that a common bile duct less than 7 mm should not be entered because there is a risk for stricture upon closure of the choledochotomy.[40] At our institution, if flushing maneuvers fail, we proceed with laparoscopic transcystic exploration. Initially, we start with either fluoroscopic-guided basket retrieval or Fogarty balloon catheters, 3F or 4F, which can be inflated and used to withdraw the stones into the abdominal cavity. If there is concern that the stone is too large to pass back through the cystic duct but small enough to pass through the ileocecal valve, we push the stone through the sphincter of Oddi. This decision is also influenced by the length, diameter, and friability of the cystic duct.

If we are unable to clear the duct in this fashion, we dilate the cystic duct with either Maryland forceps or an 8F Fogarty/angioplasty catheter, place a guidewire, and then place a 12F introducer sheath through which we can place our choledochoscope. With the choledochoscope in place, a retrieval basket can be inserted under direct vision and the stone removed. Much less commonly, when a stone is large, that is, more than 6 to 8 mm, on preoperative imaging, the transcystic approach is not appropriate and we will plan to perform a choledochotomy, preferably using a robotic approach owing to the better visualization and control.

Another approach is to perform a laparoendoscopic procedure. This process includes a cholecystectomy with IOC and intraoperative endoscopic retrograde cholangiopancreatography. A 2013 study by Liverani and colleagues[41] looked at 108 patients who underwent this treatment plan versus 54 patients who had delayed endoscopic retrograde cholangiopancreatography (endoscopic retrograde cholangiopancreatography after cholecystectomy). Of the 108 patients who underwent laparoscopic cholecystectomy, IOC and intraoperative–endoscopic retrograde cholangiopancreatography, 94 had successful removal of common bile duct stones without need for conversion to open or choledochotomy, with the rate of postendoscopic retrograde cholangiopancreatography pancreatitis being lower than those who underwent preoperative endoscopic retrograde cholangiopancreatography. Their stay was also shorter compared with patients undergoing a delayed endoscopic retrograde cholangiopancreatography, with a mean hospital time of 4.7 days compared with 6.5 days.[41] The mean operative time was 130 minutes in the one stage group and it was 95 minutes in those who underwent endoscopic retrograde cholangiopancreatography at a later time.[41] A 2020 study published by Muhammedoğlu and Kale[42] presented similar findings: shorter hospital stay, decreased cost, and less anesthesia time with a single stage laparoscopic cholecystectomy plus endoscopic retrograde cholangiopancreatography. In a meta-analysis of 629 patients across 5 randomized controlled trials, patients who underwent intraoperative endoscopic retrograde cholangiopancreatography after cholecystectomy had lower rates of endoscopic retrograde cholangiopancreatography pancreatitis, shorter hospital stay, and lower morbidity and mortality.[43] Although the evidence points to this being an ideal approach to common bile duct stones discovered intraoperatively, it is not the only approach.

Other groups compared preoperative endoscopic retrograde cholangiopancreatography plus laparoscopic cholecystectomy versus a laparoscopic cholecystectomy plus laparoscopic common bile duct exploration. One study analyzed 12 randomized controlled trials. The findings showed that those who underwent preoperative endoscopic retrograde cholangiopancreatography plus laparoscopic cholecystectomy versus a 1-stage laparoscopic cholecystectomy plus laparoscopic common bile duct exploration had a higher rate of stone clearance, lower rate of bile leak, higher rate of endoscopic retrograde cholangiopancreatography pancreatitis, and longer hospital stay. Overall, the morbidity and mortality rates were the same.[44] Another meta-analysis of 11 trials showed similar results with laparoscopic common bile duct exploration plus laparoscopic cholecystectomy being associated with a shorter hospital stay and equivalent morbidity and mortality.[45] As more surgeons become comfortable performing laparoscopic common bile duct exploration, this approach may become more common.

SUMMARY

The bad gallbladder remains one of the most common challenges a surgeon will face over the course of their career. Cholecystectomy has enjoyed an evolution from open to laparoscopic and now robotic. Several adjuncts such as IOC and intraoperative ultrasound examination have come along to help us make decisions in the operating room and decrease the need for further procedures beyond the initial surgical intervention. At the forefront of this process is our tireless pursuit of patient safety. We know all too well the devastating consequences of bile duct injury from attempting completion surgery in a heavily scarred field. At our institution it seems that the proportion of bad gallbladders certainly outweighs the straightforward ones, especially on the acute care surgery service. Therefore, it is essential that every surgeon and graduating resident who plans to practice general surgery have a systematic approach to the bad gallbladder, with a variety of options in their toolkit.

REFERENCES

1. Okamoto K, Suzuki K, Takada T, et al. Tokyo Guidelines 2018: flowchart for the management of acute cholecystitis [published correction appears in J Hepatobiliary Pancreat Sci. 2019 Nov;26(11):534]. J Hepatobiliary Pancreat Sci 2018;25(1): 55–72.

2. Ashfaq A, Ahmadieh K, Shah AA, et al. The difficult gall bladder: outcomes following laparoscopic cholecystectomy and the need for open conversion. Am J Surg 2016;212(6):1261–4.

3. Madni TD, Leshikar DE, Minshall CT, et al. The Parkland grading scale for cholecystitis. Am J Surg 2018;215(4):625–30.

4. Schuster KM, O'Connor R, Cripps M, et al. Multicenter validation of the American Association for the Surgery of Trauma grading scale for acute cholecystitis. J Trauma Acute Care Surg 2021;90(1):87–96.

5. Madni TD, Nakonezny PA, Imran JB, et al. A comparison of cholecystitis grading scales. J Trauma Acute Care Surg 2019;86(3):471–8.

6. Vaccari S, Lauro A, Cervellera M, et al. Early versus delayed approach in chole-cystectomy after admission to an emergency department. A multicenter retro-spective study. G Chir 2018;39(4):232–8.

7. Gutt CN, Encke J, Köninger J, et al. Acute cholecystitis: early versus delayed cholecystectomy, a multicenter randomized trial (ACDC study, NCT00447304). Ann Surg 2013;258(3):385–93.

8. Gurusamy KS, Davidson C, Gluud C, et al. Early versus delayed laparoscopic cholecystectomy for people with acute cholecystitis. Cochrane Database Syst Rev 2013;6:CD005440.

9. Kimura Y, Takada T, Kawarada Y, et al. Definitions, pathophysiology, and epide-miology of acute cholangitis and cholecystitis: Tokyo guidelines. J Hepatobiliary Pancreat Surg 2007;14(1):15–26.

10. Degrate L, Ciravegna AL, Luperto M, et al. Acute cholecystitis: the golden 72-h period is not a strict limit to perform early cholecystectomy. Results from 316 consecutive patients. Langenbecks Arch Surg 2013;398(8):1129–36.

11. Gomes RM, Mehta NT, Varik V, et al. No 72-hour pathological boundary for safe early laparoscopic cholecystectomy in acute cholecystitis: a clinicopathological study. Ann Gastroenterol 2013;26(4):340–5.

12. Zhu B, Zhang Z, Wang Y, et al. Comparison of laparoscopic cholecystectomy for acute cholecystitis within and beyond 72 h of symptom onset during emergency admissions. World J Surg 2012;36(11):2654–8.

13. Roulin D, Saadi A, Di Mare L, et al. Early versus delayed cholecystectomy for acute cholecystitis, are the 72 hours still the rule? A randomized trial. Ann Surg 2016;264(5):717–22.

14. Turiño SY, Shabanzadeh DM, Eichen NM, et al. Percutaneous cholecystostomy versus conservative treatment for acute cholecystitis: a cohort study. J Gastrointest Surg 2019;23(2):297–303.

15. Pavurala RB, Li D, Porter K, et al. Percutaneous cholecystostomy-tube for high-risk patients with acute cholecystitis: current practice and implications for future research. Surg Endosc 2019;33(10):3396–403.

16. Dimou FM, Adhikari D, Mehta HB, et al. Outcomes in older patients with grade III cholecystitis and cholecystostomy tube placement: a propensity score analysis. J Am Coll Surg 2017;224(4):502–11.e1.

17. Loozen CS, Oor JE, van Ramshorst B, et al. Conservative treatment of acute cholecystitis: a systematic review and pooled analysis. Surg Endosc 2017; 31(2):504–15.

18. Brazzelli M, Cruickshank M, Kilonzo M, et al. Clinical effectiveness and cost-effectiveness of cholecystectomy compared with observation/conservative man-agement for preventing recurrent symptoms and complications in adults presenting with uncomplicated symptomatic gallstones or cholecystitis: a systematic review and economic evaluation. Health Technol Assess 2014;18(55):1–101, v–vi.

19. Yun JH, Jung HI, Lee HU, et al. The efficacy of laparoscopic cholecystectomy without discontinuation in patients on antithrombotic therapy. Ann Surg Treat Res 2017;92(3):143–8.

20. Noda T, Hatano H, Dono K, et al. Safety of early laparoscopic cholecystectomy for patients with acute cholecystitis undergoing antiplatelet or anticoagulation ther-apy: a single-institution experience. Hepatogastroenterology 2014;61(134): 1501–6.

21. Sagami R, Hayasaka K, Nishikiori H, et al. Current status in the treatment of acute cholecystitis patients receiving antithrombotic therapy: is endoscopic drainage feasible?- A systematic review. Clin Endosc 2020;53(2):176–88.

22. Dissanaike S. A step-by-step guide to laparoscopic subtotal fenestrating chole-cystectomy: a damage control approach to the difficult gallbladder. J Am Coll Surg 2016;223(2):e15–8.

23. Tay WM, Toh YJ, Shelat VG, et al. Subtotal cholecystectomy: early and long-term outcomes. Surg Endosc 2020;34(10):4536–42.

24. Elshaer M, Gravante G, Thomas K, et al. Subtotal cholecystectomy for "difficult gallbladders": systematic review and meta-analysis. JAMA Surg 2015;150(2): 159–68.

25. Brunt LM, Deziel DJ, Telem DA, et al. Safe cholecystectomy multi-society practice guideline and state of the art consensus conference on prevention of bile duct injury during cholecystectomy. Ann Surg 2020;272(1):3–23.

26. van Dijk AH, Donkervoort SC, Lameris W, et al. Short- and long-term outcomes after a reconstituting and fenestrating subtotal cholecystectomy. J Am Coll Surg 2017;225(3):371–9.

27. Santos BF, Brunt LM, Pucci MJ. The difficult gallbladder: a safe approach to a dangerous problem. J Laparoendosc Adv Surg Tech A 2017;27(6):571–8.

28. Matsui Y, Hirooka S, Kotsuka M, et al. Use of a piece of free omentum to prevent bile leakage after subtotal cholecystoctomy. Surgery 2018;164(3):419–23.

29. McCoy AC, Gasevic E, Szlabick RE, et al. Are open abdominal procedures a thing of the past? An analysis of graduating general surgery residents' case logs from 2000 to 2011. J Surg Educ 2013;70(6):683–9.

30. Nebiker CA, Mechera R, Rosenthal R, et al. Residents' performance in open versus laparoscopic bench-model cholecystectomy in a hands-on surgical course. Int J Surg 2015;19:15–21.

31. Andrews S. Gallstone size related to incidence of post cholecystectomy retained common bile duct stones. Int J Surg 2013;11(4):319–21.

32. Cox MR, Budge JP, Eslick GD. Timing and nature of presentation of unsuspected retained common bile duct stones after laparoscopic cholecystectomy: a retro-spective study. Surg Endosc 2015;29(7):2033–8.

33. Flum DR, Koepsell T, Heagerty P, et al. Common bile duct injury during laparo-scopic cholecystectomy and the use of intraoperative cholangiography: adverse outcome or preventable error? Arch Surg 2001;136(11):1287–92.

34. Zang J, Yuan Y, Zhang C, et al. Elective laparoscopic cholecystectomy without intraoperative cholangiography: role of preoperative magnetic resonance cholan-giopancreatography - a retrospective cohort study. BMC Surg 2016;16(1):45.

35. Ueno K, Ajiki T, Sawa H, et al. Role of intraoperative cholangiography in patients whose biliary tree was evaluated preoperatively by magnetic resonance cholan-giopancreatography. World J Surg 2012;36(11):2661–5.

36. Lill S, Rantala A, Pekkala E, et al. Elective laparoscopic cholecystectomy without routine intraoperative cholangiography: a retrospective analysis of 1101 consec-utive cases. Scand J Surg 2010;99(4):197–200.

37. Dili A, Bertrand C. Laparoscopic ultrasonography as an alternative to intraopera-tive cholangiography during laparoscopic cholecystectomy. World J Gastroen-terol 2017;23(29):5438–50.

38. Maker AV, Kunda N. A technique to define extrahepatic biliary anatomy using ro-botic near-infrared fluorescent cholangiography. J Gastrointest Surg 2017;21(11): 1961–2.

39. Daskalaki D, Fernandes E, Wang X, et al. Indocyanine green (ICG) fluorescent cholangiography during robotic cholecystectomy: results of 184 consecutive cases in a single institution. Surg Innov 2014;21(6):615–21.

40. SAGES. Clinical spotlight review: laparoscopic common bile duct exploration - a SAGES publication. 2021. Available at: https://www.sages.org/publications/guidelines/clinical-spotlight-review-laparoscopic-common-bile-duct-exploration/. Accessed January 29, 2021.

41. Liverani A, Muroni M, Santi F, et al. One-step laparoscopic and endoscopic treatment of gallbladder and common bile duct stones: our experience of the last 9 years in a retrospective study. Am Surg 2013;79(12):1243–7.

42. Muhammedoğlu B, Kale IT. Comparison of the safety and efficacy of single-stage endoscopic retrograde cholangiopancreatography plus laparoscopic cholecystectomy versus two-stage ERCP followed by laparoscopic cholecystectomy six-to-eight weeks later: a randomized controlled trial. Int J Surg 2020;76:37–44.

43. Tan C, Ocampo O, Ong R, et al. Comparison of one stage laparoscopic cholecystectomy combined with intra-operative endoscopic sphincterotomy versus two-stage pre-operative endoscopic sphincterotomy followed by laparoscopic cholecystectomy for the management of pre-operatively diagnosed patients with common bile duct stones: a meta-analysis. Surg Endosc 2018;32(2):770–8.

44. Lyu Y, Cheng Y, Li T, et al. Laparoscopic common bile duct exploration plus cholecystectomy versus endoscopic retrograde cholangiopancreatography plus laparoscopic cholecystectomy for cholecystocholedocholithiasis: a meta-analysis. Surg Endosc 2019;33(10):3275–86.

45. Singh AN, Kilambi R. Single-stage laparoscopic common bile duct exploration and cholecystectomy versus two-stage endoscopic stone extraction followed by laparoscopic cholecystectomy for patients with gallbladder stones with common bile duct stones: systematic review and meta-analysis of randomized trials with trial sequential analysis. Surg Endosc 2018;32(9):3763–76.

46. Strasberg SM, Pucci MJ, Brunt LM, et al. Subtotal cholecystectomy-"fenestrating" vs "reconstituting" subtypes and the prevention of bile duct injury: definition of the optimal procedure in difficult operative conditions. J Am Coll Surg 2016;222(1): 89–96.

Controversies in Inguinal Hernia

Veeshal H. Patel, MD, MBA[a], Andrew S. Wright, MD[a,b],*

KEYWORDS

- Hernia • Inguinal hernia • Mesh • Hernia repair • Robotic surgery • Sports hernia

KEY POINTS

- Watchful waiting of minimally symptomatic hernias is safe, but most patients will have progressive symptoms and will eventually need hernia repair.
- Laparoscopic and open inguinal hernia repair have equivalent recurrence rates, but laparoscopic approach has less acute pain, faster return to work, and lower risk of chronic pain.
- Robotic hernia repair offers no advantage over laparoscopic repair but may help encourage the transition from open to minimally invasive surgery and is a bridge to more complex robotic abdominal wall reconstruction.
- Athletic-related groin pain ("sports hernia") is complex and needs multidisciplinary evaluation by sports medicine, hernia surgery, orthopedic surgery, and physical therapy.
- Nonmesh options for inguinal hernia repair continue to play a role in modern hernia surgery, and the Shouldice repair is the likely the best option.

INTRODUCTION

Inguinal hernias represent one of the most common pathologic conditions presenting to the general surgeon, accounting for 500,000 cases per year in the United States and more than $48 billion in health care expenditures.[1] Inguinal hernia is regarded as one of the oldest afflictions involving humanity, and observations and methods of repair are delineated as early as ancient Egypt. Notably, Leonardo da Vinci's famous drawing "Vitruvian Man" is thought to show a man with an inguinal hernia. Inguinal hernias are more common in men, with a 27% lifetime risk, when compared with women, with a 3% lifetime risk.[2] Over time the approach to hernia management and repair have gradually evolved from different techniques of open tissue repair to the introduction of mesh and eventually the widespread adoption of minimally invasive techniques.

The authors have nothing to disclose.
a Department of Surgery, University of Washington Medical School, 1959 Northeast Pacific Street Box 356410, Seattle, WA 98195, USA; b Center for VideoEndoscopic Surgery Endowed Professor, University of Washington
* Corresponding author.
E-mail address: Awright2@uw.edu
Twitter: @andrewswright (A.S.W.)

Surg Clin N Am 101 (2021) 1067–1079
https://doi.org/10.1016/j.suc.2021.06.005

Indirect inguinal hernias are resultant of failure of obliteration of the processus vaginalis, whereby a resultant hernia sac containing peritoneum passes through the internal inguinal ring. Direct inguinal hernias result from a weakness or defect in the transversalis fascia and are generally thought to be the result of developed weakness. The annual risk of hernia incarceration is not well known, but estimates are approximately 2 of 1000 cases annually.

Given the complex evolution of hernia repair and variations in practice patterns and individual surgeon technique, there remain several viable approaches and considerations in the management of a patient with an inguinal hernia. In surgical practice, several controversies persist: when to operate, the utility of a laparoscopic versus open approach, the applicability of robotic surgery, the approach to bilateral hernias, management of athletic-related groin pain ("sports hernia"), and the role of tissue-based repairs in modern hernia surgery.

INGUINAL HERNIAS: WHEN TO OPERATE OR OBSERVE

The role of inguinal hernia repair is to pre-empt incarceration while also improving quality of life. Previously, many authorities recommended routine repair of all inguinal hernias at diagnosis to prevent future risk of incarceration, strangulation, and need for emergent repair. Analysis of retrospective reviews of hernia complications shows a low estimated lifetime risk of strangulation at 0.27% (1 in 368 patients) for an 18-year-old man and 0.03% (1 in 2941 patients) for a 72-year-old man.[3] Although most surgeons agree that symptomatic hernias should be repaired, given the apparently low risk of life-threatening complications, the role of watchful waiting in asymptomatic or minimally symptomatic hernias has been extensively debated.[4]

The VA Watchful Waiting trial by Fitzgibbons and colleagues[5] compared watchful waiting with hernia repair in minimally symptomatic patients. In this seminal trial, only 2 of the 364 patients in the watchful waiting group sustained incarceration and required emergent surgery, accounting for a frequency of only 1.8 per 1000 patient years. In addition, watchful waiting did not increase the complication rate of future hernia repair. As a result of this and similar studies, many surgeons began to recommend watchful waiting in the minimally symptomatic population. This finding was ultimately used by some payers, including multiple regional councils in England's National Health Service, to restrict access to elective hernia repair on the basis that surgery for minimally symptomatic hernias was "unnecessary."

A more recent publication followed the original VA Watchful Waiting trial participants for an additional 7 years.[6] In the initial study 32% of the patients crossed over to the surgical repair group, whereas the cumulative crossover rate increased to 68% at 10 years. Crossover was considerably more common in men older than 65 years. The most common reason to undergo hernia repair was pain (54%). A similar randomized trial in the United Kingdom showed low risk to watchful waiting but that patients in the surgical repair group had improved quality of life when compared with the patients in the watchful waiting arm.[7] Crossover from the watchful waiting arm of the trial to surgery was 72% at 7 years.

Several systematic reviews and international guidelines have now been published looking at this question.[4,8] It seems clear that patients can be counseled that watchful waiting is a safe and reasonable option for minimally symptomatic hernias but that symptoms can be expected to progress, and surgery will eventually be needed in most people. As such, symptomatic inguinal hernias should be repaired given the high likelihood of progression of symptoms and the need for repair in the future. Asymptomatic or minimally symptomatic hernias should entail a discussion about the risks and benefits of repair versus watchful waiting, leading to a shared decision-making model in which the patient is empowered to make an educated choice. This discussion should be between the surgeon and patient, and not dictated by the insurer or payer.

TECHNICAL APPROACH: LAPAROSCOPIC VERSUS OPEN INGUINAL HERNIA REPAIR

Laparoscopic inguinal hernia repair was initially reported more than 30 years ago. Unlike other laparoscopic innovations such as cholecystectomy, the adoption of laparoscopic inguinal hernia has lagged and in 2017 represented only approximately 25% of inguinal hernia operations in the United States.[9] Adoption is highly surgeon dependent, and less than half of the surgeons who perform inguinal hernia repairs ever use a laparoscopic approach.[10] Adoption is also regionally variant, with the rate of utilization in the United States ranging from 10% to 48% depending on location. This variability in approach has led to significant disparities in the use of minimally invasive surgery, with laparoscopy being used less commonly in black patients[10] and women.[9] There have been several reasons proposed for the lack of adoption of laparoscopic inguinal hernia repair, including perceived lack of evidence for improved outcomes, increased cost, technical difficulty, perceived ergonomic challenges, increased operative times, and the learning curve of the procedure.[11] Economic concerns have also hampered adoption, because reimbursement is uniformly lower for laparoscopic inguinal hernia repairs than for their open equivalents.[12]

Laparoscopic totally extraperitoneal (TEP) and transabdominal preperitoneal (TAPP) repairs are the 2 most common approaches for laparoscopic inguinal hernia repair.[13] Both approaches are characterized by the use of a bridging mesh in the preperitoneal space, covering the entire myopectineal orifice consisting of the internal ring, inguinal floor, and femoral space.[14] The 2 approaches differ primarily in the initial entry and port placement. In the TAP approach the abdomen is entered as in conventional laparoscopy and the surgeon then opens the peritoneum, performs the dissection and places mesh, and then closes the peritoneum with suture or tacks. The TEP approach avoids the violation of the peritoneum but is associated with a longer learning curve for the surgeon and reduced working space. Outcomes are essentially equivalent between the 2 laparoscopic techniques.[15]

There have been several randomized controlled studies of laparoscopic and open inguinal hernia repair. Perhaps most famously, the landmark VA Multicenter trial reported in 2004 by Neumayer and colleagues[16] found that recurrence was more than twice as common in the laparoscopic group (10.1%) when compared with the open repair group (4.9%). This study was done early in the experience with laparoscopic inguinal hernia, and there are some notable issues that may make this study not generalizable to more recent experience. The size of the mesh used in this study was quite small by modern standards, and surgeons were only required to have experience with 25 prior laparoscopic hernia repairs to participate in the study.

More recent studies have shown equivalent or better results with laparoscopic inguinal hernia repair when compared with open. For example, the LEVEL trial is a randomized controlled trial (RCT) that compared the Lichtenstein and TEP approaches,[17] demonstrating that laparoscopic repair results in less early postoperative pain, faster recovery of activities of daily living, and less absence from work (1 week vs 1.4 weeks). At a mean 49-month follow-up, recurrence rates were comparable (3.8% in TEP vs 3.0% with Lichtenstein repair). A large population-based series of more than 66,000 patients showed that the laparoscopic approach was more expensive ($15,030 vs $13,303) but resulted in less use of narcotic pain medicine, reduced rate of wound complications, fewer outpatient visits, and fewer missed work hours.[18]

A recent meta-analysis of open versus laparoscopic repair of unilateral nonrecurrent inguinal hernias reviewed 12 RCTs with almost 4000 patients.[19] There were no significant differences in recurrence between laparoscopic and open repair. Laparoscopic repair had less acute pain. Importantly, laparoscopic repair also had a lower incidence of chronic pain, with an odds ratio (OR) of 0.41 (confidence interval [CI], 0.30–0.56, $P \leq .00001$).

A recent international guideline from multiple European hernia societies carefully reviewed the literature surrounding inguinal hernia.[8] It was found that direct operative costs were higher for laparoscopic approach than for open, but that this difference disappears once community costs are factored in. Furthermore, operative times were found to be equivalent between open repair with mesh and laparoscopic repair. Learning curves vary in different studies, but the general consensus seems to be a learning curve of between 50 and 100 cases.[8]

Despite initial data suggesting increased recurrence rates in the laparoscopic inguinal hernia repair, with changes in practice patterns and increased surgical experience, both approaches now have demonstrably similar recurrence rates. There are minimal perioperative complications with the laparoscopic approach, and there is significantly decreased acute pain with faster return to normal activities. Given the increased recognition of the serious morbidity of chronic pain following inguinal hernia repair, the evidence of decreased rates of chronic pain after laparoscopic repair should ideally drive further adoption.

NEW CONSIDERATIONS: ROLE OF ROBOTIC INGUINAL HERNIA REPAIR

One of the key reasons behind slow adoption of the laparoscopic hernia repair despite similar outcomes and decreased postoperative pain is the learning curve associated with laparoscopic repair. The initial learning curve of laparoscopic repair is estimated to be between 50 and 100 cases,[8] with additional improvements in complication rates and operative time continuing to occur in a linear fashion until approximately 450 cases.[20] Robotic surgery has been proposed as a novel way to increase adoption of minimally invasive inguinal hernia repair. Although there has been minimal evidence to date in support of this, proponents of robotic hernia repair point to 3D visualization, improved ergonomics, and wristed instrumentation as potential advantages of the robotic platform. In addition, the laparoscopic inguinal hernia repair is considered by many surgeons to be ergonomically challenging owing to port positioning and small working space. The potential ergonomic advantages of robotic surgery have also been proposed as an enabling technology for the adoption of minimally invasive inguinal hernia repair.

Driven primarily by marketing and social media, the adoption of robotic inguinal hernia repair has been rapid, increasing from 0.7% in 2012 to 28.8% of cases in 2018.[21] During this same period there was also a smaller increase in laparoscopic repair but a decrease in open repair, indicating that some but not all robotic adoption was driven by a movement from open to minimally invasive surgery.

There have been several case series of robotic inguinal hernia repairs. For example, the University of Pittsburgh has reported their first 300 cases[22] with acceptable short-term results. The investigators estimated that the learning curve for robotic inguinal hernia repair was 11 to 12 cases, although this was derived from a surgeon with extensive previous laparoscopic experience. In a review of 510 patients at the University of Virginia who underwent unilateral inguinal hernia repair (14% robotic, 48% laparoscopic, and 38% open), robotic hernia repair was associated with a longer operative time (105 minutes robotic, 81 minutes laparoscopic, 71 minutes open).[23]

Postoperative complications were similar (2.9% robotic, 3.3% laparoscopic, 5.2% open), and cost was significantly increased in the robotic group ($7162 robotic, $4527 laparoscopic, and $4264 open).

Using a large single-source electronic health record across 32 hospitals, Abdelmoaty and colleagues[24] looked at 734 robotic inguinal hernia repairs when compared with 1671 laparoscopic repairs. The investigators found that the robotic approach had both increased operative time (87 vs 56 minutes) and cost ($5517 vs $3269). The increased cost was primarily driven by the amortized fixed cost of the robot itself, as the variable costs (disposable equipment, mesh, etc.) were higher for laparoscopic surgery. This observation highlights the importance of different cost accounting and economic modeling approaches to analysis of robotic surgery.

To date there has been one RCT of robotic and laparoscopic inguinal hernia repair. The RIVAL trial demonstrated no differences between laparoscopic and robotic TAPP approaches in 102 patients with regard to wound complications, readmission, or pain.[25] Robotic repair was associated with a longer operative time (75.5 minutes) and cost ($3258) when compared with laparoscopic repair (40.5 minutes and $1421). There was no difference in patient quality of life or return to activity. Although many proponents of robotic surgery tout purported ergonomic advantages, in the RIVAL trial there were no overall differences in surgeon ergonomics between laparoscopic and robotic surgery as measured by the Rapid Upper Limb Assessment (RULA) tool. There was also increased surgeon frustration in the robotic cases as measured by the NASA Task Load Index Scale.

Despite the lack of evidence that robotic surgery offers any measurable advantage over laparoscopic inguinal hernia repair, it is clear from the adoption numbers that surgeons are finding value in the robotic platform. The primary advantage of the robot may be not in a comparison of laparoscopy and robotics, but in transitioning surgeons from open to MIS. Robotic inguinal hernia repair may also be a necessary stepping stone to more complex robotic abdominal wall surgery such as reoperative surgery or complex MIS abdominal wall reconstruction. The increased costs of robotic repair are concerning from a systems-level perspective but will hopefully improve with competition as new companies release robotic platforms over the coming few years.

BILATERAL VERSUS UNILATERAL HERNIA REPAIR

The presence of a unilateral inguinal hernia is a clear risk factor for development of a later contralateral hernia. Several trials have reported the rate of contralateral hernias at various follow-up intervals after index unilateral open repair. The rate of contralateral inguinal hernia formation is approximately 10%[26] at 5 years and 21% to 25% at 11 years.[27] In many cases, the contralateral hernia was likely present at the index operation, but clinically occult.

With the wider adoption of minimally invasive approaches for inguinal hernia repair, surgeons are more clearly able to evaluate for an occult contralateral hernia at the time of index surgery. In particular, occult contralateral hernias that are asymptomatic and not identified on preoperative examination are frequently encountered in the operating room during minimally invasive TAPP repair. A recent study noted that 15.8% of patients undergoing a robotic inguinal hernia repair were found to have an incidental contralateral inguinal hernia.[28]

On the one hand, repair of a contralateral hernia seems to be low risk. Repair of bilateral hernias during a TAPP repair is notable for a slightly longer operative time (25 minutes on average), but there are no significant differences in complications, time to recovery, reoperation, and recurrence rate.[13,29] On the other, the primary disadvantage to routine repair of an occult contralateral hernia is the possibility of development of chronic groin pain from the repair at a previously asymptomatic site. Weighing the relative risks and advantages, the recent HerniaSurg international guidelines suggest that it is safe and preferable to repair an occult contralateral inguinal hernia if identified intraoperatively, although they give this recommendation their weakest level of support. Given the high prevalence of an occult contralateral hernia, it is our practice to routinely discuss the possibility of bilateral repair with patients before TAPP inguinal hernia repair and to repair the contralateral side if a hernia is seen at exploration. During open or TEP inguinal hernia we do not routinely open or explore the asymptomatic contralateral side.

MANAGEMENT OF ATHLETIC-RELATED GROIN PAIN ("SPORTS HERNIA")

Athletic-related groin pain is a complex clinical scenario arising from musculoskeletal disruptions of core abdominal structures rather than a true hernia.[30] The diagnosis and management and in fact even the existence of athletic-related groin pain is controversial, and the debates over this topic could fill entire textbooks. This debate extends even to nomenclature, with little disagreement about what to call this clinical entity. The pain has been variably called athletica pubalgia, sportsman's groin, Gilmore groin, incipient hernia, inguinal disruption, core muscle injury, and numerous other terms. Most commonly this has been referred to as a "sports hernia," which adds to the confusion as by definition in this entity there is no fascial defect or true hernia. A recent review found that 33 different diagnostic terms were used across 72 studies in this area.[31]

Two recent consensus groups have attempted to standardize nomenclature. The British Hernia Society determined that this should be called "inguinal disruption,[32]" whereas the Doha group has suggested that this should be called "groin pain in athletes" with 3 major subheadings that attempt to distinguish the suggested cause of the pain[33]:

- Defined clinical entities for groin pain: Adductor-related, iliopsoas-related, inguinal-related, and pubic-related groin pain.
- Hip-related groin pain.
- Other causes of groin pain in athletes.

Much of the confusion stems from the fact there they may be several different discrete injuries that can cause groin pain in athletes. The pelvic girdle and pubic bone represent the key structures that dynamically move with exercise, permitting the lower extremities to move with the torso. Specifically with athletic injuries, often due to hyperextension or hyperabduction, one of the core muscles can partially tear or become injured, leading to instability, particularly at the fibrocartilaginous attachments to the pubic bone. This injury may be in the rectus insertion, obliques, transverse abdominus, and/or the adductors. In addition, there may be injury of the pubic bone or pubic symphysis. The "inguinal disruption" diagnosis suggested by the British Hernia Society is likely a subtype of this injury, related to disruption of the transversalis, obliques, or rectus and relating to pain in the inguinal region. There may be significant overlap with related orthopedic injuries including osteitis pubis, femoral acetabular impingement, and snapping hip syndrome. This injury itself is a site of pain, but additional compensation from remaining core muscles can lead to additional pain and injury in other locations through the pelvic girdle. There is also a school of thought that athletic groin pain may in part be neuropathic due to compression of the inguinal sensory nerves, sometimes as a sequela of musculoskeletal injury.[34]

The diagnosis and management of athletic-related groin pain can be difficult. These can be career-ending injuries for the elite college or professional athlete. Increasingly these injuries are also being recognized in high-performing recreational athletes and frequently impair return to sport. The specific type of injury affects the presentation and should also influence the choice of treatment. Patients should be evaluated by an experienced multidisciplinary team of sports medicine physicians, hernia surgeons, physical therapists, and orthopedic surgeons. Zuckerbraun and colleagues[30] have published a recent review of the many potential injuries that can cause groin pain in athletes, as well as an excellent algorithm for working through the evaluation and management of this complex process.

History and physical examination are key, along with testing of individual muscles to attempt to identify the cause. Physical examination includes evaluation for hernias, hip examination (active and passive range of motion and FADIR and FABER tests), adduction, and resisted sit-ups or abdominal crunch. Multiple injuries may be common, and in particular hip injuries may cause secondary compensatory injuries in the pelvic ring.[35]

Per the British Hernia Society consensus paper, the diagnosis of inguinal disruption (by Doha nomenclature: athletic groin pain, inguinal related) can be made if 3 of the following 5 clinical signs are present: (1) pinpoint tenderness over the pubic tubercle at the point of insertion of the conjoint tendon, (2) palpable tenderness over the deep inguinal ring, (3) pain and/or dilation of the external ring with no obvious hernia evident, (4) pain at the origin of the adductor longus tendon, and (5) dull, diffused pain in the groin, often radiating to the perineum and inner thigh or across the midline.[32]

Imaging additionally plays a role but may be difficult to interpret in the clinical context and is neither 100% sensitive nor 100% specific. Ultrasonography can help identify occult inguinal hernias that may be a cause of pain. Dedicated musculoskeletal ultrasonography can also evaluate for muscle or tendon injury, although this is highly operator dependent. MRI, specifically protocoled for groin pain, can also help elucidate the mechanism of injury. It remains important to evaluate for the various causes of pubic pain, including the hip joint, back, core muscles, and other intra-abdominal visceral pathologic conditions. Diagnostic injections may additionally play a role.

In most cases, initial treatment should be nonoperative and involve ice, anti-inflammatories, and rest. If pain continues beyond a few weeks, high-quality physical therapy is the next line. Physical therapy helps strengthen the supporting muscles to offload the pubic joint and index injury. There is good evidence that the quality of physical therapy is important and that therapy should focus on core stability and retraining of surrounding core muscles.[36] Active physical therapy with a focus on core strength and balancing exercises has a significantly higher success rate than conventional physical therapy with rest, massage, and mobilization.[37]

Percutaneous interventions such as corticosteroid injections or ilioinguinal nerve hydrodissection can serve as temporizing measures to facilitate return to activities. Although patients are often anxious to have surgery to return to sport more quickly, there is evidence that return to sport is faster with physical therapy than with surgical intervention.[38]

In selected patients who do not respond to physical therapy, surgery may be considered. Although there are no hard guidelines on how long to wait before surgery, there are suggestions that pain lasting more than 2 months may not resolve without intervention.[32] We therefore typically recommend at least 8 to 10 weeks of high-quality physical therapy before considering surgery.

There have been several proposed approaches to surgical treatment, and the choice of repair should be tailored to the athlete and the injury. Generally speaking, the quality of data in this area is poor[31] and there are no data that definitively suggest that any one surgical approach is superior. One major school of thought, led primarily by the Meyers group in Philadelphia, has argued for open groin reconstruction. Meyers and colleagues[39] have reported their personal experience in more than 5000 operations and identify at least 19 different syndromes, 26 procedures, and 121 different combinations of procedures. The investigators report that 95% of their patients undergoing operative repair return to full athletic pursuits within 3 months of surgery, although they do not report the specifics of the operative interventions or follow-up. It is difficult to know the exact components of their group's operative approach, but it seems to include suture repair of the rectus abdominus to the pubis and inguinal ligament, possible division of inguinal sensory nerves, and sometimes adductor longus tenotomies or using the adductor longus tendon to buttress the rectus repair.

Other groups prefer more limited open approaches to reinforce the inguinal floor with a "minimal" suture repair,[40] modified Bassini repair,[41] or Lichtenstein tension-free repair with mesh.[32] Some groups also feel that nerve impingement is a key feature and advocate for neurolysis, neurectomy, hydrodissection, or ablation of the ilioinguinal, iliohypogastric, and/or genitofemoral nerves, sometimes but not always combined with inguinal floor reinforcement. Still other groups advocate for a laparoscopic approach with mesh reinforcement of the area, with or without release of the inguinal ligament.[42,43] As many patients have adductor-related pain as a sole or additional injury, adductor tendon release may be performed either as a separate procedure or in conjunction with any of the aforementioned approaches.[44]

The 2 highest quality trials in surgical management of athletic-related groin pain have both shown good results with laparoscopic mesh reinforcement. Paajanen and colleagues[42] randomized 60 patients to either TEP mesh reinforcement or active physical therapy and found that 90% of patients in the surgical group returned to sport within 3 months, compared with only 27% in the nonoperative group. Pain was improved in the operative group at both 3- and 12-month follow-up. Sheen and colleagues[45] randomized patients to either laparoscopic repair or open suture repair and found that both approaches were equivalent with respect to return to sport with less initial pain in the laparoscopic group. Based on the results of these trials, we prefer a laparoscopic mesh reinforcement as the initial surgical approach in most patients who need surgery but will occasionally perform open groin reconstruction, neurolysis/neurectomy, and/or adductor tenotomy based on the location and mechanism of injury and symptoms.

THE ROLE OF TISSUE REPAIR IN MODERN HERNIA SURGERY

The vast majority of inguinal hernia repairs performed in the United States are performed with mesh, either via open or minimally invasive technique. In some ways, tissue repairs without mesh have become a lost art because surgical trainees no longer learn these operations and surgeons in practice have lost their comfort level with the art of a primary inguinal hernia repair. In a recent review of the Americas Hernia Society Quality Collaborative database, less than 4% of inguinal hernias were repaired without mesh.[46] Owing to high-profile mesh recalls, several lawsuits against companies that make mesh (and related legal advertisements on late night television and in sponsored Internet search results), and social media amplification of patients who have felt that they have been harmed by mesh, many patients now come into surgical consultation wary of any mesh-based hernia repair and asking specifically for a "no mesh" repair.

There have been numerous studies comparing various nonmesh and mesh inguinal hernia repair approaches, and there is no evidence that mesh leads to higher risk of chronic pain.[8] In one example, the Danish and Swedish Hernia Database collaboration looked at 1250 patients following Lichtenstein hernia repair compared with 630 patients with Shouldice repair and 732 with a Macy repair and found no difference in the rate of chronic pain.[47] A randomized trial of Shouldice, Lichtenstein, and TAPP inguinal hernia repairs showed that chronic pain was equivalent between the 2 open approaches and that chronic pain was least following laparoscopic repair with mesh.[48] A Cochrane review of 25 studies with 6293 participants showed that mesh reduces the risk of recurrence (relative risk 0.46; 95% CI, 0.26–0.80).[49] A separate Cochrane review showed no difference in chronic pain between the Shouldice repair and open mesh repair.[50]

Although there is no evidence that mesh increases the risk of chronic pain after inguinal hernia repair, it is still important that patients have the option of a nonmesh repair if they still desire one after a careful and informed discussion. A Cochrane review of 16 studies (2566 hernias) suggests that the Shouldice repair has a lower recurrence rate than other open techniques (OR 0.62, 95% CI 0.45–0.85).[50] The results appear to hold over time, because the recurrence risk at 18 years after Shouldice repair is as low as 2.9%.[51] The Shouldice repair is therefore likely the preferred option for nonmesh repairs at this time.[52] The Shouldice repair, however, is technically challenging with a steep learning curve, and the best results have been reported by single-center groups with high-volume experience in this technique. In addition, the Shouldice clinic itself, which has produced the best evidence for this repair, is highly restrictive in who they will operate on, and therefore it is unclear how generalizable this approach is.

The Shouldice repair is the most commonly performed nonmesh repair in the United States (77%), followed by Bassini (16%) and McVay (3.5%) repairs.[46] Other nonmesh approaches have been proposed as alternatives. The Moloney "darning" repair has been studied in 6 RCTs, and in a meta-analysis it had equivalent recurrence to mesh repair; however, there was insufficient evidence to determine the risk of chronic pain.[53] The Desarda repair is a relatively newly described alternative, in which a strip of external oblique fascia is mobilized and used as a reinforcement of the inguinal floor. Data on this approach are limited; however, one RCT has shown that recurrence after Desarda is equivalent to Lichtenstein repair at 3 years.[54] The Desarda repair may be more replicable than the Shouldice repair, but further studies are needed before this technique is adopted widely. Huynh and colleagues[55] have recently reported an intriguing case series of a minimally invasive nonmesh repair for low-risk patients with small hernias, the robotic iliopubic tract repair. This repair is based on the open iliopubic tract repair described by Nyhus, and in their phase 1 trial of 24 patients they have seen no recurrences with median 25-month follow-up.

SUMMARY

Despite the fact that the "lowly" inguinal hernia repair is one of the most common general surgical problems, or perhaps because it is so common, there remain numerous controversies about the "best" approach. This controversy has driven numerous scientific studies and international guidelines, as well as an explosion of surgeon interest and discussion on social media forums like Twitter, Facebook, and YouTube. Currently the International Hernia Collaboration on Facebook has more than 11,000 members, with frequent and active discussion on numerous hernia-related topics.[56] Although these forums can be a great tool for self-education and discussion, it is important for the surgeon to look at posts with caution. Posts and opinions may be educational and helpful but are often anecdotal and rarely evidence driven.[57] A recent review of YouTube videos of laparoscopic inguinal hernia repair videos found that only 16% had an adequate repair, whereas 46% of videos had technically unsafe maneuvers such as threatened critical structures, rough tissue handling, or dangerous fixation near the iliac vessels.[58]

Ideally, surgeons should approach each patient individually and tailor their approach based on patient factors and preferences. The informed consent process is critical, especially given increasing recognition of the risk of long-term chronic pain following hernia repair. It is therefore important that hernia surgeons have facility with multiple approaches including multiple open and minimally invasive techniques, as well as the ability to offer nonmesh repairs, or have the ability and willingness to refer patients when appropriate.

REFERENCES

1. Schroeder AD, Tubre DJ, Fitzgibbons RJ Jr. Watchful Waiting for Inguinal Hernia. Adv Surg 2019;53:293–303.
2. Kingsnorth A, LeBlanc K. Hernias: inguinal and incisional. Lancet 2003; 362(9395):1561–71.
3. Fitzgibbons RJ, Jonasson O, Gibbs J, et al. The development of a clinical trial to determine if watchful waiting is an acceptable alternative to routine herniorrhaphy for patients with minimal or no hernia symptoms. J Am Coll Surg 2003;196(5): 737–42.
4. Reistrup H, Fonnes S, Rosenberg J. Watchful waiting vs repair for asymptomatic or minimally symptomatic inguinal hernia in men: a systematic review. Hernia 2020. https://doi.org/10.1007/s10029-020-02295-3.
5. Fitzgibbons RJ Jr, Giobbie-Hurder A, Gibbs JO, et al. Watchful waiting vs repair of inguinal hernia in minimally symptomatic men: a randomized clinical trial. JAMA 2006;295(3):285–92.
6. Fitzgibbons RJ Jr, Ramanan B, Arya S, et al. Long-term results of a randomized controlled trial of a nonoperative strategy (watchful waiting) for men with minimally symptomatic inguinal hernias. Ann Surg 2013;258(3):508–15.
7. O'Dwyer PJ, Norrie J, Alani A, et al. Observation or operation for patients with an asymptomatic inguinal hernia: a randomized clinical trial. Ann Surg 2006;244(2): 167–73.
8. International guidelines for groin hernia management. Hernia 2018;22(1):1–165.
9. Thiels CA, Holst KA, Ubl DS, et al. Gender disparities in the utilization of laparoscopic groin hernia repair. J Surg Res 2017;210:59–68.
10. Vu JV, Gunaseelan V, Krapohl GL, et al. Surgeon utilization of minimally invasive techniques for inguinal hernia repair: a population-based study. Surg Endosc 2019;33(2):486–93.
11. Trevisonno M, Kaneva P, Watanabe Y, et al. A survey of general surgeons regarding laparoscopic inguinal hernia repair: practice patterns, barriers, and educational needs. Hernia 2015;19(5):719–24.
12. Kapadia S, Ozao-Choy J, de Virgilio C, et al. Laparoscopic inguinal hernia repair: undervalued by the relative value unit system. Am Surg 2020;86(10):1324–9.
13. Bittner R, Montgomery MA, Arregui E, et al. Update of guidelines on laparoscopic (TAPP) and endoscopic (TEP) treatment of inguinal hernia (International Endohernia Society). Surg Endosc 2015;29(2):289–321.

14. Claus C, Furtado M, Malcher F, et al. Ten golden rules for a safe MIS inguinal hernia repair using a new anatomical concept as a guide. Surg Endosc 2020;4: 1458–64.

15. Köckerling F, Bittner R, Jacob DA, et al. TEP versus TAPP: comparison of the perioperative outcome in 17,587 patients with a primary unilateral inguinal hernia. Surg Endosc 2015;29(12):3750–60.

16. Neumayer L, Giobbie-Hurder A, Jonasson O, et al. Open mesh versus laparoscopic mesh repair of inguinal hernia. N Engl J Med 2004;350(18):1819–27.

17. Langeveld HR, van't Riet M, Weidema WF, et al. Total extraperitoneal inguinal hernia repair compared with Lichtenstein (the LEVEL-Trial): a randomized controlled trial. Ann Surg 2010;251(5):819–24.

18. Rana G, Armijo PR, Khan S, et al. Outcomes and impact of laparoscopic inguinal hernia repair versus open inguinal hernia repair on healthcare spending and employee absenteeism. Surg Endosc 2020;34(2):821–8.

19. Bullen NL, Massey LH, Antoniou SA, et al. Open versus laparoscopic mesh repair of primary unilateral uncomplicated inguinal hernia: a systematic review with meta-analysis and trial sequential analysis. Hernia 2019;23(3):461–72.

20. Schouten N, Simmermacher RK, van Dalen T, et al. Is there an end of the "learning curve" of endoscopic totally extraperitoneal (TEP) hernia repair? Surg Endosc 2013;27(3):789–94.

21. Sheetz KH, Claflin J, Dimick JB. Trends in the Adoption of Robotic Surgery for Common Surgical Procedures. JAMA Netw Open 2020;3(1):e1918911.

22. Tam V, Rogers DE, Al-Abbas A, et al. Robotic inguinal hernia repair: a large health system's experience with the first 300 cases and review of the literature. J Surg Res 2019;235:98–104.

23. Charles EJ, Mehaffey JH, Tache-Leon CA, et al. Inguinal hernia repair: is there a benefit to using the robot? Surg Endosc 2018;32(4):2131–6.

24. Abdelmoaty WF, Dunst CM, Neighorn C, et al. Robotic-assisted versus laparoscopic unilateral inguinal hernia repair: a comprehensive cost analysis. Surg Endosc 2019;33(10):3436–43.

25. Prabhu AS, Carbonell A, Hope W, et al. Robotic inguinal vs transabdominal laparoscopic inguinal hernia repair: The RIVAL randomized clinical trial. JAMA Surg 2020;155(5):380–7.

26. Chung L, Norrie J, O'Dwyer PJ. Long-term follow-up of patients with a painless inguinal hernia from a randomized clinical trial. Br J Surg 2011;98(4):596–9.

27. van Veen RN, Wijsmuller AR, Vrijland WW, et al. Long-term follow-up of a randomized clinical trial of non-mesh versus mesh repair of primary inguinal hernia. Br J Surg 2007;94(4):506–10.

28. Jarrard JA, Arroyo MR, Moore BT. Occult contralateral inguinal hernias: what is their true incidence and should they be repaired? Surg Endosc 2019;33(8): 2456–8.

29. Griffin KJ, Harris S, Tang TY, et al. Incidence of contralateral occult inguinal hernia found at the time of laparoscopic trans-abdominal pre-peritoneal (TAPP) repair. Hernia 2010;14(4):345–9.

30. Zuckerbraun BS, Cyr AR, Mauro CS. Groin pain syndrome known as sports hernia: A Review. JAMA Surg 2020;155(4):340–8.

31. Serner A, van Eijck CH, Beumer BR, et al. Study quality on groin injury management remains low: a systematic review on treatment of groin pain in athletes. Br J Sports Med 2015;49(12):813.

32. Sheen AJ, Stephenson BM, Lloyd DM, et al. 'Treatment of the Sportsman's groin': British Hernia Society's 2014 position statement based on the Manchester Consensus Conference. Br J Sports Med 2014;48(14):1079–87.

33. Weir A, Brukner P, Delahunt E, et al. Doha agreement meeting on terminology and definitions in groin pain in athletes. Br J Sports Med 2015;49(12):768–74.

34. Comin J, Obaid H, Lammers G, et al. Radiofrequency denervation of the inguinal ligament for the treatment of 'Sportsman's Hernia': a pilot study. Br J Sports Med 2013;47(6):380–6.

35. Hammoud S, Bedi A, Voos JE, et al. The recognition and evaluation of patterns of compensatory injury in patients with mechanical hip pain. Sports Health 2014; 6(2):108–18.

36. Ellsworth AA, Zoland MP, Tyler TF. Athletic pubalgia and associated rehabilitation. Int J Sports Phys Ther 2014;9(6):774–84.

37. Abouelnaga WA, Aboelnour NH. Effectiveness of active rehabilitation program on sports hernia: randomized control trial. Ann Rehabil Med 2019;43(3):305–13.

38. King E, Ward J, Small L, et al. Athletic groin pain: a systematic review and meta-analysis of surgical versus physical therapy rehabilitation outcomes. Br J Sports Med 2015;49(22):1447–51.

39. Meyers WC, McKechnie A, Philippon MJ, et al. Experience with "sports hernia" spanning two decades. Ann Surg 2008;248(4):656–65.

40. Muschaweck U, Berger L. Minimal Repair technique of sportsmen's groin: an innovative open-suture repair to treat chronic inguinal pain. Hernia 2010;14(1): 27–33.

41. Gilmore J. Groin pain in the soccer athlete: fact, fiction, and treatment. Clin Sports Med 1998;17(4):787–93, vii.

42. Paajanen H, Syvähuoko I, Airo I. Totally extraperitoneal endoscopic (TEP) treatment of sportsman's hernia. Surg Laparosc Endosc Percutan Tech 2004;14(4): 215–8.

43. Lloyd DM, Sutton CD, Altafa A, et al. Laparoscopic inguinal ligament tenotomy and mesh reinforcement of the anterior abdominal wall: a new approach for the management of chronic groin pain. Surg Laparosc Endosc Percutan Tech 2008;18(4):363–8.

44. Atkinson HD, Johal P, Falworth MS, et al. Adductor tenotomy: its role in the management of sports-related chronic groin pain. Arch Orthop Trauma Surg 2010; 130(8):965–70.

45. Sheen AJ, Montgomery A, Simon T, et al. Randomized clinical trial of open suture repair versus totally extraperitoneal repair for treatment of sportsman's hernia. Br J Surg 2019;106(7):837–44.

46. AlMarzooqi R, Tish S, Huang LC, et al. Review of inguinal hernia repair techniques within the Americas Hernia Society Quality Collaborative. Hernia 2019; 23(3):429–38.

47. Bay-Nielsen M, Nilsson E, Nordin P, et al. Chronic pain after open mesh and sutured repair of indirect inguinal hernia in young males. Br J Surg 2004;91(10): 1372–6.

48. Köninger J, Redecke J, Butters M. Chronic pain after hernia repair: a randomized trial comparing Shouldice, Lichtenstein and TAPP. Langenbecks Arch Surg 2004; 389(5):361–5.

49. Lockhart K, Dunn D, Teo S, et al. Mesh versus non-mesh for inguinal and femoral hernia repair. Cochrane Database Syst Rev 2018;9(9):Cd011517.

50. Amato B, Moja L, Panico S, et al. Shouldice technique versus other open techniques for inguinal hernia repair. Cochrane Database Syst Rev 2012;2012(4): Cd001543.
51. Martín Duce A, Lozano O, Galván M, et al. Results of Shouldice hernia repair after 18 years of follow-up in all the patients. Hernia 2021. https://doi.org/10.1007/s10029-021-02422-8.
52. Bendavid R, Mainprize M, Iakovlev V. Pure tissue repairs: a timely and critical revival. Hernia 2019;23(3):493–502.
53. Finch DA, Misra VA, Hajibandeh S. Open darn repair vs open mesh repair of inguinal hernia: a systematic review and meta-analysis of randomised and non-randomised studies. Hernia 2019;23(3):523–39.
54. Szopinski J, Dabrowiecki S, Pierscinski S, et al. Desarda versus Lichtenstein technique for primary inguinal hernia treatment: 3-year results of a randomized clinical trial. World J Surg 2012;36(5):984–92.
55. Huynh D, Fadaee N, Al-Aufey B, et al. Robotic iliopubic tract (r-IPT) repair: technique and preliminary outcomes of a minimally invasive tissue repair for inguinal hernia. Hernia 2020;24(5):1041–7.
56. Ghanem O, Logghe HJ, Tran BV, et al. Closed Facebook™ groups and CME credit: a new format for continuing medical education. Surg Endosc 2019; 33(2):587–91.
57. Bernardi K, Milton AN, Hope W, et al. Are online surgical discussion boards a safe and useful venue for surgeons to ask for advice? A review of the International Hernia Collaboration Facebook Group. Surg Endosc 2020;34(3):1285–9.
58. Huynh D, Fadaee N, Gök H, et al. Thou shalt not trust online videos for inguinal hernia repair techniques. Surg Endosc 2020. https://doi.org/10.1007/s00464-020-08035-z.

Management of Incidentalomas

Keely Reidelberger, BS, MS[a], Abbey Fingeret, MD, MHPTT[b],*

KEYWORDS

- Incidental Meckel diverticulum • Adrenal incidentaloma • Incidental thyroid nodule
- Incidental solitary pulmonary nodule • Incidental small bowel intussusception
- Asymptomatic gallstones • Incidental appendectomy

KEY POINTS

- Resection of incidental Meckel diverticulum should be considered for healthy children and young adults, a palpable abnormality, or a diverticulum larger than 2 cm.
- Adrenalectomy is indicated for incidentaloma with indeterminate or suspicious radiographic appearance, size greater than 4 cm, rapid growth, or secretion.
- Incidental thyroid nodules most commonly are benign and should be considered for fine-needle aspiration biopsy based on sonographic risk, size, and patient risk factors.
- Most incidental solitary pulmonary nodules are benign and can be monitored with surveillance imaging unless high-risk features are present.

INTRODUCTION

Incidental findings are common in the evaluation of surgical patients. Understanding the appropriate assessment and management of these frequent occurrences is important for the provision of comprehensive quality care. This review details the epidemiology, considerations, and recommendations for management of common incidental manifestations in surgical patients, including Meckel diverticulum, adrenal incidentaloma, thyroid nodule, solitary pulmonary nodule, small bowel intussusception, gallstones, and incidental appendectomy.

INCIDENTAL MECKEL DIVERTICULUM

In normal embryologic development, the omphalomesenteric duct completely obliterates. A Meckel diverticulum represents a persistent remnant of the omphalomesenteric duct that normally involutes between the fifth and sixth weeks of embryologic

[a] University of Nebraska Medical Center College of Medicine, 986880 Nebraska Medical Center, Omaha, NE 68198-6880, USA; [b] Department of Surgery, Division of Surgical Oncology, University of Nebraska Medical Center, 986880 Nebraska Medical Center, Omaha, NE 68198-6880, USA
* Corresponding author.
E-mail address: abbey.fingeret@unmc.edu
Twitter: @DrFingeret (A.F.)

Surg Clin N Am 101 (2021) 1081–1096
https://doi.org/10.1016/j.suc.2021.06.006
0039-6109/21/© 2021 Elsevier Inc. All rights reserved.

development.[1] The diverticulum arises on the antimesenteric border of the small bowel at the mid to distal ileum (**Fig. 1**). Although generally, rare with an estimated prevalence of 1% to 3%, it is the most common congenital anomaly of the gastrointestinal tract.[2–5] Meckel diverticulae may cause pathology with abdominal pain, gastrointestinal bleeding, or obstruction or more frequently is clinically silent, particularly in adults. Gastrointestinal bleeding may occur from native intestinal or heterotopic mucosa—most commonly gastric, followed by pancreatic or colonic.[6] The rule of 2s classically has been used to describe the anatomic and pathologic findings of Meckel diverticulum: 2% of the population, male predominance of 2 to 1, 2 feet from the ileocecal valve, and 2 inches long with pathologic presentation before the age of 2 years.[7] A Meckel diverticulum may be an incidental finding on imaging or during laparotomy or laparoscopy for an alternate indication.[8,9] When an incidental Meckel diverticulum is identified, the surgeon needs to make a determination of the potential risks of resection versus the future risks of bleeding or other complication.

To determine whether to resect an incidental Meckel diverticulum, first the natural history must be delineated. The potential for an asymptomatic Meckel diverticulum to progress to complication is challenging to quantify. Given the rates of disease in infants, toddlers, and children compared with adults, it has been postulated that the incidence of symptoms decreases with age, although the male prevalence remains greater than the female prevalence.[10] From population-based studies, the incidence of complications from Meckel diverticulum requiring surgery is estimated at 4.2% to

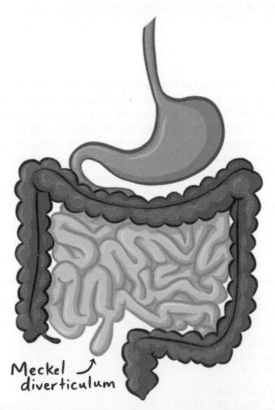

Fig. 1. A Meckel diverticulum arising from the antimesenteric border of the distal ileum.

6.2%.[7,10] The size and composition of the diverticulum also may influence progression to symptoms, with 1 study finding that patients with a diverticulum greater than 2 cm or heterotopic mucosa had a higher likelihood of symptomatic disease.[11]

If a Meckel diverticulum is identified incidentally on imaging for a patient who is not undergoing abdominal exploration, further imaging or elective resection is not recommended.[3,5,7,11,12] For those with an incidental finding of Meckel diverticulum at the time of abdominal exploration via laparoscopy or laparotomy for an alternate indication, the decision to resect should be patient-centered based on the risk of future complications. The existing data are from retrospective studies, case series, and systematic reviews because prospective studies are lacking in this area. There is controversy regarding recommendations to resect, with some investigators advocating against elective resection and others in favor.[4,6,7,12–15] Resection should be considered selectively for otherwise healthy children and young adults, those with a palpable abnormality, or adults less than 50 years of age with a diverticulum greater than 2 cm.[11,16,17]

Resection may be performed by simple diverticulectomy with division of the diverticulum at its base or alternatively with small bowel resection and sewn or stapled anastomosis via either laparoscopy or laparotomy.[18–22] Small bowel resection should be considered if luminal narrowing may result from diverticulectomy or if there is a palpable abnormality near the base of the diverticulum.[22] Outcomes of elective resection of an incidental Meckel diverticulum generally are excellent with low overall morbidity and mortality, although in 1 study complications were more prevalent in those undergoing elective resection at 5.3% than those who did not at 1.3%.[5] Complications from incidental resection are difficult to differentiate from the index procedure, so estimates of 2% to 20% morbidity may not be attributed directly to the diverticulectomy, although complication rates for elective Meckel resection are approximately 2%.[10] If an incidental Meckel diverticulum is left in situ, patient counseling of the finding and potential symptoms is indicated.

ADRENAL INCIDENTALOMA

Adrenal incidentaloma, a mass of the adrenal gland visualized on imaging for an alternate indication, is a common finding and may prompt further evaluation (**Fig. 2A**). Adrenal masses may arise from the medulla or the layers of the adrenal cortex—zona glomerulosa, zona fasciculata, and zona reticularis (**Fig. 2B**). The detection of adrenal masses has increased with the expansion of cross-sectional imaging. Incidental adrenal masses greater than 1 cm in diameter are found on 5% to 7% of all abdominal CT examinations, in older patients at up to 10%, and in obese or hypertensive patients up to 12%.[23–25] Incidental adrenal masses are found at similar rates in autopsy studies, from 1% to 9%.[23] Bilateral adrenal incidentalomas occur in up to 15% of patients who are identified to have an incidental adrenal finding on imaging[26]; although most incidental adrenal masses are benign and nonfunctional, up to 10% secrete excess hormones with 6.4% secreting cortisol, 3.1% catecholamines, 0.6% aldosterone, and rarely androgens—highlighting the importance of biochemical testing.[27]

Fortunately, incidentally discovered malignancy in the adrenal gland is an uncommon diagnosis. In this setting of an incidentaloma, the frequency of primary adrenal malignancy is 2% to 5%, and the frequency of metastatic disease with an undiagnosed primary cancer is 0.7% to 2.5%.[28,29] Up to 13% of patients with a known malignancy have an adrenal mass identified and 26% to 36% of these lesions are metastatic disease.[24,30] In historical autopsy studies, patients with a known malignancy had a prevalence of adrenal metastases as high as 27%.[31] The management

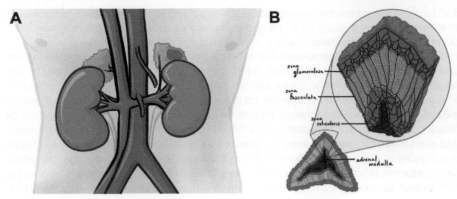

Fig. 2. (*A*) An adrenal adenoma. (*B*) Anatomy of the adrenal gland.

of an adrenal incidentaloma depends on the likelihood of malignancy and the functional status.

The size of the incidentally discovered adrenal lesion, whether by computed tomography (CT) or magnetic resonance imaging (MRI), is predictive of malignancy. Adrenal incidentaloma greater than 4 cm or those displaying rapid growth characteristics are indicative of primary or secondary malignancy in 71% of cases.[32] More than 90% of cases of adrenocortical carcinoma are greater than 4 cm at the time of presentation. Studies have shown that using a threshold of 4 cm for resection yielded a 93% sensitivity in detecting adrenocortical carcinoma but had limited specificity.[26,33] Although useful in directing intervention for large masses, size should be used in concert with other clinical and radiographic characteristics to guide management of smaller lesions. Adrenalectomy is recommended for incidental adrenal masses greater than 4 cm or exhibiting rapid growth, because smaller adrenal mass size at time of diagnosis of adrenocortical carcinoma is associated with a more favorable prognosis.[26,33–35]

In addition to size, CT characteristics of intracellular lipid content and vascular enhancement patterns can be used to differentiate benign adenoma from malignancy; 70% of adrenal adenomas contain significant intracellular lipid with densitometry of less than 10 Hounsfield units attenuation and may allow for differentiation from malignant lesions with a sensitivity of 71% and a specificity of 98%.[36–39] A lesion displaying low attenuation densitometry on nonenhanced CT with other characteristics, including homogeneity and smooth borders, is more likely to be a benign adenoma.[40] Up to 30% of adenomas do not have low attenuation by nonenhanced CT, making them indistinguishable from malignant lesions based on Hounsfield units.[41,42]

For incidental adrenal lesions of higher attenuation, contrast-enhanced CT with delayed imaging for washout delineating vascular enhancement pattern should be performed.[43] Adenomas typically display immediate contrast enhancement and then washout rapidly. Malignant lesions exhibit delayed contrast washout due to capillary leak.[44] An absolute contrast washout of 50% at 10 minutes is 96% to 100% sensitive and 98% to 100% specific for differentiating adenoma from carcinoma, pheochromocytoma, and metastases.[38,41,42,45–48]

Incidental adrenal masses that have heterogeneity, irregular borders, calcifications, a density of greater than 10 Hounsfield units, or less than 50% washout are indeterminate for benignity and should be considered for resection.[48–51] Biopsy with fine-needle aspiration (FNA) or core needle biopsy rarely is indicated for adrenal incidentalomas.

For patients with a known history of malignancy who are not candidates for metastatectomy and in whom adrenal gland mass represents the only site of metastatic disease or the safest potential metastasis to biopsy, then percutaneous image–guided biopsy could be considered after biochemical evaluation to exclude pheochromocytoma. Biopsy to exclude adrenocortical carcinoma is not useful to distinguish from benign adrenal adenoma.

Adrenalectomy may be indicated based on size or imaging characteristics. Even for lesions with planned resection, biochemical work-up is paramount for safe preparation for surgery and postoperative management. For adrenal incidentalomas that do not meet resection criteria by appearance, the presence of excess hormone secretion is an independent surgical indication.[52] Biochemical work-up should proceed to assess for hypercortisolism, hyperaldosteronism, hyperandrogenism, and catecholamine excess. For Cushing syndrome, testing may include a low-dose dexamethasone suppression test, midnight salivary cortisol levels, or a 24-hour urinary free cortisol measurement. Androgen secretion can be determined with measurement of dehydroepiandrosterone sulfate, although this is extremely rare. For hyperaldosteronism, the plasma aldosterone concentration should be obtained, and a ratio of plasma renin activity calculated. If the aldosterone-to-renin ratio is elevated, even in the presence of an adrenal adenoma on imaging, further evaluation with adrenal venous sampling should be considered. The presence or absence of adrenal lesions on crosssectional imaging can demonstrate a significant amount of discordance with adrenal venous sampling. In 1 study, CT was accurate in only 53% of patients, incorrectly excluding 22% from adrenalectomy and leading to unnecessary adrenalectomy in 25%.[53] Another study found CT and MRI discordant with adrenal venous sampling localization in 37.8% of patients, and, if operative intervention were based on imaging alone, would have led to inappropriate adrenalectomy in 18.5% and inappropriate medical management in 19.1% of cases.[54] Given the discordant findings of CT and MRI in primary hyperaldosteronism, surgical resection without adrenal venous sampling is recommended only for young, good-risk surgical candidates with a solitary unilateral lesion greater than 1 cm.[55] Evaluation for pheochromocytoma should proceed with plasma metanephrines as a screening test. If equivocal, confirmatory testing can be performed with 24-hour urinary catecholamine levels.[56] Patients found to have excess hormone secretion should be evaluated for adrenalectomy by a high-volume surgeon.[57]

INCIDENTAL THYROID NODULE

Thyroid nodules are common, with a prevalence of greater than 50% by the seventh decade of life, and most are identified incidentally. In the American Thyroid Association Management Guidelines for Adult Patients with Thyroid Nodules, a thyroid nodule is defined as a discrete lesion within the thyroid gland that is palpably or ultrasonographically distinct from surrounding thyroid parenchyma (**Fig. 3**).[58] Thyroid malignancy is found in 4% to 6.5% of thyroid nodules.[59–62] For thyroid nodules incidentally discovered on PET CT that are fluorodeoxyglucose (FDG) avid, the malignancy risk is up to 34.8%.[58,63]

The evaluation of an incidental thyroid nodule is aimed at determining whether the nodule is autonomously functioning, causing clinical or subclinical hyperthyroidism, and then evaluating for malignancy. A thorough history of hyperthyroid or hypothyroid symptoms, compressive or invasive symptoms of globus sensation, or voice changes; personal history of ionizing radiation exposure; and family history of thyroid nodules or malignancy should be obtained. Laboratory evaluation with serum thyroid-stimulating

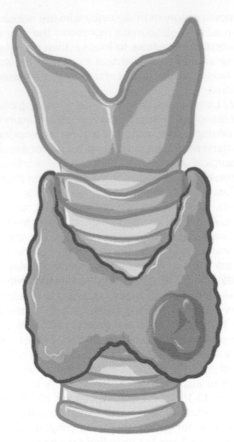

Fig. 3. A thyroid nodule.

hormone (TSH) level should be performed. If TSH is suppressed, the evaluation should proceed with measurement of TSH-receptor antibodies or a thyroid scintigraphy. If euthyroid or hypothyroid, a dedicated thyroid ultrasound should be performed with assessment of the thyroid to confirm the presence and characteristics of the nodule or nodules and assess the central and lateral neck lymph node compartments for lymphadenopathy.[58,64]

Thyroid nodule malignancy risk is variable based on sonographic appearance; therefore, size threshold for FNA biopsy is dependent on sonographic characteristics. FNA should be performed with ultrasound guidance. Very-low-risk nodules with cystic, partially cystic, or spongiform appearance may be observed or considered for FNA if greater than 2 cm. Low-risk partially cystic or solid nodules with isoechoic or hyperechoic appearance and no high-risk features should be considered for FNA at 1.5 cm. Intermediate-risk and high-risk nodules that are hypoechoic or have suspicious sonographic characteristics are recommended for FNA at 1 cm. Suspicious characteristics include microcalcifications, rim calcifications, taller-than-wide shape, irregular borders, extrathyroidal extension, and thyroid nodules in the setting of lymphadenopathy suspicious for thyroid cancer metastases.[58,65] FNA should be performed for PET CT–FDG avid thyroid nodules greater than 1 cm. Biopsy of nodules less than 1 cm may be considered for high-risk patients with a personal history of radiation or family history of thyroid malignancy.[66,67] For nodules that do not meet criteria for FNA, surveillance should occur at 6 months to 12 months.[66]

Management of incidental thyroid nodules is dependent on sonographic appearance and FNA cytology results. Thyroid nodule cytology is reported using a standardized diagnostic model, the Bethesda system (**Table 1**).[68] Patients with nondiagnostic cytology (Bethesda I) should undergo repeat FNA. For patients with benign cytology (Bethesda II), radiofrequency ablation or thyroidectomy may be considered if symptomatic.[69] Patients with indeterminate cytology (Bethesda III and IV) may have further evaluation with molecular markers or be considered hemithyroidectomy for definitive diagnosis. For patients with suspicious or malignant cytology (Bethesda V and VI), active surveillance may be considered if low risk features or proceed to hemithyroidectomy or total thyroidectomy.[70]

INCIDENTAL SOLITARY PULMONARY NODULE

Incidental pulmonary nodules are detected in asymptomatic patients undergoing imaging for purposes other than lung cancer screening. These nodules are defined as lesions surrounded by normal lung and measure less than 3 cm.[71-73] The prevalence of incidental pulmonary nodules is estimated as 25% of healthy adults.[72] Malignancy is uncommon, with as few as 1% of nodules containing cancer, even in patients with a smoking history and high risk of malignancy.[74] Thus, a vast majority of incidental pulmonary nodules have a benign etiology. The goal of the evaluation of a patient with an incidental pulmonary nodule is to assess for malignancy adequately while limiting morbidity of evaluation and unnecessary follow-up examinations.[75] The size and morphology of a solitary pulmonary nodule are the most important factors that determine malignancy risk. The use of high-resolution imaging with CT sections of 1 mm is necessary to adequately evaluate morphology.

The most common cause of a benign pulmonary nodule is an infectious granuloma—responsible for up to 80% of cases.[76] Common organisms producing infectious granulomas are endemic fungi and mycobacteria. The classical description of an infectious granuloma is a well-circumscribed and calcified nodule. Benign pulmonary hamartomas are responsible for an estimated 10% of incidental pulmonary nodules.[77] These nodules may appear with calcifications resembling popcorn or may have a heterogeneous appearance of fat, muscle, or connective tissue.[78] Other benign

Table 1		
Bethesda system diagnostic categories for reporting thyroid cytopathology		
Bethesda Class	**Diagnostic Category**	**Malignancy Risk (%)**
I	Nondiagnostic (unsatisfactory)	5–10
II	Benign	0–3
III	Atypia of undetermined significance or follicular lesion of undetermined significance	10–30
IV	Follicular neoplasm (or suspicious for follicular neoplasm)	25–40
V	Suspicious for malignancy	50–75
VI	Malignant	97–99

Data from: Cibas ES, Ali SZ. The 2017 Bethesda system for reporting thyroid cytopathology. Thyroid 2017; 27: 1341.

etiologies of incidental pulmonary nodules include pulmonary arteriovenous malformations, hemangiomas, leiomyomas, and fibromas.

Although rare, an incidental pulmonary nodule may have a malignant etiology, such as a primary lung cancer, neuroendocrine tumor, or metastasis. Primary lung cancer is the most common adenocarcinoma, followed by squamous cell carcinoma (SCC), and non–small cell lung carcinoma (NSCLC).[72] The location of the nodule is relevant as adenocarcinoma and NSCLC are more likely to occur peripherally, whereas SCC more frequently is found centrally. Metastatic cancer often is identified on imaging for restaging and infrequently considered an incidental finding.

Incidental pulmonary nodules can be considered by their size and appearance to determine risk profile. Solitary nodules less than 6 mm with low-risk appearance do not require follow-up, those 6 mm to 8 mm are recommended for 6-month to 12-month interval CT follow-up, and those greater than 8 mm should be considered for follow-up CT at 3 months, PET CT, or tissue sampling.[75] Patients with higher-risk nodule morphology should be considered for 12-month follow-up for solitary nodules less than 6 mm.[75]

INCIDENTAL SMALL BOWEL INTUSSUSCEPTION

Intussusception, or telescoping of the bowel into itself, may present with symptoms of abdominal pain or obstruction or be found incidentally in an asymptomatic patient. The invagination of the bowel into the adjacent lumen may cause obstruction or bowel edema, ischemia, or perforation (**Fig. 4**). Incidental intussusception may be spontaneously reducing or transient.[79] Although intussusception is most common in the first 3 years of life, it can occur at any age.[80] In children, intussusception most frequently is idiopathic, although in adults, it is associated more often with a pathologic lead point.[81] In adults, more than half of symptomatic intussusception is due to a malignant etiology.[82]

In children, incidental asymptomatic intussusception may be managed with observation and is likely to resolve spontaneously if the intussusceptum is a short segment less than 3.5 cm.[83] Short segment intussusceptum in adults also is associated with a higher likelihood of spontaneous reduction.[84] Due to the higher likelihood of malignant pathology in adults, resection should be considered. Although intussusception may be an incidental finding on imaging, a thorough history may reveal subacute or chronic symptoms of partial bowel obstruction. If malignancy is suspected, an oncologic resection should be performed. Historically, operative reduction of the intussusception was not recommended prior to resection.[85] Contemporarily, preoperative or

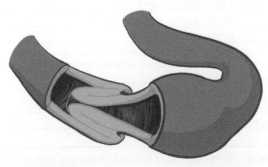

Fig. 4. Small bowel intussusception.

intraoperative reduction may be considered if it will improve patient optimization for surgery or decrease morbidity while maintaining oncologic principles.[86]

Asymptomatic Gallstones

In the United States, cholelithiasis is highly prevalent, with estimates of more than 14 million adult women and 6 million adult men affected.[87] A majority of patients with gallstones are asymptomatic. For these patients, prophylactic cholecystectomy is not indicated unless high-risk features are present because there is no benefit to survival or quality of life.[88] Patients should be counseled regarding symptoms of biliary colic, cholecystitis, choledocholithiasis, cholangitis, and pancreatitis and prompted to seek care if they acquire these symptoms.

Patients with high risk for complications of symptomatic cholelithiasis or potential for gallbladder carcinoma should be considered for prophylactic cholecystectomy, including gallbladder calcification or porcelain gallbladder, gallbladder adenoma or polyp, or a gallstone larger than 3 cm.[89–92] Patients with hereditary spherocytosis should be considered for prophylactic cholecystectomy, particularly at the time of splenectomy, if indicated.[93,94] Similarly, patients with sickle cell disease are recommended to have prophylactic cholecystectomy if asymptomatic cholelithiasis is identified, because increased risk of perioperative complications is associated with urgent cholecystectomy for acute cholecystitis in this population.[95–97]

INCIDENTAL APPENDECTOMY

The lifetime incidence of acute appendicitis is estimated at 7%.[98,99] The highest incidence occurs prior to the fourth decade of life but still may occur in elderly patient populations, who may have higher rates of perforation, morbidity, and mortality[100–104] Incidental appendectomy refers to removal of the noninflamed appendix at the time of another indicated abdominal procedure and has been evaluated during a variety of operations including cholecystectomy, hysterectomy, and urologic procedures.[98,102,103] Overall, incidental appendectomy has not been shown to be cost-effective for most adults, particularly for older patients.[105,106] Incidental appendectomy may be cost-effective for adult patients under 25 years to 55 years, depending on the cost for those undergoing elective laparoscopic or open procedures.[107,108]

Despite potential cost efficacy in younger adults and generally safe operative risk profile, the effects of incidental appendectomy may not be understood fully. The impact of appendectomy on the gut microbiota potentially is deleterious. Incidental prophylactic appendectomy is associated with a profound microbial dysbiosis in the long term.[109] The intestinal microbiome has been linked to anastomotic healing, diverticulitis, and colorectal neoplasms.[110]

SUMMARY

Incidental findings in surgery are common. Evaluation and management are patient-centered with a focus on comprehensive quality care that limits morbidity. Recommended management evolves as diagnostic imaging and treatment modalities improve.

CLINICS CARE POINTS

- Resection of incidental Meckel's diverticulum should be considered for healthy children and young adults, a palpable abnormality, or a diverticulum larger than two centimeters.

- Adrenalectomy is indicated for incidentaloma with indeterminate or suspicious radiographic appearance, size greater than four centimeters, rapid growth, or secretion.
- Incidental thyroid nodules are most commonly benign and should be considered for fine needle aspiration biopsy based on sonographic risk, size, and patient risk factors.
- Most incidental solitary pulmonary nodules are benign and can be monitored with surveillance imaging unless high risk features are present.

DISCLOSURE

The authors have nothing to disclose. This research did not receive any specific grant from funding agencies in the public, commercial, or not-for-profit sectors.

REFERENCES

1. Yahchouchy EK, Marano AF, Etienne JC, et al. Meckel's diverticulum. J Am Coll Surg 2001;192(5):658–62.
2. Hansen CC, Soreide K. Systematic review of epidemiology, presentation, and management of Meckel's diverticulum in the 21st century. Medicine (Baltimore) 2018;97(35):e12154.
3. Sagar J, Kumar V, Shah DK. Meckel's diverticulum: a systematic review. J R Soc Med 2006;99(10):501–5.
4. Ueberrueck T, Meyer L, Koch A, et al. The significance of Meckel's diverticulum in appendicitis–a retrospective analysis of 233 cases. World J Surg 2005;29(4): 455–8.
5. Zani A, Eaton S, Rees CM, et al. Incidentally detected Meckel diverticulum: to resect or not to resect? Ann Surg 2008;247(2):276–81.
6. Francis A, Kantarovich D, Khoshnam N, et al. Pediatric Meckel's Diverticulum: Report of 208 Cases and Review of the Literature. Fetal Pediatr Pathol 2016; 35(3):199–206.
7. Soltero MJ, Bill AH. The natural history of Meckel's Diverticulum and its relation to incidental removal. A study of 202 cases of diseased Meckel's Diverticulum found in King County, Washington, over a fifteen year period. Am J Surg 1976;132(2):168–73.
8. Thurley PD, Halliday KE, Somers JM, et al. Radiological features of Meckel's diverticulum and its complications. Clin Radiol 2009;64(2):109–18.
9. Elsayes KM, Menias CO, Harvin HJ, et al. Imaging manifestations of Meckel's diverticulum. AJR Am J roentgenology 2007;189(1):81–8.
10. Cullen JJ, Kelly KA, Moir CR, et al. Surgical management of Meckel's diverticulum. An epidemiologic, population-based study. Ann Surg 1994;220(4): 564–8, discussion 568-569.
11. Park JJ, Wolff BG, Tollefson MK, et al. Meckel diverticulum: the Mayo Clinic experience with 1476 patients (1950-2002). Ann Surg 2005;241(3):529–33.
12. Bani-Hani KE, Shatnawi NJ. Meckel's diverticulum: comparison of incidental and symptomatic cases. World J Surg 2004;28(9):917–20.
13. Kashi SH, Lodge JP. Meckel's diverticulum: a continuing dilemma? J R Coll Surg Edinb 1995;40(6):392–4.
14. Leijonmarck CE, Bonman-Sandelin K, Frisell J, et al. Meckel's diverticulum in the adult. Br J Surg 1986;73(2):146–9.
15. Aarnio P, Salonen IS. Abdominal disorders arising from 71 Meckel's diverticulum. Ann Chir Gynaecol 2000;89(4):281–4.

16. Peoples JB, Lichtenberger EJ, Dunn MM. Incidental Meckel's diverticulectomy in adults. Surgery 1995;118(4):649–52.

17. Robijn J, Sebrechts E, Miserez M. Management of incidentally found Meckel's diverticulum a new approach: resection based on a Risk Score. Acta Chir Belg 2006;106(4):467–70.

18. Shalaby RY, Soliman SM, Fawy M, et al. Laparoscopic management of Meckel's diverticulum in children. J Pediatr Surg 2005;40(3):562–7.

19. Chan KW, Lee KH, Mou JW, et al. Laparoscopic management of complicated Meckel's diverticulum in children: a 10-year review. Surg Endosc 2008;22(6): 1509–12.

20. Chan KW, Lee KH, Wong HY, et al. Laparoscopic excision of Meckel's diverticulum in children: what is the current evidence? World J Gastroenterol 2014; 20(41):15158–62.

21. Ezekian B, Leraas HJ, Englum BR, et al. Outcomes of laparoscopic resection of Meckel's diverticulum are equivalent to open laparotomy. J Pediatr Surg 2019; 54(3):507–10.

22. Rivas H, Cacchione RN, Allen JW. Laparoscopic management of Meckel's diverticulum in adults. Surg Endosc 2003;17(4):620–2.

23. Terzolo M, Stigliano A, Chiodini I, et al. AME position statement on adrenal incidentaloma. Eur J Endocrinol 2011;164(6):851–70.

24. Bovio S, Cataldi A, Reimondo G, et al. Prevalence of adrenal incidentaloma in a contemporary computerized tomography series. J Endocrinol Invest 2006; 29(4):298–302.

25. Barzon L, Scaroni C, Sonino N, et al. Incidentally discovered adrenal tumors: endocrine and scintigraphic correlates. J Clin Endocrinol Metab 1998;83(1): 55–62.

26. Angeli A, Osella G, Ali A, et al. Adrenal incidentaloma: an overview of clinical and epidemiological data from the National Italian Study Group. Horm Res 1997;47(4–6):279–83.

27. Cawood TJ, Hunt PJ, O'Shea D, et al. Recommended evaluation of adrenal incidentalomas is costly, has high false-positive rates and confers a risk of fatal cancer that is similar to the risk of the adrenal lesion becoming malignant; time for a rethink? Eur J Endocrinol 2009;161(4):513–27.

28. Aron D, Terzolo M, Cawood TJ. Adrenal incidentalomas. Best Pract Res Clin Endocrinol Metab 2012;26(1):69–82.

29. Bittner JGt, Brunt LM. Evaluation and management of adrenal incidentaloma. J Surg Oncol 2012;106(5):557–64.

30. Song JH, Chaudhry FS, Mayo-Smith WW. The incidental adrenal mass on CT: prevalence of adrenal disease in 1,049 consecutive adrenal masses in patients with no known malignancy. AJR Am J Roentgenol 2008;190(5):1163–8.

31. Abrams HL, Spiro R, Goldstein N. Metastases in carcinoma; analysis of 1000 autopsied cases. Cancer 1950;3(1):74–85.

32. Frilling A, Tecklenborg K, Weber F, et al. Importance of adrenal incidentaloma in patients with a history of malignancy. Surgery 2004;136(6):1289–96.

33. Mantero F, Terzolo M, Arnaldi G, et al. A survey on adrenal incidentaloma in Italy. Study Group on Adrenal Tumors of the Italian Society of Endocrinology. J Clin Endocrinol Metab 2000;85(2):637–44.

34. Henley DJ, van Heerden JA, Grant CS, et al. Adrenal cortical carcinoma–a continuing challenge. Surgery 1983;94(6):926–31.

35. Iniguez-Ariza NM, Kohlenberg JD, Delivanis DA, et al. Clinical, Biochemical, and Radiological Characteristics of a Single-Center Retrospective Cohort of 705 Large Adrenal Tumors. Mayo Clin Proc Innov Qual Outcomes 2018;2(1):30–9.

36. Lee MJ, Hahn PF, Papanicolaou N, et al. Benign and malignant adrenal masses: CT distinction with attenuation coefficients, size, and observer analysis. Radiology 1991;179(2):415–8.

37. Korobkin M, Giordano TJ, Brodeur FJ, et al. Adrenal adenomas: relationship between histologic lipid and CT and MR findings. Radiology 1996;200(3):743–7.

38. Caoili EM, Korobkin M, Francis IR, et al. Adrenal masses: characterization with combined unenhanced and delayed enhanced CT. Radiology 2002;222(3):629–33.

39. Boland GW, Lee MJ, Gazelle GS, et al. Characterization of adrenal masses using unenhanced CT: an analysis of the CT literature. AJR Am J Roentgenol 1998;171(1):201–4.

40. Arnaldi G, Boscaro M. Adrenal incidentaloma. Best Pract Res Clin Endocrinol Metab 2012;26(4):405–19.

41. Pena CS, Boland GW, Hahn PF, et al. Characterization of indeterminate (lipid-poor) adrenal masses: use of washout characteristics at contrast-enhanced CT. Radiology 2000;217(3):798–802.

42. Caoili EM, Korobkin M, Francis IR, et al. Delayed enhanced CT of lipid-poor adrenal adenomas. AJR Am J Roentgenol 2000;175(5):1411–5.

43. Mayo-Smith WW, Boland GW, Noto RB, et al. State-of-the-art adrenal imaging. Radiographics 2001;21(4):995–1012.

44. Blake MA, Cronin CG, Boland GW. Adrenal imaging. AJR Am J Roentgenol 2010;194(6):1450–60.

45. Korobkin M, Brodeur FJ, Francis IR, et al. CT time-attenuation washout curves of adrenal adenomas and nonadenomas. AJR Am J Roentgenol 1998;170(3):747–52.

46. Johnson PT, Horton KM, Fishman EK. Adrenal mass imaging with multidetector CT: pathologic conditions, pearls, and pitfalls. Radiographics 2009;29(5):1333–51.

47. Park BK, Kim CK, Kim B, et al. Comparison of delayed enhanced CT and chemical shift MR for evaluating hyperattenuating incidental adrenal masses. Radiology 2007;243(3):760–5.

48. Blake MA, Kalra MK, Sweeney AT, et al. Distinguishing benign from malignant adrenal masses: multi-detector row CT protocol with 10-minute delay. Radiology 2006;238(2):578–85.

49. Hamrahian AH, Ioachimescu AG, Remer EM, et al. Clinical utility of noncontrast computed tomography attenuation value (hounsfield units) to differentiate adrenal adenomas/hyperplasias from nonadenomas: Cleveland Clinic experience. J Clin Endocrinol Metab 2005;90(2):871–7.

50. Delivanis DA, Bancos I, Atwell TD, et al. Diagnostic performance of unenhanced computed tomography and (18) F-fluorodeoxyglucose positron emission tomography in indeterminate adrenal tumours. Clin Endocrinol (Oxf) 2018;88(1):30–6.

51. Szolar DH, Korobkin M, Reittner P, et al. Adrenocortical carcinomas and adrenal pheochromocytomas: mass and enhancement loss evaluation at delayed contrast-enhanced CT. Radiology 2005;234(2):479–85.

52. Nieman LK. Approach to the patient with an adrenal incidentaloma. J Clin Endocrinol Metab 2010;95(9):4106–13.

53. Young WF, Stanson AW, Thompson GB, et al. Role for adrenal venous sampling in primary aldosteronism. Surgery 2004;136(6):1227–35.

54. Kempers MJ, Lenders JW, van Outheusden L, et al. Systematic review: diagnostic procedures to differentiate unilateral from bilateral adrenal abnormality in primary aldosteronism. Ann Intern Med 2009;151(5):329–37.

55. Mulatero P, Stowasser M, Loh KC, et al. Increased diagnosis of primary aldosteronism, including surgically correctable forms, in centers from five continents. J Clin Endocrinol Metab 2004;89(3):1045–50.

56. Canu L, Van Hemert JAW, Kerstens MN, et al. CT Characteristics of Pheochromocytoma: Relevance for the Evaluation of Adrenal Incidentaloma. J Clin Endocrinol Metab 2019;104(2):312–8.

57. Anderson KL Jr, Thomas SM, Adam MA, et al. Each procedure matters: threshold for surgeon volume to minimize complications and decrease cost associated with adrenalectomy. Surgery 2018;163(1):157–64.

58. Haugen BR, Alexander EK, Bible KC, et al. 2015 American Thyroid Association Management Guidelines for Adult Patients with Thyroid Nodules and Differentiated Thyroid Cancer: The American Thyroid Association Guidelines Task Force on Thyroid Nodules and Differentiated Thyroid Cancer. Thyroid 2016;26(1): 1–133.

59. Kwong N, Medici M, Angell TE, et al. The Influence of Patient Age on Thyroid Nodule Formation, Multinodularity, and Thyroid Cancer Risk. J Clin Endocrinol Metab 2015;100(12):4434–40.

60. Lin JD, Chao TC, Huang BY, et al. Thyroid cancer in the thyroid nodules evaluated by ultrasonography and fine-needle aspiration cytology. Thyroid 2005; 15(7):708–17.

61. Hegedus L. Clinical practice. The thyroid nodule. N Engl J Med 2004;351(17): 1764–71.

62. Steele SR, Martin MJ, Mullenix PS, et al. The significance of incidental thyroid abnormalities identified during carotid duplex ultrasonography. Arch Surg 2005;140(10):981–5.

63. Soelberg KK, Bonnema SJ, Brix TH, et al. Risk of malignancy in thyroid incidentalomas detected by 18F-fluorodeoxyglucose positron emission tomography: a systematic review. Thyroid 2012;22(9):918–25.

64. Tan GH, Gharib H. Thyroid incidentalomas: management approaches to nonpalpable nodules discovered incidentally on thyroid imaging. Ann Intern Med 1997;126(3):226–31.

65. Alexander EK, Marqusee E, Orcutt J, et al. Thyroid nodule shape and prediction of malignancy. Thyroid 2004;14(11):953–8.

66. Brito JP, Ito Y, Miyauchi A, et al. A Clinical Framework to Facilitate Risk Stratification When Considering an Active Surveillance Alternative to Immediate Biopsy and Surgery in Papillary Microcarcinoma. Thyroid 2016;26(1):144–9.

67. Brito JP, Singh-Ospina N, Gionfriddo MR, et al. Restricting ultrasound thyroid fine needle aspiration biopsy by nodule size: which tumors are we missing? A population-based study. Endocrine 2016;51(3):499–505.

68. Cibas ES, Ali SZ. The 2017 Bethesda System for Reporting Thyroid Cytopathology. Thyroid 2017;27(11):1341–6.

69. Bernardi S, Giudici F, Cesareo R, et al. Five-Year Results of Radiofrequency and Laser Ablation of Benign Thyroid Nodules: A Multicenter Study from the Italian Minimally Invasive Treatments of the Thyroid Group. Thyroid 2020;30(12): 1759–70.

70. Castro MR, Morris JC, Ryder M, et al. Most patients with a small papillary thyroid carcinoma enjoy an excellent prognosis and may be managed with minimally invasive therapy or active surveillance. Cancer 2015;121(18):3364–5.

71. MacMahon H, Naidich DP, Goo JM, et al. Guidelines for Management of Incidental Pulmonary Nodules Detected on CT Images: From the Fleischner Society 2017. Radiology 2017;284(1):228–43.

72. Gould MK, Donington J, Lynch WR, et al. Evaluation of individuals with pulmonary nodules: when is it lung cancer? Diagnosis and management of lung cancer, 3rd ed: American College of Chest Physicians evidence-based clinical practice guidelines. Chest 2013;143(5 Suppl):e93S–120S.

73. Ost D, Fein AM, Feinsilver SH. Clinical practice. The solitary pulmonary nodule. N Engl J Med 2003;348(25):2535–42.

74. McWilliams A, Tammemagi MC, Mayo JR, et al. Probability of cancer in pulmonary nodules detected on first screening CT. N Engl J Med 2013;369(10):910–9.

75. Bueno J, Landeras L, Chung JH. Updated Fleischner Society Guidelines for Managing Incidental Pulmonary Nodules: Common Questions and Challenging Scenarios. Radiographics 2018;38(5):1337–50.

76. Ost D, Fein A. Management strategies for the solitary pulmonary nodule. Curr Opin Pulm Med 2004;10(4):272–8.

77. Ost D, Fein A. Evaluation and management of the solitary pulmonary nodule. Am J Respir Crit Care Med 2000;162(3 Pt 1):782–7.

78. Hochhegger B, Nin CS, Alves GR, et al. Multidetector Computed Tomography Findings in Pulmonary Hamartomas: A New Fat Detection Threshold. J Thorac Imaging 2016;31(1):11–4.

79. Kornecki A, Daneman A, Navarro O, et al. Spontaneous reduction of intussusception: clinical spectrum, management and outcome. Pediatr Radiol 2000; 30(1):58–63.

80. Mandeville K, Chien M, Willyerd FA, et al. Intussusception: clinical presentations and imaging characteristics. Pediatr Emerg Care 2012;28(9):842–4.

81. Navarro O, Daneman A. Intussusception. Part 3: Diagnosis and management of those with an identifiable or predisposing cause and those that reduce spontaneously. Pediatr Radiol 2004;34(4):305–12, quiz 369.

82. Marinis A, Yiallourou A, Samanides L, et al. Intussusception of the bowel in adults: a review. World J Gastroenterol 2009;15(4):407–11.

83. Munden MM, Bruzzi JF, Coley BD, et al. Sonography of pediatric small-bowel intussusception: differentiating surgical from nonsurgical cases. AJR Am J Roentgenol 2007;188(1):275–9.

84. Lvoff N, Breiman RS, Coakley FV, et al. Distinguishing features of self-limiting adult small-bowel intussusception identified at CT. Radiology 2003;227(1): 68–72.

85. Wang N, Cui XY, Liu Y, et al. Adult intussusception: a retrospective review of 41 cases. World J Gastroenterol 2009;15(26):3303–8.

86. Honjo H, Mike M, Kusanagi H, et al. Adult intussusception: a retrospective review. World J Surg 2015;39(1):134–8.

87. Peery AF, Crockett SD, Murphy CC, et al. Burden and Cost of Gastrointestinal, Liver, and Pancreatic Diseases in the United States: Update 2018. Gastroenterology 2019;156(1):254–272 e211.

88. Ransohoff DF, Gracie WA, Wolfenson LB, et al. Prophylactic cholecystectomy or expectant management for silent gallstones. A decision analysis to assess survival. Ann Intern Med 1983;99(2):199–204.

89. Leitzmann MF, Giovannucci EL, Rimm EB, et al. The relation of physical activity to risk for symptomatic gallstone disease in men. Ann Intern Med 1998;128(6): 417–25.

90. Leitzmann MF, Rimm EB, Willett WC, et al. Recreational physical activity and the risk of cholecystectomy in women. N Engl J Med 1999;341(11):777–84.

91. Muszynska C, Lundgren L, Lindell G, et al. Predictors of incidental gallbladder cancer in patients undergoing cholecystectomy for benign gallbladder disease: Results from a population-based gallstone surgery registry. Surgery 2017; 162(2):256–63.

92. Alshahri TM, Abounozha S. Best evidence topic: Does the presence of a large gallstone carry a higher risk of gallbladder cancer? Ann Med Surg (Lond) 2021; 61:93–6.

93. Sandler A, Winkel G, Kimura K, et al. The role of prophylactic cholecystectomy during splenectomy in children with hereditary spherocytosis. J Pediatr Surg 1999;34(7):1077–8.

94. Caprotti R, Franciosi C, Romano F, et al. Combined laparoscopic splenectomy and cholecystectomy for the treatment of hereditary spherocytosis: is it safe and effective? Surg Laparosc Endosc Percutan Tech 1999;9(3):203–6.

95. Ramdath A, Zeineddin A, Nizam W, et al. Outcomes after Cholecystectomy in Patients with Sickle Cell Disease: Does Acuity of Presentation Play a Role? J Am Coll Surg 2020;230(6):1020–4.

96. Muroni M, Loi V, Lionnet F, et al. Prophylactic laparoscopic cholecystectomy in adult sickle cell disease patients with cholelithiasis: A prospective cohort study. Int J Surg 2015;22:62–6.

97. de'Angelis N, Abdalla S, Carra MC, et al. Low-impact laparoscopic cholecystectomy is associated with decreased postoperative morbidity in patients with sickle cell disease. Surg Endosc 2018;32(5):2300–11.

98. Santoshi N, Gaitonde K, Patil N, et al. Incidental appendectomy during radical cystectomy–is it necessary? Urology 2002;59(5):678–80.

99. Prystowsky JB, Pugh CM, Nagle AP. Current problems in surgery. Appendicitis. Curr Probl Surg 2005;42(10):688–742.

100. Al-Omran M, Mamdani M, McLeod RS. Epidemiologic features of acute appendicitis in Ontario, Canada. Can J Surg 2003;46(4):263–8.

101. Addiss DG, Shaffer N, Fowler BS, et al. The epidemiology of appendicitis and appendectomy in the United States. Am J Epidemiol 1990;132(5):910–25.

102. Warren JL, Penberthy LT, Addiss DG, et al. Appendectomy incidental to cholecystectomy among elderly Medicare beneficiaries. Surg Gynecol Obstet 1993; 177(3):288–94.

103. Dilek ON, Guler O, Guler AA, et al. Prophylactic appendectomy: is it worth to be done? Acta Chir Belg 2001;101(2):65–7.

104. Hui TT, Major KM, Avital I, et al. Outcome of elderly patients with appendicitis: effect of computed tomography and laparoscopy. Arch Surg 2002;137(9): 995–8, discussion 999-1000.

105. Sugimoto T, Edwards D. Incidence and costs of incidental appendectomy as a preventive measure. Am J Public Health 1987;77(4):471–5.

106. Wang HT, Sax HC. Incidental appendectomy in the era of managed care and laparoscopy. J Am Coll Surg 2001;192(2):182–8.

107. Newhall K, Albright B, Tosteson A, et al. Cost-effectiveness of prophylactic appendectomy: a Markov model. Surg Endosc 2017;31(9):3596–604.

108. Albright JB, Fakhre GP, Nields WW, et al. Incidental appendectomy: 18-year pathologic survey and cost effectiveness in the nonmanaged-care setting. J Am Coll Surg 2007;205(2):298–306.
109. Sanchez-Alcoholado L, Fernandez-Garcia JC, Gutierrez-Repiso C, et al. Incidental Prophylactic Appendectomy Is Associated with a Profound Microbial Dysbiosis in the Long-Term. Microorganisms 2020;8(4):609–19.
110. Skowron KB, Shogan BD, Rubin DT, et al. The New Frontier: the Intestinal Microbiome and Surgery. J Gastrointest Surg 2018;22(7):1277–85.

Controversies in Vascular Surgery

Kellie R. Brown, MD, DFSVS, Shahriar Alizadegan, MD*

KEYWORDS

- Controversies • Vascular • Aortic aneurysm • Deep venous thrombosis • IVC filter
- Carotid endarterectomy • Carotid stent

KEY POINTS

This article is a brief review of some of the current controversies in vascular surgery, based on the current management recommendations and available evidence for practice. Current evidence in the management of carotid artery disease, aortic aneurysms, acute deep venous thrombosis, and inferior vena cava filter placement is reviewed.

TREATMENT OF CAROTID ARTERY DISEASE
Carotid Endarterectomy, Stenting, or Best Medical Management?

The first surgical reconstruction of a symptomatic carotid stenosis was performed by Raul Carrea in 1951 using an internal to external carotid transposition.[1] The first formal carotid endarterectomy (CEA) was done by DeBakey in 1953.[2] Since that time the original procedure has undergone some modifications including patch angioplasty and shunting (either routine or selective), both of which have been shown to decrease the risk of perioperative stroke, whereas patch angioplasty has been shown to decrease the risk of restenosis. The rise of endovascular approaches to the treatment of carotid artery occlusive disease has created controversy around which technique, open CEA or endovascular carotid artery stenting (CAS), is most appropriate. Percutaneous carotid intervention was first described by Klaus Mathias,[3] who performed a carotid angioplasty for stenosis. The first CAS was performed in 1989 to treat an intimal flap after angioplasty[4] and since that time CAS has gained acceptance as treatment of carotid stenosis in certain patients.

Several randomized controlled trials (RCTs) for CAS versus CEA have been published, many of which have been criticized for design flaws. The first of these was the CAVATAS trial, which randomized symptomatic patients with greater than 50% stenosis who were at low or moderate operative risk to endovascular versus open surgical repair.[5] The trial was conducted prior to the availability of embolic protection

Division of Vascular and Endovascular Surgery, The Medical College of Wisconsin, 8701 Watertown Plank Road, Milwaukee, WI 53226, USA
* Corresponding author.
E-mail address: salizadegan@mcw.edu

Surg Clin N Am 101 (2021) 1097–1110
https://doi.org/10.1016/j.suc.2021.06.007
0039-6109/21/© 2021 Elsevier Inc. All rights reserved.

devices (EPDs) and dedicated CASs, so many of these patients had angioplasty alone and no embolic protection. They found that the 30-day risk of death/any stroke was 10% in both arms. This was criticized for a high event rate in the operative group. The SAPPHIRE study randomized 334 patients with greater than 70% asymptomatic stenosis who were high risk for surgery to CAS with EPDs or CEA.[6] The trial was stopped early for low enrollment. The 30-day death/stroke/myocardial infarction (MI) rate was not significantly different in CAS versus CEA (5.8% vs 12.6%, respectively), with CAS having a lower rate of MI. Critics of this trial pointed out that high-risk asymptomatic patients may be better off with medical management, but this trial provided at least some evidence that high-risk patients may benefit from CAS.

The SPACE trial evaluating CAS versus CEA in symptomatic patients also was terminated early due to slow enrollment but found no difference in ipsilateral stroke or death rates at 30 days.[7] The EVA-3S trial was stopped early due to a significantly higher rate of stroke/death in the CAS arm (9.6 vs 3.9, respectively, with CEA) and was largely criticized for including centers with insufficient experience in CAS.[8] The International Carotid Stenting Study (ICSS) published their 5-year results in 2014 and showed no difference fatal or nondisabling strokes between CAS or CEA (6.4% vs 6.5%, respectively); however, the rate of nondisabling strokes favored CEA.[9]

The 2010 CREST trial was designed to answer some of the criticisms of the previous trials, with mandatory use of EPDs and participation by only sufficiently experienced operators. The investigators randomized 2502 symptomatic and asymptomatic patients and followed them for a mean of 2.5 years. The primary endpoint was a composite of stroke, MI, or death within 30 days or any ipsilateral stroke within 4 years of randomization. They reported no difference in the primary endpoint between CAS or CEA (7.2% vs 6.8%, respectively), with a higher risk of stroke with CAS (4.1 vs 2.3, respectively; $P = .01$) and a higher risk of MI with CEA (2.3% vs 1.1%, respectively; $P = .03$).[10] It was suggested that quality of life was more affected by stroke than by MI, leading the current guidelines to suggest CEA is preferred to CAS for reduction of all-cause stroke and mortality in a majority of patients undergoing carotid intervention. CREST did find an interaction between age and treatment efficacy favoring CAS for those under age 70 and CEA for those older than age 70, which was confirmed with a pooled analysis of the EVA-3S, ICSS, SPACE, and the symptomatic CREST cohort.[11]

Several trials have aimed at evaluating CEA versus CAS in standard-risk, asymptomatic patients. ACT-1 enrolled 1453 average-risk, asymptomatic patients with greater than or equal to 70% stenosis and randomized them 3:1, with 1089 patients in the CAS arm and 364 in the CEA arm. All patients were less than 79 years old. The 30-day risks of stroke/death were not different (2.9% CAS vs 1.7% CEA; $P = .33$) and overall 5-year stroke-free survival was not different. The conclusion was that CAS was not inferior to CEA.[12] The SPACE -2 trial similarly looked at average-risk patients with asymptomatic carotid stenosis but added a third arm of best medical therapy (BMT) alone.[13] This trial was stopped early due to slow enrollment, and enrolled only 513 patients instead of the 3550 planned. Their results showed no difference between any group in rates of any stroke (CEA 3.9%, CAS 4.1, and BMT 0.9%; $P = .26$). The low enrollment limited the power to show any method superior to the other. There are 2 more trials of CEA and CAS ongoing, CREST 2 and ACST-2, which may alter guidelines once their results are available; however, the current Society for Vascular Surgery guidelines[14] advocate CAS only for symptomatic patients with greater than or equal to 50% stenosis who have high anatomic risk (distal lesion, prior ipsilateral neck surgery, neck irradiation, prior cranial nerve injury, or tracheal stoma) or high physiologic risk factors (severe uncorrectable coronary artery disease, congestive heart failure, or chronic obstructive pulmonary disease).

More recently, transcarotid artery revascularization (TCAR) has emerged as a treatment option for patients with carotid artery disease. This technique combines direct common carotid artery access with reversal of flow during CAS placement to provide CEA-like neuroprotection in a less invasive approach. TCAR attempts to minimize the potential for cerebral embolization by eliminating the need for aortic arch manipulation and by providing reversal of flow while crossing and intervening on the carotid lesion. There are several factors that are necessary for patients to be eligible for TCAR (**Box 1**).[15]

Results from the prospective, single-arm, multicenter ROADSTER trial enrolled 208 patients who were at high risk for CEA, 75% were asymptomatic.[16] The 30-day periprocedural stroke rate was 1.4%, and the combined stroke/death/MI rate was 3.5%. This represents the lowest reported stroke rate for any prospective multicenter trial of CAS. One-year follow-up demonstrated a low ongoing ipsilateral stroke rate (0.6%) and overall mortality rate (4.2%).[17] The early results of the open-label, single-arm, postapproval registry recently were published. This detailed the early outcomes for 632 patients undergoing TCAR and revealed a 30-day stroke/death rate of 2.3%, and stroke/death/MI rate of 3.2%.[17]

Results of a recent systematic review and meta-analysis of TCAR evaluated 4012 patients in 9 nonrandomized studies.[18] The 30-day stroke/death rate for TCAR was 1.9% and stroke/death/MI rate was 2.7%. Within this analysis, 2 studies suggested TCAR was associated with a lower risk of stroke and death compared with transfemoral CAS at 30 days (1.33% vs 2.55%, respectively), and 4 studies suggested that TCAR was associated with a lower risk of cranial nerve injury than CEA (0.54% vs 1.84%, respectively); however, no difference in 30-day risk of stroke, death, or MI was seen between TCAR and CEA in this study.

Thus, the decision between whether to use CEA, CAS, or TCAR for treatment of carotid stenosis has not been settled completely. In addition, there have been significant advances in medical therapy for stroke prevention in the years since the first trials for CEA versus BMT were published, and the risk of stroke in patients with carotid artery disease has decreased. There are some investigators who believe that asymptomatic carotid artery stenosis, even severe stenosis, is best treated with aggressive medical management. Abbot[19] published an analysis of the BMT arms from the major asymptomatic CEA trials that demonstrated the risk of stroke in the BMT arm in modern trials

---

Box 1
Anatomic inclusion and ineligibility criteria for transcarotid artery revascularization

Transcarotid revascularization anatomic criteria[15]
    Symptomatic patients with greater than 50% common carotid artery or internal carotid artery stenosis
    Asymptomatic patients with greater than 80% common carotid artery or internal carotid artery stenosis
    Target vessel diameter of 4 mm to 9 mm
    Carotid bifurcation at least 5 cm above clavicle

Transcarotid ineligibility criteria
    Contraindication to antiplatelet or anticoagulation
    Uncorrected bleeding disorders
    Allergy to nitinol
    Lesions in the ostium of the common carotid artery

is lower than the event rate published for ACAS and other earlier studies that established CEA as the standard for asymptomatic disease. The event rate with intervention also has decreased (because those arms all include BMT as well), however, so it is not clear whether asymptomatic carotid disease is best treated by BMT alone with modern medical therapy. There is hope that with CREST-2, which is randomizing both CEA and CAS against modern BMT, the answer will be known.

ABDOMINAL AORTIC ANEURYSM

The first open abdominal aortic aneurysm (AAA) repair was performed by Carrell in 1948, followed by Dubost in 1951. Voorhees described the first aortic replacement with synthetic material in 1952. Techniques of open aortic aneurysm repair continued to be advanced by DeBakey and Cooley throughout the mid-twentieth century[20]; however, operative techniques remained essentially unchanged until the development of the first endovascular repair by Parodi,[21] in 1990.

Endovascular aneurysm repair (EVAR) was approved by US Food and Drug Administration in 1999. Since that time, endovascular repair has surpassed open repair and currently is the most common repair technique for AAAs.

Elective Repair: Open or Endovascular?

The accepted size criteria for AAA repair is 5.5 cm in men and 5 cm in women. Risk of annual rupture at this size was estimated at 2.2% in the UK Small Aneurysm Trial. This annual rupture risk increases to 11% at 5.9 cm (**Table 1**).[22] Female sex, larger initial AAA diameter, smoking, lower forced expiration volume of in the first second of expiration, and higher mean blood pressure were independently associated with increased risk of rupture in this trial.[23]

The OVER trial, which randomized 881 patients to open or EVAR, reported that EVAR had a lower perioperative mortality (0.5% vs 3.0%, respectively; $P = .004$), lower hospital stay (3 days vs 7 days, respectively), and lower intensive care unit (ICU) stay (1 day vs 4 days, respectively) than open repair.[24] At 2 years, however, there was no difference in mortality (7% vs 9.8%, respectively; $P = .13$), and no difference was demonstrated in major morbidity, procedure failure, secondary intervention, aneurysm-related hospitalizations, quality of life, or erectile function.[25] In midterm follow-up (mean 5.2 years), there was no difference in survival, number of secondary therapeutic procedures, postrepair hospitalizations, quality of life, or erectile dysfunction. Aneurysm rupture after repair was uncommon but occurred only in the endovascular repair group.[24] In long-term follow-up (14 years), there was no difference in overall survival; however, there were more secondary interventions in the EVAR group.[25] The immediate perioperative survival advantage for EVAR was sustained for the first 3 years of follow-up, after which there was no significant difference in

Table 1 Annual rupture risk of abdominal aortic aneurysm[22]	
Abdominal Aortic Aneurysm Diameter (cm)	Rupture Risk (%)
3.0–3.9	0.3
4.0–4.9	0.5–1.5
5.0–5.9	1–11
6.0–6.9	11–22
>7	>30

survival. This immediate survival advantage along with significant advances in technology has led to EVAR as the first choice for elective aneurysm repair in patients with suitable anatomy. The UK National Institute for Health and Care Excellence (NICE), however, recently published guidelines recommending open repair over EVAR for elective aneurysms.[26]

Primarily in response to the NICE publication, Antoniou and colleagues[27] published a meta-analysis involving 7 RCTs involving a total of 2983 patients undergoing open or EVAR. They reported significantly lower odds of perioperative mortality for EVAR (odds ratio [OR] 0.36) but no difference in long term all-cause mortality. Aneurysm-related mortality however, favored open repair after 4 years.[27]

This report demonstrates the importance and role of risk distribution over time. A patient who undergoes open repair has most of the risk perioperatively, whereas a patient who undergoes EVAR has lower perioperative risk but has a higher risk for reintervention and aneurysm related mortality over time. In practice, many factors need to be considered when considering elective aneurysm repair. In older or high-risk patients with a shorter life expectancy, endovascular repair seems preferable, because these patients cumulatively have a lower chance of reaching the point of rupture or need for reintervention. In younger and healthier patients, open repair may be preferable.

The authors believe that both options have value and that, after consideration of all short-term and long-term risks, the treatment plan should be tailored to a patient's personalized needs.[27]

Ruptured Abdominal Aortic Aneurysm: Open or Endovascular?

A ruptured AAA (rAAA) is a true vascular emergency, historically associated with up to 80% mortality.[28] There has been a 50% decline in the incidence of rAAA in the United States over the past 20 years.[29] Early diagnosis and treatment of AAA through screening programs have contributed to this decline. The first open rAAA was repaired with a homograft by Henry Bahnson in1953.[20] The technique of open repair for ruptured aneurysms has remained essentially unchanged since first proposed and refined in the latter half of the past century. Endovascular repair for ruptured aneurysms was introduced in 1994.[30] Since that time, the prevalence of EVAR for ruptured aneurysm has gained acceptance. One major advantage of endovascular repair for rAAA is the ability to perform the entire procedure under local anesthesia in a hemodynamically unstable patient.[31]

Several RCTs were conducted early in the world experience with EVAR for rupture, none of which showed a difference in mortality. The ECAR study, published in 2015, randomized 158 hemodynamically stable patients with confirmed rAAA who were suitable for either EVAR or open aneurysm repair (OAR).[32] They found no difference between EVAR and OAR in 30-day mortality (18% vs 24%, respectively; $P = .24$) or 1-year mortality (30% vs 35%, respectively; $P = .30$). Although they found a decreased ICU stay for EVAR, the overall hospital length of stay was similar. Another prospective, multicenter RCT from Amsterdam randomizing 116 patients had similar findings, with no difference in 30-day mortality (EVAR 21% vs OAR 25%; $P = .66$) and found no difference in mortality between the groups in up to 6 years of follow-up.[33] Criticisms of these studies were that they randomized only hemodynamically stable patients and therefore did not reflect real-world practice.

The IMPROVE trial attempted to reflect real-world practice by randomizing 613 patients with a clinical diagnosis of rAAA prior to imaging.[34] If patients were randomized to the open arm, they underwent open repair immediately. If randomized to the endovascular arm, patients underwent CTA to evaluate anatomy. If suitable, they underwent EVAR. If not, they were repaired open. They were evaluated on an intent-to-treat basis. Of the 316 patients randomized to EVAR, 174 had suitable anatomy, and 275 had confirmed ruptures. Of the 297 randomized to open repair, 261 had confirmed ruptures. They reported no difference in 30-day mortality for all patients (EVAR 35.4% vs OAR 37.4%; $P = .62$) or among confirmed ruptures (EVAR 36.4% vs OAR 40.6%; $P = .31$). They did find that length of stay was shorter for the endovascular group and that a higher percentage of EVAR patients were discharged directly to home (EVAR 94% vs OAR 77%; $P<.001$). A long-term follow-up, published in 2017, revealed improved mortality at 3 years for EVAR (EVAR 48% vs OAR 56%; $P = .053$) but no difference at 7 years.[35]

Although these trials demonstrated the feasibility of EVAR for rAAA, and some benefit in length of stay and discharge destination, they did not show a significant mortality benefit. Endovascular technology, however, has improved significantly since the time of these trials, and there are some more recent data that show benefit.

Mehta and colleagues[36] published a report of 283 patients who underwent rAAA repair from 2002 to 2011; 120 patients underwent EVAR and 163 underwent OAR. These patients were followed-up for 5 years. The EVAR group had a significantly lower 30-day mortality (24% vs 44%, respectively; $P<.005$) and a better cumulative 5-year survival (37% vs 26%, respectively; $P<.005$).[36]

A recent meta-analysis included 136 studies with a total of 267,259 patients undergoing either EVAR (58,273) or OAR (208,986) for rAAA.[37] The pooled perioperative mortality after EVAR was 0.245 and after OAR was 0.378 ($P<.001$). The perioperative mortality after both EVAR or OAR improved over time, and the advantage of EVAR with respect to perioperative mortality has become more pronounced over time. The investigators concluded that if patients with rAAA can be treated with EVAR, they will have decreased mortality compared with patients treated with open repair.

This question also has been studied on a population level. Saleta and colleagues[38] published a retrospective cohort study evaluating all rAAA repairs done in Ontario, Canada, from 2003 to 2016. This cohort included 2692 patients, 261 of whom had EVAR, and 2431 of whom had open repair. They found that EVAR was associated with a lower 30-day all-cause mortality (hazard ratio 0.49; $P<.01$). There was no difference in the mortality from 31 days to 5 years, but the mortality benefit realized in the first 30 days persisted beyond 4.5 years.

Finally, a recent propensity matched study using the Vascular Quality Initiative database also looked at this question.[39] A total of 4929 patients undergoing rAAA repair in the Vascular Quality Initiative from 2003 to 2018 (2749 in EVAR and 2180 in OAR) were evaluated. Raw analysis found a significant benefit to EVAR. After propensity matching, there were 724 matched pairs. Analysis demonstrated persistent benefit for EVAR in 30-day mortality (18% EVAR vs 32% OAR; $P<.001$), any complication (35% EVAR vs 68% OAR; $P<.001$), and 1-year survival (73% EVAR vs 59% OAR; $P<.001$). The investigators also demonstrated a temporal trend for decreased mortality with EVAR, as was found in the meta-analysis.

Therefore, although the initial randomized trials failed to find conclusive evidence of an advantage to EVAR for rAAA, several recent studies have found good evidence for benefit. EVAR for rAAA, however, requires immediately available expertise, equipment and supplies. Although the endovascular technique affords significant advantages in appropriate patients in centers where EVAR is available on an emergent basis, immediate control of the bleeding and repair of the aorta is imperative. Therefore, it may be preferable to perform open repair at a nearby center rather than involve a long transfer time to a center well equipped for endovascular repair.[40]

Recent Society for Vascular Surgery guidelines recommend a door-to-intervention time of less than 90 minutes. Based on current evidence, the authors recommend an attempt at EVAR for all ruptured aneurysms with suitable anatomy in centers that are appropriately equipped and staffed for EVAR in the emergent setting. The authors believe, however, that immediate open repair by a qualified surgeon is preferable to a long transfer for the purpose of EVAR.

EXTENSIVE DEEP VENOUS THROMBOSIS
Anticoagulation or Thrombolysis?

The best management strategy for extensive VTE has been subject to debate since the introduction of thrombolysis. Advocates of broader use of thrombolysis consider benefits of early lysis to include the prevention of post-thrombotic syndrome (PTS) and the improvement of quality of life. The initial data seemed to support this approach. The CAVENT trial enrolled 209 patients and randomized them to catheter-directed thrombolysis (CDT) plus therapeutic anticoagulation (101 patients) versus anticoagulation alone (108 patients) and followed them for 5 years. There was no difference in PTS incidence at 6 months' follow-up (30.3% vs 32.2%, respectively; $P = .77$) but by 24 months the CDT arm had less PTS (41.1% vs 55.6%, respectively; $P = .047$).[50] At 5 years, the reduction in PTS with CDT was pronounced (43% vs 71%, respectively; $P<.0001$). The number needed to treat to prevent PTS in 1 patient at 5 years was 4. Bleeding complications were reported in 20 patients in the CDT group (19.8%); only 5 (5.9%) were considered clinically relevant. There were no bleeding complications in the control group. There was no difference in recurrent VTE between the groups during follow-up.[51]

A subsequent Cochrane review published in 2016 evaluated 17 RCTs with 1103 participants.[52] Results were combined as any thrombolysis compared with standard anticoagulation. The investigators found that complete clot lysis occurred more often with lysis at early follow-up (RR 4.91; $P = .004$) and intermediate follow-up (RR 2.44; $P = .002$). They also found that lysis was associated with significantly less PTS (RR 0.66; $P<.0001$). Lysis was associated, however, with an increased risk of bleeding complications (RR 2.23; $P = .0006$). This analysis included trials with both systemic thrombolysis and CDT and found that results were similar with both therapies. Due to the low number of participants in many of these trials, the evidence was found to be only of moderate quality; however, the investigators stated they felt confident with the results.[52]

Technology continued to progress, and the wide dissemination of pharmaco-mechanical thrombolysis (PMT), which is the combination of catheter or device-mediated mechanical thrombus maceration/aspiration and instillation of lysis, made another RCT necessary. In 2017, the ATTRACT trial was published.[53] This trial randomized 692 patients with acute DVT to PMT plus anticoagulation (337 patients) versus anticoagulation alone (355 patients) with a primary outcome of PTS between 6 months and 24 months of follow-up. The investigators found no difference in PTS (47% PMT vs 48% control; $P = .56$) or recurrent VTE (12% PMT vs 8% control; $P = .09$). PMT had a higher risk of major bleeding within 10 days (1.7% vs 0.3%, respectively, of patients; $P = .049$).[53] Subsequent subgroup analysis did suggest, however, a reduction in moderate to severe PTS in those patients with iliofemoral DVT (18% PMT vs 24% control; $P = .04$). Finally, the CAVA trial evaluated 184 patients with acute DVT randomized to ultrasound-accelerated CDT (USCDT) versus standard anticoagulation alone and found no difference in PTS at 1 year (USCDT 29% vs control 35%; $P = .42$).[54]

Therefore, for uncomplicated DVT, the authors currently recommend therapeutic anticoagulation alone. Thrombolytic therapy should be used selectively, in low-risk patients with extensive iliofemoral DVT who are symptomatic or in those who present with phlegmasia and a risk for ischemia or compartment syndrome.

INFERIOR VENA CAVA FILTERS
Who, Where, and When?

Pulmonary embolism (PE) is one of the major preventable causes of mortality. This potentially lethal condition is secondary to venous thromboembolism (VTE). The indications for anticoagulation to prevent or treat VTE and PE are well established.[41] In certain clinical conditions however, anticoagulation is contraindicated or has failed. Inferior vena cava (IVC) filter is an option for these patients that may prevent PE and decrease mortality.

The first commercially available IVC filter was used in 1973 and for many years thereafter permanent IVC filters were used routinely in patients with deep venous thrombosis (DVT) or PE who could not be anticoagulated, to prevent subsequent PE. Retrievable filters were made available in 2004, primarily for use in patients with a temporary risk for PE.[42]

Although placement of IVC filters has increased steadily over the years, since the availability of retrievable filters, the increase has been primarily in those patients who do not currently have a DVT or PE (prophylactic filter placement), a practice that remains controversial. On a population level, although in 2010 the filter placement in the United States outpaced that of Europe 25:1, the number of annual VTE-related deaths remained similar.[43] This is striking, in that the large number of filters placed did not reduce incidence of death from PE on a population basis.

A recent meta-analysis reviewed the literature on the results of IVC filter placement in preventing death in patients at risk for PE.[44] The investigators included 11 studies (6 randomized and 5 observational) involving 2055 patients with filters and 2149 controls. The meta-analysis found that IVC filters did significantly reduce the risk for PE (OR 0.50; 95% CI, 0.33–0.75) but increased the risk for DVT (OR 1.70; 95% CI, 1.17–2.48) and failed to significantly change PE-related mortality (OR 0.51; 95% CI, 0.25–1.05) or all-cause mortality (OR 0.91; 95% CI, 0.70–1.19). When the analysis was limited to only the 6 RCTs, the results were similar. Therefore, although filters did decrease PE, they did not prevent death and increased the risk for DVT.

There are 2 populations where prophylactic filter use has gained some traction: trauma and bariatric surgery. This, however, also remains controversial. In the trauma population, there have been several controlled trials to evaluate this practice. A 2014 meta-analysis evaluating prophylactic filter placement in trauma patients included 8 controlled studies involving 432 patients with filter placement and 4160 patients without.[45] They found a reduction of PE (relative risk [RR] 0.20; 95% CI, 0.06–0.70) and fatal PE (RR 0.09; 95% CI, 0.01–0.81) but found no significant difference in the incidence of DVT (RR 1.76; 95% CI, 0.50–6.19) or mortality (RR 0.70; 0.40–1.23). The number needed to treat to prevent 1 additional PE with IVC filters was estimated to range from 109 to 962, depending on the baseline PE risk.[45] The investigators concluded that the quality of evidence is low but does support prophylactic IVC filter use in trauma; however, which patients benefit most is yet to be determined.

More recently, Haut and colleagues[46] published the results of an RCT involving 240 severely injured trauma patients (mean injury severity score 27) with a contraindication for immediate anticoagulation. Patients were randomized to early filter placement versus no filter placement, with anticoagulation when clinically safe. The investigators

Table 2
Societal guidelines for placement of inferior vena cava filter

Guideline	Recommendations
CHEST/ACCP guidelines[1,2]	• In patients with acute VTE and contraindication to AC, recommend the use of an IVC filter • In patients with high-risk/massive PE, consider IVC filter in addition to anticoagulation • In patients with recurrent VTE despite adequate AC, IVC filter is an option of last resort
SIR guidelines[30]	IVC filters are indicated in patients with PE or IVC, iliac, femoral, or popliteal DVT and 1 or more of the following: • Contraindication to AC • Complication of AC • Failure of AC • Inability to achieve/maintain adequate AC • Thrombus progression despite adequate AC • High-risk/massive PE with residual DVT • Free-floating caval or iliac DVT • Severe cardiopulmonary disease and DVT Prophylactic IVC filters (no documented DVT/PE) are indicated in the following settings: • Severe trauma, closed head injury, spinal cord injury, multiple long-bone or pelvic fractures • Patients at high risk for VTE (immobilized, ICU patient, and so forth)
AHA guidelines[38]	• Adult patients with any confirmed acute PE (or proximal DVT) with contraindications to anticoagulation or with active bleeding complication should receive an IVC filter • For patients with recurrent acute PE despite therapeutic anticoagulation, it is reasonable to place an IVC filter • Placement of an IVC filter may be considered for patients with acute PE and very poor cardiopulmonary reserve, including those with high-risk/massive PE

Abbreviations: AC, anticoagulation; ACCP, American College of Chest Physicians; AHA, American Heart Association; SIR, Society of Interventional Radiology.

found no difference in PE or death at 90 days (filter 13.9% vs no filter 14.4%; $P = .98$). 67% of patients had prophylactic anticoagulation started within 7 days of admission. When the analysis was limited to the 33% of patients who did not receive any anticoagulation for at least 7 days, PE was found in 14.7% of the group with no filter (1 fatal), and none of the patients who received a filter. There were complications of filters as well, with 5.7% requiring more than one attempt to remove, 1 patient who required surgical removal, and 31.5% who were lost to follow-up; therefore, the filters were not removed. The investigators concluded that early prophylactic filter placement was not effective and should be used only in those patients who still are unable to have prophylactic anticoagulation after 7 days.

Bariatric surgery patients are another population in which prophylactic filter placement is thought to possibly be useful, because PE is 1 of the leading causes of death after bariatric surgery. Reddy and colleagues[47] recently published an analysis of the National Inpatient Sample with regard to prophylactic filter placement. They analyzed a total of 258,480 patients who underwent bariatric surgery from 2005 to 2015 and created propensity matched controls for the 1047 patients who had prophylactic filters placed. This analysis found that IVC filter placement was associated with an increased risk of in-hospital death or PE (1.4% vs 0.4%, respectively; P = .19), increased risk of DVT (1.8% vs 0.3%, respectively; P<.01), longer length of stay (3 days vs 2 days, respectively; P<.01), and increased charges ($63,000 vs $37,000; P<.01). A meta-analysis evaluating 7 studies involving 102,767 patients undergoing bariatric surgery, with weighted average incidences of DVT (0.9%), PE (1.6%), and mortality (1.0%), for a follow-up ranging from 3 weeks to 3 months, found IVC filters were associated with a higher risk of DVT (RR 2.81; P = .007) but no significant difference in PE (RR 1.02; P = .9) or mortality (RR 3.27; P = .1).[48] Finally, a propensity matched cohort study involving the Michigan Bariatric Surgery Collaborative also found prophylactic IVC filter placement prior to bariatric surgery was associated with higher rates of PE (0.84% vs 0.46%, respectively; OR 2.0; 95% CI, 0.6–6.5), DVT (1.2% vs 0.37%, respectively; OR 3.3; 95% CI, 1.1–10.1), venous thromboembolism (1.9% vs 0.74%, respectively; OR 2.7; 95% CI, 1.1–6.3), serious complications (5.8% vs 3.8%, respectively; OR 1.6; 95% CI, 1.0–2.4), permanently disabling complications (1.2% vs 0.37%; OR 4.3; 95% CI, 1.2–15.6), and death (0.7% vs 0.09%, respectively; OR 7.0; 95% CI, 0.9–57.3).[49] Thus, it seems that prophylactic filter placement in bariatric surgery patients currently is not supported by the literature.

Current indications for IVC filter placement (**Table 2**) include absolute contraindication for anticoagulation, failure of anticoagulation, anticoagulation-related complications, and progression of thrombus despite anticoagulation. Prophylactic IVC filter placement remains controversial. It may benefit those trauma patients who are unable to have anticoagulation for more than 7 days after injury. The benefit in bariatric patients is yet to be determined and may increase risk of harm.

SUMMARY

This article highlights some of the management controversies in vascular surgery. There has been significant change in management strategies to provide safe, less invasive, and more durable outcomes. Introduction of endovascular techniques has been a crucial factor in expanding the boundaries of vascular surgery techniques; however, the availability of medical, endovascular, and open surgical management creates controversy in management decisions that hopefully will be addressed by ongoing vigorous research.

CLINICS CARE POINTS

- Advances in medical therapy has decresed risk of events in both BMT and after carotid interventions.
- Carotid artery stenting is only recommended for symptomatic patient and certain anatomic criteria.
- Carotid endarterectomy is the preferred treatment strategy for severe asymptomatic stenosis and symptomatic patients with good surgical risk.
- Open and endovascular repair should be considered in elective repair of AAA. Treatment plan should be tailored on patient's personalized needs.
- EVAR is the preferred technique in repair of rAAA in facilities with available expertise and equipment in patients with suitable anatomy
- IVC filters reduce PE risk but increase the risk of DVT.
- There is paucity of evidence indicating a significant change in PE related mortality with use of IVC filters.

- Patients with IVC filters should be followed up closely and filters should be removed as soon as the condition leading to their placement has resolved.

- Uncomplicated DVT should be treated with anticoagulation alone.

- Thrombolytic therapy should be only used in selected cases with low bleeding risk and extensive iliafemoral DVT and phlegmasia or compartment syndrome.

REFERENCES

1. Friedman SG. The first carotid endarterectomy. J Vasc Surg 2014;60(6): 1703–8.e84.
2. Debakey ME, Crawford ES, Cooley DA, et al. Cerebral arterial insufficiency: one to 11-year results following arterial reconstructive operation. Ann Surg 1965; 161(6):921–45.
3. Mathias K. Ein neuartiges Katheter-System zur perkutanen transluminalen Angioplastie von Karotisstenosen [A new catheter system for percutaneous transluminal angioplasty (PTA) of carotid artery stenoses]. Fortschr Med 1977;95(15): 1007–11.
4. Castriota F, Martins EC, Liso A, et al. Technical evolution of carotid stents. Interv Cardiol Rev 2008;3:74.
5. CAVATAS Investigators. Endovascular versus surgical treatment in patients with carotid stenosis in the Carotid and Vertebral Artery Transluminal Angioplasty Study (CAVATAS): a randomised trial. Lancet 2001;357(9270):1729–37.
6. Yadav JS, Wholey MH, Kuntz RE, et al, for the Stenting and Angioplasty with Protection in Patients at High Risk for Endarterectomy Investigators. Protected carotid-artery stenting versus endarterectomy in high-risk patients. N Engl J Med 2004;351:1493–501.
7. SPACE Collaborative Group, Ringleb PA, Allenberg J, Brückmann H, et al. Hacke 30 day results from the SPACE trial of stent-protected angioplasty versus carotid endarterectomy in symptomatic patients: a randomised non-inferiority trial. Lancet 2006;368(9543):1239–47.
8. Mas JL, Chatellier G, Beyssen B, et al. Endarterectomy versus stenting in patients with symptomatic severe carotid stenosis. N Engl J Med 2006;355(16):1660–71.
9. Bonati LH, Dobson J, Featherstone RL, et al. Long-term outcomes after stenting versus endarterectomy for treatment of symptomatic carotid stenosis: the International Carotid Stenting Study (ICSS) randomised trial. Lancet 2015;385(9967): 529–38.
10. Brott TG, Hobson RW 2nd, Howard G, et al. Stenting versus endarterectomy for treatment of carotid-artery stenosis [published correction appears in N Engl J Med. 2010 Jul 29;363(5):498] [published correction appears in N Engl J Med. 2010 Jul 8;363(2):198]. N Engl J Med 2010;363(1):11–23.
11. Howard G, Roubin GS, Jansen O, et al. Association between age and risk of stroke or death from carotid endarterectomy and carotid stenting: a meta-analysis of pooled patient data from four randomised trials [published correction appears in Lancet. 2016 Mar 26;387(10025):1276]. Lancet 2016;387(10025): 1305–11.
12. Rosenfield K, Matsumura JS, Chaturvedi S, et al. Randomized trial of stent versus surgery for asymptomatic carotid stenosis. N Engl J Med 2016;374(11):1011–20.
13. Reiff T, Eckstein HH, Mansmann U, et al. Angioplasty in asymptomatic carotid artery stenosis vs. endarterectomy compared to best medical treatment: One-year

interim results of SPACE-2 [published online ahead of print, 2019 Mar 15]. Int J Stroke 2019;15(6). 1747493019833017.

14. Ricotta JJ, Aburahma A, Ascher E, et al. Updated Society for Vascular Surgery guidelines for management of extracranial carotid disease: executive summary [published correction appears in J Vasc Surg. 2012 Mar;55(3):894]. J Vasc Surg 2011;54(3):832–6.

15. Wu WW, Liang P, O'Donnell TFX, et al. Anatomic eligibility for transcarotid artery revascularization and transfemoral carotid artery stenting. J Vasc Surg 2019; 69(5):1452–60.

16. Kwolek CJ, Jaff MR, Leal JI, et al. Results of the ROADSTER multicenter trial of transcarotid stenting with dynamic flow reversal. J Vasc Surg 2015;62(5): 1227–34.

17. Kashyap VS, Schneider PA, Foteh M, et al. Early outcomes in the ROADSTER 2 study of transcarotid artery revascularization in patients with significant carotid artery disease. Stroke 2020;51(9):2620–9.

18. Naazie IN, Cui CL, Osaghae I, et al. A systematic review and meta-analysis of transcarotid artery revascularization with dynamic flow reversal versus transfemoral carotid artery stenting and carotid endarterectomy. Ann Vasc Surg 2020; 69:126–36.

19. Abbott AL. Medical (nonsurgical) intervention alone is now best for prevention of stroke associated with asymptomatic severe carotid stenosis: results of a systematic review and analysis. Stroke 2009;40(10):e573–83.

20. Bahnson HT. Considerations in the excision of aortic aneurysms. Ann Surg 1953; 138(3):377–86.

21. Parodi JC. Endoluminal treatment of arterial diseases using a stent-graft combination: reflections 20 years after the initial concept. J Endovasc Surg 2007;4:3.

22. The UK Small Aneurysm Trial Participants: Mortality results for randomised controlled trial of early elective surgery or ultrasonographic surveillance for small abdominal aortic aneurysms. Lancet 1998;352:1649–55.

23. Brown LC, Powell JT. Risk factors for aneurysm rupture in patients kept under ultrasound surveillance. UK Small Aneurysm Trial Participants. Ann Surg 1999; 230(3):289–97.

24. Lederle FA, Freischlag JA, Kyriakides TC, et al. Outcomes following endovascular vs open repair of abdominal aortic aneurysm: a randomized trial. JAMA 2009; 302(14):1535–42.

25. Lederle FA, Freischlag JA, Kyriakides TC, et al. Long-term comparison of endovascular and open repair of abdominal aortic aneurysm. N Engl J Med 2012; 367(21):1988–97.

26. Abdominal aortic aneurysm: diagnosis and management. London: National Institute for Health and Care Excellence (UK); 2020 Mar 19 (NICE Guideline, No. 156.). Available at: https://www.nice.org.uk/guidance/ng156.

27. Antoniou GA, Antoniou SA, Torella F. Editor's choice - endovascular vs. open repair for abdominal aortic aneurysm: systematic review and meta-analysis of updated peri-operative and long-term data of randomised controlled trials. Eur J Vasc Endovasc Surg 2020;59(3):385–97.

28. Budd JS, Finch DR, Carter PG. A study of the mortality from ruptured abdominal aortic aneurysms in a district community. Eur J Vasc Surg 1989;3(4):351–4.

29. Sidloff D, Stather P, Dattani N, et al. Aneurysm global epidemiology study: public health measures can further reduce abdominal aortic aneurysm mortality. Circulation 2014;129:747–53.

30. Yusuf SW, Whitaker SC, Chuter TA, et al. Emergency endovascular repair of leaking aortic aneurysm. Lancet 1994;344(8937):1645.

31. Armstrong RA, Squire YG, Rogers CA, et al. Type of anesthesia for endovascular abdominal aortic aneurysm repair. J Cardiothorac Vasc Anesth 2019;33(2): 462–71.

32. Desgranges P, Kobeiter H, Katsahian S, et al. ECAR (Endovasculaire ou Chirurgie dans les Anévrysmes aorto-iliaques Rompus): A French randomized controlled trial of endovascular versus open surgical repair of ruptured aorto-iliac aneurysms. Eur J Vasc Endovasc Surg 2015;50(3):303–10.

33. Reimerink JJ, Hoornweg LL, Vahl AC, et al. Endovascular repair versus open repair of ruptured abdominal aortic aneurysms. A multicenter randomized controlled trial. Ann Surg 2013;258:248–56.

34. IMPROVE Trial Investigators. Endovascular or open repair strategy for ruptured abdominal aortic aneurysm: 30 day outcomes from IMPROVE randomized trial. BMJ 2014;348:f7661.

35. IMPROVE Trial Investigators. Comparative clinical effectiveness and cost effectiveness of endovascular strategy v open repair for ruptured abdominal aortic aneurysm: three year results of the IMPROVE randomized trial. BMJ 2017;359: j4859.

36. Mehta M, Byrne J, Darling RC 3rd, et al. Endovascular repair of ruptured infrarenal abdominal aortic aneurysm is associated with lower 30-day mortality and better 5-year survival rates than open surgical repair. J Vasc Surg 2013;57(2): 368–75.

37. Kontopodis N, Galanakis N, Antoniou SA, et al. Meta-analysis and meta-regression analysis of outcomes of endovascular and open repair for ruptured abdominal aortic aneurysm. Eur J Vasc Endovasc Surg 2020;59:399–410.

38. Saleta K, Jussain MA, de Mestral C, et al. Population -based long-term outcomes of open versus endovascular aortic repair of ruptured abdominal aortic aneurysms. J Vasc Surg 2020;71:1867–78.

39. Wang LJ, Lochan S, Al-Nouri O, et al. Endovascular repair of ruptured abdominal aortic aneurysm is superior to open repair: propensity-matched analysis in the vascular quality initiative. J Vasc Surg 2020;72:498–507.

40. Livesay JJ, Talledo OG. Endovascular aneurysm repair is not the treatment of choice in most patients with ruptured abdominal aortic aneurysm. Tex Heart Inst J 2013;40(5):556–9.

41. Kearon C, Akl EA, Ornelas J, et al. Antithrombotic therapy for VTE disease: CHEST guideline and expert panel report [published correction appears in Chest. 2016 Oct;150(4):988]. Chest 2016;149(2):315–52.

42. Muneeb A, Dhamoon AS. Inferior vena cava filter. In: StatPearls. Treasure Island, FL: StatPearls Publishing; 2020.

43. Wang SL, Lloyd AJ. Clinical review: Inferior vena cava filters in the age of patient-centered outcomes. Ann Med 2013;45(7):474–81.

44. Bikdeli B, Chatterjee S, Desai NR, et al. Inferior vena cava filters to prevent pulmonary embolism: systematic review and meta-analysis. J Am Coll Cardiol 2017; 70(13):1587–97.

45. Haut ER, Garcia LJ, Shihab HM, et al. The effectiveness of prophylactic inferior vena cava filters in trauma patients. A systematic review and meta-analysis. JAMA Surg 2014;149(2):194–202.

46. Ho KM, Rao S, Honeybul S, et al. A multicenter trial of vena cava filters in severely injured patients. N Engl J Med 2019;381:328–37.
47. Reddy S, Zack CJ, Lakhter V, et al. Prophylactic inferior vena cava filters prior to bariatric surgery. J Am Coll Cardiol Intv 2019;12(12):1153–60.
48. Kaw R, Pasupuleti V, Overby DW, et al. Inferior vena cava filters and postoperative outcomes in patients undergoing bariatric surgery: a meta-analysis. Surg Obes Relat Dis 2014;10(4):725–33.
49. Birkmeyer NJ, Finks JF, English WJ, et al, Michigan Bariatric Surgery Collaborative. Risks and benefits of prophylactic inferior vena cava filters in patients undergoing bariatric surgery. J Hosp Med 2013;8(4):173–7.
50. Enden T, Haig Y, Kløw NE, et al. Long-term outcome after additional catheter-directed thrombolysis versus standard treatment for acute iliofemoral deep vein thrombosis (the CaVenT study): a randomised controlled trial. Lancet 2012; 379(9810):31–8.
51. Haig Y, Enden T, Grøtta O, et al. Post-thrombotic syndrome after catheter-directed thrombolysis for deep vein thrombosis (CaVenT): 5-year follow-up results of an open-label, randomised controlled trial. Lancet Haematol 2016;3(2): e64–71.
52. Watson L, Broderick C, Armon MP. Thrombolysis for acute deep vein thrombosis. Cochrane Database Syst Rev 2016;11(11):CD002783.
53. Vedantham S, Goldhaber SZ, Julian JA, et al. Pharmacomechanical catheter-directed thrombolysis for deep-vein thrombosis. N Engl J Med 2017;377(23): 2240–52.
54. Notten P, Ten Cate-Hoek AJ, Arnoldussen CWKP, et al. Ultrasound-accelerated catheter-directed thrombolysis versus anticoagulation for the prevention of post-thrombotic syndrome (CAVA): a single-blind, multicentre, randomised trial. Lancet Haematol 2020;7(1):e40–9.

Controversies in Surgery
Trauma

Stephanie Bonne, MD*, Fariha Sheikh, MD

KEYWORDS

- REBOA • Rib fixation • Thoracotomy • Trauma laparoscopy • Resuscitation

KEY POINTS

- Resuscitative endovascular balloon occlusion of the aorta is a procedure that involves vascular occlusion to limit hemorrhage to avoid thoracotomy.
- Emergency thoracotomy can be used to salvage patients meeting strict criteria with penetrating and blunt trauma.
- Balanced resuscitation in trauma patients is preferred for lower morbidity and mortality in the setting of hemorrhagic shock.
- Laparoscopy has a role in trauma surgery and can prevent the occurrence of nontherapeutic laparotomy.
- Rib fixation has demonstrated the ability to improve length of stay and mechanical ventilation in flail chest trauma.

INTRODUCTION

Trauma surgery is a constantly evolving field of practice as new surgical technology becomes available, and we learn more about the physiologic response to injury and inflammation. As changes develop, there may be varying opinions, and at time, controversies, about the optimal management for certain injuries. For example, although research remains ongoing in the area of resuscitative endovascular balloon occlusion of the aorta (REBOA) and rib fixation, some of these controversies are closer to having more definitive conclusions. Controversies on resuscitation and the use of laparoscopy in trauma patients have promising answers that are in practice, such as the use of balanced resuscitation and the use of laparoscopy in the stable trauma patient to evaluate for potential intraabdominal or diaphragm injuries. This chapter navigates through each topic and offers the current recommendations that are in use.

Department of Surgery, Division of Trauma and Surgical Critical Care, Rutgers, New Jersey Medical School, 150 Bergen Street, Newark, NJ 07103, USA
* Corresponding author.
E-mail address: Slb391@njms.rugters.edu

Surg Clin N Am 101 (2021) 1111–1121
https://doi.org/10.1016/j.suc.2021.06.008
0039-6109/21/© 2021 Elsevier Inc. All rights reserved.

Resuscitative Endovascular Balloon Occlusion of the Aorta

Indication/patient selection

Currently a popular topic in the management of traumatic hemorrhage, resuscitative endovascular balloon occlusion of the aorta REBOA was initially introduced during the Korean War as a means of hemorrhage control. Now, more than 50 years later, REBOA has entered a resurgence as a potential means of minimizing hemorrhage while bridging to definitive control. The overall intent of the device is to limit distal hemorrhage and progressive shock while preserving some degree of perfusion to the myocardium and brain.[1-3]

Patient selection plays a large role in determining whether REBOA is safe and would be successful in the intended goal. Use is indicated in patients with hemorrhagic shock secondary to traumatic injuries located below the diaphragm. When considering whether a patient is an optimal candidate for REBOA versus resuscitative thoracotomy (RT), patients with shock due to thoracic hemorrhage should be ruled out for REBOA because impending collapse will need to be controlled by clamping the thoracic aorta. Patients who are actively undergoing cardiopulmonary resuscitation (CPR) should be considered for RT for penetrating injuries less than 15 minutes of down time and signs of life. There are varying practices regarding resuscitative thoracotomy for blunt injuries, with some centers advocating for zone 1 REBOA placement, other centers using thoracotomy, and still other centers not further resuscitating the patient in blunt arrest. For patients with abdominal and pelvic trauma that do not respond or are transient responders to resuscitation, those with systolic blood pressure (SBP) less than 80 may benefit from either REBOA catheter placement or RT to control hemorrhage. Patients who are able to maintain SBP greater than 80 with resuscitation can be transferred to the operating room for either definitive management or prepelvic packing. It is important to note that current recommendations do not apply to the pediatric or geriatric patients, as studies are lacking for those populations.[4,5]

Technique and placement positions

When the decision is made to insert an REBOA catheter, it is important that the person or team involved in positioning the catheter will also be involved in the definitive control of hemorrhage. Ideally ultrasound guidance should be used for safe percutaneous insertion of a femoral catheter; however, it is not required, and a blind percutaneous or cutdown technique may also be used; this can also be initiated by placing an arterial catheter and then upsize to a 7-Fr REBOA catheter.[6,7]

Before placing the catheter, an estimation of the landing zone or the intended placement of the balloon located at the distal end of the catheter must occur. REBOA placement should not be used in zone II, which lies between the celiac plexus and the renal arteries. Zone I placement can be estimated at the sternal notch (approximately 46 cm) and for zone III at the xiphoid process (approximately 28 cm). After the balloon is tested and the catheter along with the peel-away sheath that is then removed, the balloon is inflated. Most commercially available catheters have an arterial transduction port proximal and distal to the balloon, allowing for 2 arterial tracings to be compared. When the balloon is inflated, the proximal arterial tracing should remain intact or increase and represents the blood pressure being experienced by the brain and upper extremities. This distal port should be flat and represents the blood pressure (or lack thereof) being experienced by the lower extremities and in the case of zone 1 placement, the bowel and kidneys. The balloon is inflated slowly as to avoid overinflation, and monitoring for an increase in blood pressure indicates that the occlusion if effective. The patient should then be prepped for more definitive hemorrhage control, and the balloon should not be inflated for longer than 30 minutes due to risk of distal ischemia.[8,9]

Pros/cons

Although there are ongoing studies investigating the general benefits of REBOA, the immediate benefits of this relatively minimally invasive procedure are clear. If deployed correctly and expeditiously, REBOA has the ability to occlude the aorta and stop distal hemorrhage. In doing so, there is preservation of flow and a degree of perfusion to the heart and brain. Insertion can be accomplished in minimum time, and the patient can be spared a thoracotomy. A secondary benefit of avoiding a thoracotomy is also decreasing the risk of injury to the health care team, as this emergency procedure can often be associated with accidental needlesticks and exposure to blood-borne diseases. For enhanced benefit, REBOA utilization in a hybrid room with fluoroscopic capability enables the prospect of immediate embolization of the injured vessels after balloon inflation.[10]

The overall complication rate from REBOA is reported to be on average 35%. As alluded to earlier, a major potential complication from REBOA use is the ischemia, which can occur as a consequence of aortic occlusion. This ischemia can be inclusive of the kidneys, liver, intestine, and extremities and may also be followed by subsequent reperfusion injury. The risk of limb ischemia is not always related to aortic occlusion, as the femoral sheath can also traumatize and/or occlude the vessel, especially when catheters are larger than 8 Fr. One must also be vigilant when inflating the balloon to avoid arterial rupture. It is recommended to start slowly with small increments of volume of 8 mL in zone I and 2 mL in zone III inflation. Furthermore, when using the device, it should be placed by either a surgeon or an interventionalist who would be familiar with techniques used in catheter insertion, the complications that can arise, and the ability to proceed to definitive hemorrhage control.[11,12]

Regarding the duration of REBOA balloon inflation, a time limit of 30 minutes is the most common recommendation. However, studies specify that zone I occlusion has a higher risk of ischemia, and deflation should occur at 15 minutes when possible. Animal studies have demonstrated clear demise if that balloon is left inflated for 45 minutes in zone I, thus it is imperative to be mindful of the duration of balloon inflation when using REBOA.[13]

Success

Overall survival rates after implementation of REBOA are 30% to 37%, but this varies significantly based on patient and injury factors. REBOA placement within zone I is associated with a 2-fold higher mortality than zone III placements. Other predictors of increased mortality include a Glasgow Coma Scale score less than 13, ongoing CPR at the time of REBOA placement, higher Injury Severity Scores, and age greater than 59 years. Conversely, hospitals with a higher volume of REBOA use have higher survival rates when compared with low-volume centers. Perhaps, the largest pitfall to REBOA use is the learning curve for both individual practitioners and centers and the necessity for high volume to have relative success. Familiarity with the device, appropriate patient selection, and shorter time to complete aortic occlusion are all proposed reasons as to the relative success in facilities that use REBOA more frequently.[14–16]

Emergency Department Thoracotomy

Indication

Emergency department thoracotomy (EDT) is the epitome of a potentially life-saving procedure, yet the decision to perform this procedure must be made quickly and also carries the immense possibility of being futile. Guidelines have been established through national trauma societies to guide physicians as to the criteria that may lead to a potential positive outcome from performing an EDT. A procedure that was once done widely is now done selectively based on criteria.

Because of the difficulty in performing a randomized controlled trial to evaluate the benefits of EDT, we must then rely on quantitative data to depict the outcomes of this controversial procedure. Data obtained from patients who have undergone EDT have led to general guidelines that indicate that patients with penetrating injuries who are undergoing CPR for less than 15 minutes or those with blunt trauma who are undergoing CPR for less than 10 minutes are possible candidates for EDT. Contraindications for EDT include patients without signs of life (respiratory or motor effort, systolic blood pressure >60, pupillary activity cardiac electrical activity) who undergo CPR for greater than 15 minutes for penetrating trauma or greater than 10 minutes for blunt trauma. Furthermore, patients with penetrating injuries to the neck or extremities with greater than 5 minutes of CPR are typically deemed nonsalvageable.[17]

Key steps

Once the decision is made to proceed with EDT, communication must be had with the resuscitative team to ensure that all members of the team are practicing in safe conditions. A left anterolateral thoracotomy incision is made in a curvilinear fashion, and the Finochietto rib retractor is placed and opened to spread the ribs for adequate exposure to the chest. The lung is then retracted, and the pericardium is grasped anterior to the phrenic nerve and incised to evaluate for tamponade. The aorta is then clamped to preserve proximal perfusion and prevent distal hemorrhage. Further interventions can be to repair or occlude cardiac lacerations, pulmonary lacerations, or clamping the hilum if an air embolus is suspected. Intracardiac epinephrine can be injected directly into the left ventricle, and open cardiac massage or internal defibrillation can be performed. Once the patient's injuries and clinical status are further delineated, the patient is either then taken to the operating room for definitive therapy or declared dead if the injuries are nonsalvageable.[18,19]

Potential complications

One can surmise that the atmosphere in which an EDT is being performed is quite chaotic due to the urgency and tenuous clinical status, and this puts all team members involved in the resuscitative efforts at risk for needle sticks or even lacerations from the blade being used to make the incision. It is imperative for all staff to wear protective equipment but also to be clear with communication as the procedure ensues. Closed loop communication is vitally important. Distinct roles should be delegated, and instruments should be passed off in a safe manner. Not only are staff at risk for injury from instruments, but if the ribs are cracked and divided the edges create an additional surface that can cause harm.

The patient can also be injured further by lack of adequate exposure and experience. Care must be taken not to transect the phrenic nerve when creating the pericardiotomy. The aorta can be injured if a clamp other than a vascular clamp is used that can damage the tissue. Similarly, the esophagus can be injured if it is inadvertently clamped instead of or in addition to the aorta. In terms of performing the steps adequately, if the aorta itself is not completely clamped, for example, if the pleura is not separated, the distal exsanguination will continue and the patient will not be salvaged. If the procedure is carried out to the success of maintaining an adequate blood pressure, bleeding will occur from the transected inferior mammary artery and will require ligation to minimize further hemorrhage.[20,21]

Success

The overall mortality associated with patients who arrive to the trauma already in arrest is extremely high. For patients with penetrating thoracic injuries who arrive in shock and undergo EDT, the survival is 35%. Patients arriving in shock with penetrating wounds outside of the thoracic cavity who undergo EDT have a survival rate of 15%. Blunt injuries fare far worse with a 2% survival for patients after EDT that arrive in shock. It is important to emphasize that only 1% of patients survive after EDT if the patients arrive with no vital signs.[22] For those who do survive in the short term, there are even lower levels of long-term survival and neurologic recovery.

An evaluation of all trauma patients older than 18 years who underwent EDT over a 5-year period with data submitted to the American College of Surgeons Trauma Quality Improvement Program showed that the overall survival for patients who underwent EDT was approximately 10%, but overall use of EDT has decreased slightly. This may be due to a combination of the guidelines indicating which patients would be suitable candidates for this maximally invasive heroic procedure and the use of REBOA. However, patient survival over that time period also improved by 2%. Those who have a higher chance of survival, aside from patients who sustained penetrating trauma, are patients younger than 60 years and patients who were not undergoing CPR on arrival. Nonetheless, the basis on which patients would benefit from EDT is guided not only by which patients are mostly likely to survive but also those who would have a meaningful recovery if they survived.[15,23]

Blood Products and Resuscitation

Goals

Uncontrolled hemorrhage in the first 2 to 3 hours after presentation is the primary cause of preventable deaths in trauma patients with reportedly up to 50,000 deaths per year in the United States that can be prevented with hemorrhage control and proper resuscitation. In the acutely unstable trauma patient, hemorrhage control and resuscitation are needed simultaneously. Over time, various questions and practice patterns have gained popularity, and questions regarding resuscitation have been addressed.[24]

The basis for resuscitation in the setting of any unstable patient is to restore perfusion and optimize oxygen delivery to vital organs. Studies have demonstrated that there is a direct correlation between oxygen delivery and survival in patients. But how much resuscitation is enough? What products are ideal for resuscitation? How can we monitor resuscitation? During World War I and World War II, patients were being resuscitated with crystalloid and whole blood. With the Vietnam War, resuscitation moved toward relying heavily on crystalloid; however, it was evident that an abundance of crystalloid can damage the lungs and result in acute respiratory distress syndrome. Thus, although the overall intravascular volume loss was mitigated, the overall outcome was poor due to pulmonary congestion and edema. Furthermore, aggressive use of crystalloid can alter intestinal mobility, liver function, and cardiac function. Since then, the concepts of damage control surgery and a shift back toward administering blood products early on as opposed to crystalloid has taken effect.[25,26]

In 2005, the concept of component therapy resuscitation gained recognition and was found to have several benefits. Component therapy involves resuscitation that uses a balance of packed red blood cells and fresh frozen plasma, in addition to a proportional use of platelet repletion. The volume that is lost during hemorrhage consists not only of red blood cell but also clotting factors and platelets, without which the clotting cascade would not be functional. If resuscitation consists solely of packed red blood cells, the clotting components would be diluted and their function declines.[25,27]

Permissive hypotension

Permissive hypotension has also been used to optimize the patient's clinical status before definitive control of hemorrhage. This concept is based on the theory of meeting a minimal threshold to maintain perfusion to organs while also preserving clot formation on areas of injury. If the systolic blood pressure is pushed to greater than a general cutoff of 80, then there is the potential of disrupting the developing clot and perpetuating hemorrhage. Furthermore, there is less risk of generalized edema and acute respiratory distress syndrome (ARDS). There were studies published in the 1990s that demonstrated an increase in survival for patients who were managed with delayed resuscitation and permissive hypotension. However, although later studies did support this method of resuscitation for blunt trauma patients, there was no difference in survival for patients with penetrating trauma. In addition, patients with traumatic brain injuries need to maintain adequate perfusion pressure to salvage brain tissue. Lastly, the early studies that focused on permissive hypotension were primarily using crystalloid for resuscitation rather than colloid, which may have added to the survival benefit of limiting resuscitative fluid.[28]

Use of viscoelastic tests to guide resuscitation

Thromboelastography (TEG) was developed in 1948 and uses the viscoelasticity of blood to evaluate real-time clotting development and stability, thereby guiding what blood components are needed to optimize hemostasis. Rotational thromboelastometry (ROTEM), similarly elucidates each component of clot integrity. Before checking TEG and ROTEM values, resuscitation with hemostatic products was guided by laboratory values that focused on international normalized ratio (INR), partial thromboplastin time (PTT), and fibrin; however, there is concern that simply using these markers may lead to unnecessary transfusion of products. A randomized controlled trial by Gonzalez and colleagues compared resuscitation led by TEG versus coagulation markers and found that although there was no difference in the amount of red cells that were transfused, the group that underwent resuscitation led by TEG values was transfused less plasma and platelets. As stated earlier, the risk of massive resuscitation, whether it be with blood products or not, is the risk of fluid overload and lung injury. The potential benefit of using a TEG-guided resuscitation is obtaining real-time data on the clotting ability to transfuse more precise amounts of blood components, thus limiting the risk of overresuscitation. Current studies are ongoing and further information is needed to truly assess the benefits of using viscoelastic tests for patients with large-volume blood loss.[29,30]

Role of Laparoscopy

Indications and patient selection

Exploratory laparotomy provides maximal exposure for trauma patients, but there is risk for iatrogenic injury, postoperative bowel obstruction, ileus, and long-term wound issues including loss-of-domain hernia and intestinal fistula. Patients can also have cardiorespiratory complications in up to 20% of cases.[31,32] Nontherapeutic laparotomies are those in which there are no injuries found that require intervention, and the rate is approximately 25% in trauma. The decision to move toward exploratory laparotomy for trauma can be guided with the use of additional tools such as the Focused Abdominal Sonography for Trauma examination, diagnostic peritoneal lavage, local wound exploration, and computed tomography (CT) imaging. As helpful as they are with guidance, these adjuncts have a rate of delayed laparotomy rate of up to 6.8% and are associated with increased morbidity.[33]

Highly-selected trauma patients are candidates for minimally invasive surgery and carry many of the same benefits as general surgical procedures. Choosing the right candidate for diagnostic laparoscopy in the setting of trauma relies on much of the basic principles in trauma. Hemodynamically unstable patients require laparotomy. Patients who present with tachycardia, hypotension, or peritonitis necessitate exploration without the delay of further imaging outside of a potential chest radiograph.[34,35] Other contraindications to diagnostic laparoscopy include anterior wounds with a bullet found posteriorly on the radiograph, evisceration of abdominal organs, previous operations creating a frozen abdomen, and inability to tolerate insufflation such as patients with increased intracranial pressure.

The patient with hemodynamic stability, left thoracoabdominal trauma, or potential diaphragm or blunt hollow viscous injury can benefit from diagnostic laparoscopy. In doing so, the intraabdominal anatomy is visualized, the bowel is run in its entirety and solid organs and diaphragm can be evaluated and if there are no injuries requiring intervention, then the risks and complications associated with a nontherapeutic laparotomy can be avoided in 55% of cases. Furthermore, some investigators have reported moving toward laparoscopic evaluation after failed nonoperative management to first offer a minimally invasive approach to what may only be a potential injury.[36]

Indications for converting to laparotomy

Reported conversion rates in trauma patients range from as low as 13% to as high as 94%. Hemodynamic instability in the trauma patient should always be an indication for conversion to laparotomy. Additional conversion can occur due to difficult anatomy or inadequate visualization. Surgeon expertise also effects the need for conversion to laparotomy, as many of the encountered injuries require a complex laparoscopic skillset. If a surgeon can safely repair a diaphragm injury laparoscopically, it can be done, but the repair quality is more important than the size of the incision, so an open approach is appropriate when necessary.[37]

Pros and cons of diagnostic laparoscopy for trauma

As stated earlier, the primary benefit of performing a laparoscopic evaluation of intraabdominal injury over a laparotomy is the potential to avoid a nontherapeutic laparotomy. Although seemingly harmless, the potential complication rate from a nontherapeutic laparotomy is as high as 9%. These complications can range from bowel obstructions, hernia, wound infections, pneumonia, venous thromboembolism, and cardiac arrest.[38] The missed injury rate for laparoscopy is approximately 0.5%, which makes it a reliable alternative to laparotomy and nonoperative management. Delayed diagnosis in patients undergoing nonoperative management can lead to significant mortality and morbidity if missed even by as little as 5 hours.[39]

There are potential complications to be aware from laparoscopy, as well. There may be difficulty with equipment malfunction, which can delay potential diagnoses. Patient may develop hemodynamic instability with gas insufflation and can subsequently develop cardiovascular collapse and emboli. Access into the abdomen may be difficult or can cause iatrogenic injuries if there is difficulty with the placement of a Veress needle. Injury to the omentum or bowel can occur with whatever method of entry is used. Port site hernias are a baseline risk with laparoscopy, although likely smaller than a hernia that would be associated with a laparotomy incision.[32,37]

Rib Plating

Indications, patient selection, and timing

Rib fractures occur in 10% to 26% of blunt trauma patients, and they carry high morbidity. Patients with rib fractures, regardless of the presence of additional injuries, are at risk for pneumonia, hemothorax, empyema, pneumothorax, and ARDS. The risk of mortality correlates with the increase in number of fractures and can be as high as 34% with 8 fractured ribs. Because of the severity of outcomes, the concept of open reduction and internal fixation of the fractured ribs with plates has been implemented to mitigate the morbidity.[40]

Thus far, data have been focused on the plating of ribs fractures that involve a flail chest. Flail chest is a situation in which 3 or more contiguous ribs are fractured in 2 or more areas, which can cause paradoxic movement of the chest. Flail chest alone is associated with a high rate of respiratory failure and mortality. Although pain control and pulmonary therapy are the mainstay for rib fracture management, rib plating offers the potential benefit of optimizing pain control, stabilizing an otherwise unstable chest wall, and in turn, improving lung expansion. Earlier use of rib plating was centered around patients with flail who were on the ventilator, but this has since expanded to nonvented patients.

Current recommendations and data remain more prevalent for patients with radiographical or clinical flail chest, and study findings have overlapped with advances in critical care medicine, making it relatively difficult to discern early on whether patients were benefitting from the plating or improved intensive care unit (ICU) care. Clinical practice guidelines conditionally recommend plating for patients with flail chest, whereas other recommendations also include patients with displaced rib fractures or those with persistent pain due to nonunion of fractured ribs and respiratory compromise.[41] Fixation of ribs 3 through 10 is currently supported due to the thought that ribs 1, 2, 11, and 12 do not offer significant stability to the chest wall.[42,43] There has also been some suggestion that in patients with pulmonary contusion, there may not be a benefit of fixation, as the damage has already occurred; however, this is limited to a single study.[44] There is evidence clearly supporting early fixation within the first 24 to 72 hours of injury once resuscitation is complete to move forward with fixation, as early fixation is associated with decreased length of hospital stay, length of mechanical ventilation, and decreased risk of pneumonia. Contraindications to plating are hemodynamic instability and patients with severe traumatic brain injury or other significant traumatic disease burden that would require ventilator dependence such as cervical spine injury.[45,46]

Adjuncts to rib fixation

Before rib fixation, obtaining appropriate imaging does aid in operative planning. CT imaging can delineate the number and location of fractures and can then help in planning for the ideal incision. Incisions can be made transverse or longitudinally depending on the number of ribs intending to repair and can be placed anteriorly or posteriorly depending on the location of fractures. In addition, one can determine whether plating is necessary for fractures located under the scapula or even close to the spine.

Video-assisted thoracoscopic surgery is often times performed at the time of rib fixation, although it is not essential. The benefits of performing a VATS during rib plating procedures is that it allows full evaluation of the chest cavity for additional injuries that need to be repaired, and it offers the opportunity to remove residual hematoma or associated collections. Nerve blocks can also be performed at the same time under direct visualization, in addition to cryoablation.[47,48]

Outcomes

Although earlier studies were based on single center data with relatively few patients, studies have become more robust and now include randomized controlled trials to truly evaluate the benefits of rib fixation. In addition, although initially surgical technique varied between types of fixation, such as wire fixation versus plating, the technique has become relatively uniform with plating. Guidelines were developed based on matching patient selection and surgical technique. Findings have been consistent with patients with flail chest that rib fixation does aid in decreasing length of hospital stay, ICU, and days of mechanical ventilation. Thus far, studies have not been able to truly assess the effect of rib fixation on pain.[49,50]

The debate is ongoing as to whether rib fixation of nonflail rib fractures is beneficial. Currently there is a multicenter randomized controlled trial being conducted in the Netherlands that is studying the benefit of rib plating versus nonoperative management of simple rib fractures or in other words nonflail chest anatomy.[46]

DISCLOSURE

The authors have nothing to disclose.

REFERENCES

1. DuBose JJ, Scalea TM, Brenner M, et al. The AAST prospective Aortic Occlusion for Resuscitation in Trauma and Acute Care Surgery (AORTA) registry: Data on contemporary utilization and outcomes of aortic occlusion and resuscitative balloon occlusion of the aorta (REBOA). J Trauma Acute Care Surg 2016;81(3):409–19.
2. Davidson AJ, Russo RM, DuBose JJ, et al. Potential benefit of early operative utilization of low profile, partial resuscitative endovascular balloon occlusion of the aorta (P-REBOA) in major traumatic hemorrhage. Trauma Surg Acute Care Open 2016;1(1):e000028.
3. Manley JD, Mitchell BJ, DuBose JJ, et al. A modern case series of resuscitative endovascular balloon occlusion of the aorta (REBOA) in an out-of-hospital, combat casualty care setting. J Spec Oper Med 2017;17(1):1–8.
4. Bulger EM, Perina DG, Qasim Z, et al. Clinical use of resuscitative endovascular balloon occlusion of the aorta (REBOA) in civilian trauma systems in the USA, 2019: a joint statement from the American College of Surgeons Committee on Trauma, the American College of Emergency Physicians, the National Association of Emergency Medical Services Physicians and the National Association of Emergency Medical Technicians. Trauma Surg Acute Care Open 2019;4(1):e000376.
5. Biffl WL, Fox CJ, Moore EE. The role of REBOA in the control of exsanguinating torso hemorrhage. J Trauma Acute Care Surg 2015;78(5):1054–8.
6. Linnebur M, Inaba K, Haltmeier T, et al. Emergent non-image-guided resuscitative endovascular balloon occlusion of the aorta (REBOA) catheter placement: A cadaver-based study. J Trauma Acute Care Surg 2016;81(3):453–7.
7. Brenner M, Hoehn M, Pasley J, et al. Basic endovascular skills for trauma course: bridging the gap between endovascular techniques and the acute care surgeon. J Trauma Acute Care Surg 2014;77(2):286–91.
8. Ibrahim JA, Safcsak K, Smith HG. Repeatability of REBOA as an unforeseen tool. Am Surg 2017;83(7):e264–5.
9. Stannard A, Eliason JL, Rasmussen TE. Resuscitative endovascular balloon occlusion of the aorta (REBOA) as an adjunct for hemorrhagic shock. J Trauma 2011;71(6):1869–72.
10. Borger van der Burg BLS, Kessel B, DuBose JJ, et al. Consensus on resuscitative endovascular balloon occlusion of the Aorta: A first consensus paper using a Delphi method. Injury 2019;50(6):1186–91.
11. Ribeiro Junior MAF, Feng CYD, Nguyen ATM, et al. The complications associated with resuscitative endovascular balloon occlusion of the aorta (REBOA). World J Emerg Surg 2018;13:20.

12. Morrison JJ, Galgon RE, Jansen JO, et al. A systematic review of the use of resuscitative endovascular balloon occlusion of the aorta in the management of hemorrhagic shock. J Trauma Acute Care Surg 2016;80(2):324–34.

13. Davidson AJ, Russo RM, Reva VA, et al. The pitfalls of resuscitative endovascular balloon occlusion of the aorta: Risk factors and mitigation strategies. J Trauma Acute Care Surg 2018;84(1):192–202.

14. Theodorou CM, Anderson JE, Brenner M, et al. Practice, practice, practice! Effect of resuscitative endovascular balloon occlusion of the aorta volume on outcomes: Data From the AAST AORTA Registry. J Surg Res 2020;253:18–25.

15. Moore LJ, Brenner M, Kozar RA, et al. Implementation of resuscitative endovascular balloon occlusion of the aorta as an alternative to resuscitative thoracotomy for noncompressible truncal hemorrhage. J Trauma Acute Care Surg 2015;79(4):523–30, discussion 530-522.

16. Kinslow K, Shepherd A, McKenney M, et al. Resuscitative endovascular balloon occlusion of aorta: a systematic review. Am Surg 2021. 3134820972985.

17. Aseni P, Rizzetto F, Grande AM, et al. Emergency department resuscitative thoracotomy: indications, surgical procedure and outcome. A narrative review. Am J Surg 2021;221(5):1082–92.

18. Burlew CC, Moore EE, Moore FA, et al. Western trauma association critical decisions in trauma: resuscitative thoracotomy. J Trauma Acute Care Surg 2012;73(6):1359–63.

19. Seamon MJ, Haut ER, Van Arendonk K, et al. An evidence-based approach to patient selection for emergency department thoracotomy: A practice management guideline from the Eastern Association for the Surgery of Trauma. J Trauma Acute Care Surg 2015;79(1):159–73.

20. Suliburk JW. Complications of emergency center thoracotomy. Tex Heart Inst J 2012;39(6):876–7.

21. Kostick N, Gray S, Huynh D. Resuscitative thoracotomy for multiple gunshot wounds with cardiac tamponade despite pericardial window. Cureus 2020;12(12):e11907.

22. Rhee PM, Acosta J, Bridgeman A, et al. Survival after emergency department thoracotomy: review of published data from the past 25 years. J Am Coll Surg 2000;190(3):288–98.

23. Joseph B, Khan M, Jehan F, et al. Improving survival after an emergency resuscitative thoracotomy: a 5-year review of the trauma quality improvement program. Trauma Surg Acute Care Open 2018;3(1):e000201.

24. Chang R, Holcomb JB. Optimal fluid therapy for traumatic hemorrhagic shock. Crit Care Clin 2017;33(1):15–36.

25. Moore EE, Moore HB, Chapman MP, et al. Goal-directed hemostatic resuscitation for trauma induced coagulopathy: Maintaining homeostasis. J Trauma Acute Care Surg 2018;84(6S Suppl 1):S35–40.

26. Hardaway RM. Wound shock: a history of its study and treatment by military surgeons. Mil Med 2004;169(4):265–9.

27. Armand R, Hess JR. Treating coagulopathy in trauma patients. Transfus Med Rev 2003;17(3):223–31.

28. Nirula R, Maier R, Moore E, et al. Scoop and run to the trauma center or stay and play at the local hospital: hospital transfer's effect on mortality. J Trauma 2010;69(3):595–9, discussion 599-601.

29. Gonzalez E, Moore EE, Moore HB, et al. Goal-directed hemostatic resuscitation of trauma-induced coagulopathy: a pragmatic randomized clinical trial comparing a viscoelastic assay to conventional coagulation assays. Ann Surg 2016;263(6):1051–9.

30. Drumheller BC, Stein DM, Moore LJ, et al. Thromboelastography and rotational thromboelastometry for the surgical intensivist: A narrative review. J Trauma Acute Care Surg 2019;86(4):710–21.

31. Koto MZ, Matsevych OY, Mosai F, et al. Laparoscopy for blunt abdominal trauma: a challenging endeavor. Scand J Surg 2019;108(4):273–9.

32. Kindel T, Latchana N, Swaroop M, et al. Laparoscopy in trauma: An overview of complications and related topics. Int J Crit Illn Inj Sci 2015;5(3):196–205.

33. Sosa JL, Arrillaga A, Puente I, et al. Laparoscopy in 121 consecutive patients with abdominal gunshot wounds. J Trauma 1995;39(3):501–4, discussion 504-506.

34. Zantut LF, Ivatury RR, Smith RS, et al. Diagnostic and therapeutic laparoscopy for penetrating abdominal trauma: a multicenter experience. J Trauma 1997;42(5):825–9, discussion 829-831.

35. Sosa JL, Baker M, Puente I, et al. Negative laparotomy in abdominal gunshot wounds: potential impact of laparoscopy. J Trauma 1995;38(2):194–7.

36. Poole GV, Thomae KR, Hauser CJ. Laparoscopy in trauma. Surg Clin North Am 1996;76(3):547–56.

37. Matsevych O, Koto M, Balabyeki M, et al. Trauma laparoscopy: when to start and when to convert? Surg Endosc 2018;32(3):1344–52.

38. Shamim AA, Zeineddin S, Zeineddin A, et al. Are we doing too many non-therapeutic laparotomies in trauma? An analysis of the National Trauma Data Bank. Surg Endosc 2020;34(9):4072–8.

39. Justin V, Fingerhut A, Uranues S. Laparoscopy in blunt abdominal trauma: for whom? When? and Why? Curr Trauma Rep 2017;3(1):43–50.

40. Flagel BT, Luchette FA, Reed RL, et al. Half-a-dozen ribs: the breakpoint for mortality. Surgery 2005;138(4):717–23, discussion 723-715.

41. Cacchione RN, Richardson JD, Seligson D. Painful nonunion of multiple rib fractures managed by operative stabilization. J Trauma 2000;48(2):319–21.

42. Tanaka H, Yukioka T, Yamaguti Y, et al. Surgical stabilization of internal pneumatic stabilization? A prospective randomized study of management of severe flail chest patients. J Trauma 2002;52(4):727–32, discussion 732.

43. Marasco SF, Davies AR, Cooper J, et al. Prospective randomized controlled trial of operative rib fixation in traumatic flail chest. J Am Coll Surg 2013;216(5):924–32.

44. Voggenreiter G, Neudeck F, Aufmkolk M, et al. Operative chest wall stabilization in flail chest–outcomes of patients with or without pulmonary contusion. J Am Coll Surg 1998;187(2):130–8.

45. de Moya M, Nirula R, Biffl W. Rib fixation: Who, What, When? Trauma Surg Acute Care Open 2017;2(1):e000059.

46. Wijffels MME, Prins JTH, Polinder S, et al. Early fixation versus conservative therapy of multiple, simple rib fractures (FixCon): protocol for a multicenter randomized controlled trial. World J Emerg Surg 2019;14:38.

47. Fokin AA, Hus N, Wycech J, et al. Surgical stabilization of rib fractures: indications, techniques, and pitfalls. JBJS Essent Surg Tech 2020;10(2):e0032.

48. Schots JP, Vissers YL, Hulsewe KW, et al. Addition of video-assisted thoracoscopic surgery to the treatment of flail chest. Ann Thorac Surg 2017;103(3):940–4.

49. Beks RB, Reetz D, de Jong MB, et al. Rib fixation versus non-operative treatment for flail chest and multiple rib fractures after blunt thoracic trauma: a multicenter cohort study. Eur J Trauma Emerg Surg 2019;45(4):655–63.

50. Fokin AA, Wycech J, Weisz R, et al. Outcome analysis of surgical stabilization of rib fractures in trauma patients. J Orthop Trauma 2019;33(1):3–8.

Moving?

Make sure your subscription moves with you!

To notify us of your new address, find your **Clinics Account Number** (located on your mailing label above your name), and contact customer service at:

Email: journalscustomerservice-usa@elsevier.com

800-654-2452 (subscribers in the U.S. & Canada)
314-447-8871 (subscribers outside of the U.S. & Canada)

Fax number: 314-447-8029

Elsevier Health Sciences Division
Subscription Customer Service
3251 Riverport Lane
Maryland Heights, MO 63043

*To ensure uninterrupted delivery of your subscription, please notify us at least 4 weeks in advance of move.